T0230614

VARIORUM COLLECTED STUDIES SERIES

The Hospitaller State on Rhodes and its Western Provinces, 1306–1462

Anthony Luttrell

The Hospitaller State on Rhodes and its Western Provinces, 1306–1462

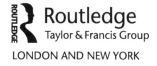

Routledge
Taylor & Francis Group

LONDON AND NEW YORK

First published 1999 in the Variorum Collected Studies Series by Ashgate Publishing

Published 2017 by Routledge
2 Park Square, Milton Park, Abingdon, Oxon, OX14 4RN
711 Third Avenue, New York, NY 10017, USA

Routledge is an imprint of the Taylor & Francis Group, an informa business

British Library Cataloguing-in-Publication Data
Luttrell, Anthony, 1932–
     The Hospitaller State on Rhodes and its Western Provinces, 1306–1462.
     (Variorum Collected Studies Series: CS655)
     1. Knights of Malta. 2. Orders of knighthood and chivalry–Greece–Rhodes–
     History. 3. Rhodes (Greece : Island)–History.
     I. Title.
     271. 7' 912' 09495' 87

US Library of Congress Cataloging-in-Publication Data
Library of Congress Catalog Card Number is pre-assigned as

ISBN 13: 978-0-86078-796-9 (hbk)

CONTENTS

This volume contains x + 340 pages

PUBLISHER'S NOTE

The articles in this volume, as in all others in the Variorum Collected Studies Series, have not been given a new, continuous pagination. In order to avoid confusion, and to facilitate their use where these same studies have been referred to elsewhere, the original pagination has been maintained wherever possible.

Each article has been given a Roman number in order of appearance, as listed in the Contents. This number is repeated on each page and is quoted in the index entries.

PREFACE

The volume of recent publication on the military-religious orders has been extraordinary, but the quality is somewhat uneven and the need remains for detailed studies based upon the documents and on archive research. A number of the papers reprinted in this volume focus on the establishment of the Hospitallers on Rhodes and elsewhere in the East, on Cyprus and at Bodrum for example, and on their settlement and government on Rhodes itself; one item concerns the background to the Hospitallers' move to Rhodes during the period following the Latins' loss of Acre in 1291. Other studies treat the Western provinces and priories from which the Hospital derived the manpower, resources and political support essential to its operations in the Levant; these papers attempt in particular to establish statistically, if crudely, the extent of the Order's commanderies, the number of its brethren and the amounts of money which the Western provinces sent to the Eastern Convent. Two articles deal with the Hospitallers' spiritual life and their medical activities.

A major theme of these studies is the creation on Rhodes of an 'island order state', an institution which the Hospital transferred to Malta in 1530 and continued to operate with a primarily naval function until 1798. Following their acquisition of Rhodes, the Hospitallers created there an island society and economy which permitted them to survive and to carry out their military mission; that involved securing the cooperation of the Greek population and creating local wealth and manpower which would be available when needed. The Order also maintained, largely to convince its Western supporters of its devotion to the holy war against the infidel, an outpost on the Anatolian mainland which until 1402 was at Smyrna and from 1407 onwards at Bodrum. The Hospital's Rhodian metropolis could not, however, be made self-sufficient and it depended heavily on its Western 'colonies'. The Order's most lucrative single source of wealth was the sugar from its plantations in Cyprus, but its real hinterland lay in the priories of its European provinces which were organized to recruit brethren, to exploit their properties and privileges, and to create a surplus of cash to export to Rhodes through a Western treasurer, who was often established at Avignon. A system of seniority and promotions attracted men to serve in Rhodes and rewarded them with commanderies in the West.

Parts of this story have already been presented in three earlier Variorum

Collected Studies volumes of 1978, 1982 and 1992. The contributions reprinted here are largely based on the fragments of the Rhodian archives now preserved in Malta and on other archive sources in the Vatican and elsewhere in the West. Some additions and corrections are listed in the 'Addenda et Corrigenda' section at the end of this volume. That final section also brings up to date the list given in the 1992 publication of items which are not reproduced in any of the Variorum Collected Studies volumes. From item XVIII the gazetteer and documents have been omitted. Item XV has been translated from the Catalan original, and item V had to be reset owing to omissions and other errors in the original publication.

I am extremely grateful, once again, to all those who have generously permitted the reproduction of work and, above all, to John Smedley and the staff of Ashgate for their help and collaboration.

This volume is dedicated to the memory of Kenneth Setton, who died in 1995, in recognition of his friendship and support across many years.

Bath   ANTHONY LUTTRELL
December 1998

I

The Genoese at Rhodes: 1306-1312

Rhodes was one of the larger islands of the Eastern Mediterranean. It was strategically placed both on the sea routes from East to West and, in particular, on those from the Black Sea to Egypt. Its invasion in 1306 was initially a joint venture launched from Cyprus by the Hospitallers of the Order of Saint John and a small group of Genoese who had interests on the island [1]. Rhodes had escaped permanent Latin occupation after the Western conquest of Constantinople in 1204. Greek rule in the imperial capital had been restored in 1261 but Byzantine control of Rhodes became increasingly tenuous. In 1302 the Turkish victory at Bapheos left the Emperor Andronikos II searching for support among competing Latin powers and even, between 1304 and 1307, negotiating for an alliance with the Mongols [2]. For those at Constantinople, Rhodes and the lesser islands close to it were a distant and marginal preoccupation; they were often devastated by the Anatolian Turks whose maritime razzias and slave raids depopulated them, apparently with the intention of creating a deserted buffer zone. Possession of some Aegean islands was disputed between individuals or families from Venice and Genoa,

---

[1] Genoese interest in Rhodes awaits detailed study: C. JONA, *Genova e Rodi agli albori del Rinascimento*, in «Atti della Società Ligure di Storia Patria», LXIV, 1935, published some sixty documents for the years 1424 to 1506. The present notes and amendments are preliminary and incomplete; they attempt no prosopographical analysis of the families involved. Advice on certain points was kindly given by Julian Chrysostomides and Elizabeth Zachariadou to whom I am most grateful.

[2] A. LAIOU, *Constantinople and the Latins: the Foreign Policy of Andronicus II 1282-1328*, Cambridge Mass., 1972. Turkish activities on and around Rhodes before 1306 await a specialized study not attempted here.

whose citizens had long frequented them as traders, as pirates and occasionally as inhabitants or settlers. Various Genoese and Venetians had established themselves, if only briefly, on Rhodes[3]. The potential value of Rhodes was also appreciated in the West where from about 1290 onwards there were occasional suggestions for a permanent Latin occupation of the island for use as a crusading outpost. Rhodes was envisaged as a base from which to enforce the papal blockade of Egypt and Syria by controlling Latin traders taking war materials to those countries, and especially by preventing the lucrative traffic in slaves from the Black Sea who were vital to the Mamluk regime[4].

In 1303 Andronikos II brought in the Catalan company from Sicily to confront the Turks in Anatolia but their leader, Roger de Flor, soon turned against the empire itself. The Sicilians and Catalans who then became active in the East showed some interest in certain Aegean islands. According to the chronicle of Ramon Muntaner, at Christmas 1304 Andronikos appointed Roger de Flor as *megas dux*, that is as imperial Admiral with overall command of the naval forces, and early in 1305 the emperor gave him the Kingdom of Anatolia and «all the islands of Romania»[5]. Though he was on the spot, Muntaner may have misunderstood the precise meaning and intention behind these titles which probably did not confer jurisdiction over the islands[6], but the Catalans clearly believed in their own claims. Thus on 10 May 1305 Roger de Flor's successor, Berenguer d'Entença, formally entitled himself *magnus dux [...]*

---

[3] The most detailed and recent treatment is A. SAVVIDES, *Rhodes from the End of the Gabalas Rule to the Conquest by the Hospitallers: A. D. c. 1250-1309*, in «Byzantinos Domos», II, 1988. Savvides provides many sources but relies on a work by C. Papachristodolou (1972) based on only a few outdated sources and on another by G. Martines (1979) which lacks references; some of their assertions derive from the fantasies of Karl Hopf which still await systematic revision on the basis of the original sources.

[4] A. LUTTRELL, *The Hospitallers in Cyprus, Rhodes, Greece and the West: 1291-1440*, London, 1978, I, p. 282; II, p. 165; S. SCHEIN, *Fideles Crucis: the Papacy, the West, and the Recovery of the Holy Land 1274-1314*, Oxford, 1991, pp. 97-98, 177-178, 223.

[5] RAMON MUNTANER, *Crònica*, in «Les quatre grans cròniques», ed. F. SOLDEVILA, Barcelona, 1971, pp. 847 (cap. 199), 855 (cap. 212).

[6] Cf. A. LAIOU cit., pp. 132, 144.

imperii Romanie ac dominus Natulii ac insularum eiusdem imperii [7]. In 1304 Roger de Flor ravaged the islands of Chios, Lesbos and Lemnos, while in January 1305 he attempted to defend Chios, which he claimed as his own, against thirty Turkish ships; in the following spring King Federigo of Sicily's half-brother Sancho of Aragon also attacked various unidentified Aegean islands [8].

The Catalans had rapidly become the major threat to Andronikos who was compelled to turn to one of the two main Latin parties for help against them. The Genoese had occupied Rhodes in 1248 only to be dislodged in the following year by the Greeks of Nicaea [9]. In 1278 the *dominus* of Rhodes was the Levantine Genoese Giovanni dello Cavo, a corsair who became an imperial captain and was later made Admiral of the Byzantine fleet [10]. In the following years Rhodes probably returned to a Byzantine control exercized

---

[7] Text in A. RUBIÓ I LLUCH, *Diplomatari de l'Orient català: 1301-1409*, Barcelona, 1947, pp. 15-16.

[8] A. LAIOU cit., pp. 136, 138, 144-145, 147, 152, 154.

[9] M. BALARD, *La Romanie génoise (XII*[e] *- début du XV*[e] *siècle)*, I, Genoa-Rome, 1978, p. 41. In about 1271 a Nicetas Leon of Rhodes or *Nichetas Malareoltas de Rode* attacked certain Venetians in the Gulf of Corinth: text in G. TAFEL-G. THOMAS, *Urkunden zur älteren Handels-und Staatsgeschichte der Republik Venedig*, 3 vols., Venice, 1856-1857, III, pp. 161, 167, 170, 236, 268, 269. A. SAVVIDES cit., p. 207, states that he was Genoese but the name suggests a Greek. The imperial *capitaneus* in control of Rhodes in February 1273 was named Criviciotas: texts in G. TAFEL-G. THOMAS cit., III, pp. 173, 196-197, 208, 258. For an analysis of this text and its chronology, G. MORGAN, *The Venetian Claims Commission of 1278*, in «Byzantinische Zeitschrift», LXIX, 1976.

[10] In 1278 there was a *Iohanne de Cavo Genuensis Namphi et Rhodi insulae dominus*, that is a Genoese from Anaphe, perhaps with a Greek mother, who ruled Rhodes: text in A. FERRETTO, *Codice diplomatico delle relazioni fra la Liguria, la Toscana e la Lunigiana ai tempi di Dante: 1265-1321*, in «Atti della Società Ligure di Storia Patria», XXXI, fasc. 2, 1903, pp. 244-246, n. 1. Contrary to what has been written, the grammar makes it clear that Giovanni was from Anaphe and lord of only one island, Rhodes. MARINO SANUDO, *Istoria del Regno di Romania*, in «Chroniques Gréco-Romanes inédites ou peu connues», ed. C. HOPF, Berlin, 1873, p. 132, described him as *Zuan da Cavo*, a native of Anaphe who in about 1282 was Admiral of six imperial galleys which defeated the Venetians. A Venetian text of March 1278 showed that in 1277 *Johannes de lo Cavo* alias *de Capite*, who was the emperor's *homo* and had been active as a corsair at least since about 1271, had robbed Venetian shipping in the Gulf of Corinth with eleven (but G. MORGAN cit., p. 413, suggests two) *ligna* armed at Ania opposite Samos and one *lignum* armed at Butrinto, and had committed many other robberies while in imperial service: texts in G. TAFEL-G. THOMAS cit., III, pp. 162-163, 184, 185, 194, 207, 220, 224-226, 229, 230, 241, 247, 252, 259, 263, 272-273.

rather loosely from Constantinople[11]. When Andronikos called in the Catalan company in 1303 the position of the Genoese within the empire was weakened in consequence, but the emperor was soon obliged to employ them to oppose the Catalans. Some Genoese did trade in the Black Sea, in Egypt or in Cyprus; they carried slaves from Kaffa to Alexandria; they made profits as imperial sea captains with their own private agenda; or they combined such activities. Individuals, part merchant and part pirate, were accustomed to operating within a confused and fluctuating, virtually anarchic, maritime milieu in which they variously opposed Greeks and Turks, Venetians and Catalans, and sometimes fellow Genoese. Commercial and corsair interests cut across boundaries between Latin and Greek and between Christian and Muslim. A few Genoese adventurers received imperial titles or island lordships[12]. For example, Chios was granted, probably in 1308 or 1309, to Benedetto Zaccaria of Genoa, who already held Phocaea on the mainland nearby; he was to hold it from the emperor[13]. A few years earlier Karpathos and other nearby islands between Rhodes and Crete had been granted to Andrea Moresco, a Genoese sea captain in imperial service.

Venetian interest in the islands around Rhodes was also considerable[14]. Venetian ships and merchants had occasionally used

---

[11] A. SAVVIDES cit., pp. 214-216, 230-231, follows earlier writers in supposing that from 1282/3 onwards Rhodes was governed by Andrea Moresco, that he «drove the Turks away», that Michael VIII who died in 1282 made him his Admiral, and that he used Rhodes as a base for countless raids, but there seems to be no evidence for such claims before 1304. The coins discussed in G. SCHLUMBERGER, *Numismatique de Rhodes avant la conquête de l'île par les Chevaliers Saint-Jean*, in «Revue Archéologique», XXXI, 1876, give no such indication. The idea that Giovanni de lo Cavo was succeeded on Rhodes by Moresco in 1282 circa appeared in K. HOPF, *Veneto-Byzantinische Analekten*, new ed., Amsterdam, 1964, p. 117, which stated that he was on Crete in 1279. The text, in *Leonardo Marcello notaio in Candia: 1278-1281*, ed. M. CHIAUDANO - A. LOMBARDO, Venice, 1960, p. 102, shows only that an Andrea *Marasco*, a *habitator* in Candia, «affirmed» his son Marco to a barber on 16 October 1280. The absence of indications as to who did rule Rhodes between 1282 and 1306 may reflect a power vacuum there.

[12] A. LAIOU cit., pp. 147-157 et *passim*; M. BALARD cit., I, pp. 62-64.

[13] For this dating, E. ZACHARIADOU, *Trade and Crusade. Venetian Crete and the Emirates of Menteshe and Aydin: 1300-1415*, Venice, 1983, pp. 7-8.

[14] What follows revises A. LUTTRELL cit., I, 283; V, pp. 196-197.

Rhodes as a harbour and a commercial base. In 1234 Venice had concluded a treaty with the ruler of Rhodes, Leon Gabalas, which promised trading rights, a church, a fondaco and a *curia* for Venetian citizens there [15]. In 1283 the Venetian Pancrazio Malipiero attacked
Kos, some way north-west of Rhodes, with twenty-five galleys but he
was defeated there by the Greek inhabitants, who supported the emperor, and by their Turkish allies [16]; and in the following year Giacomo Tiepolo led another Venetian expedition against Kos [17]. Developments and institutions on Kos had long been somewhat distinct
from the those on Rhodes [18]. In 1300 there were Venetians who held
estates on Kos, at least one of which had been granted *in affictum*
by the commune of Crete; some Venetians from Crete were leasing
lands on Kos to Greeks through contracts involving vine planting
and other improvements [19]. By their peace treaty with Andronikos
II of 1302 the Venetians were to keep four unnamed islands they
had recently taken from Byzantium but were to hand back all the
others [20]. Kos may have been one of the four, since in 1302 a Venetian force was sent from Crete to Kos to occupy the castle, though
the expedition was captured by some Greeks from Monemvasia;
at the same time the Venetians were holding hostages from Kos
on Crete [21]. In 1305 Niccolò Venier freed his slave Vaxili of Kos on
condition that he remained on Venier's *casale* of *Açupadhe* on Kos [22].
At Rhodes the Venetians were less firmly established, though there

[15] Text in G. TAFEL-G. THOMAS cit., II, pp. 320-322.

[16] Date established in R.-J. LOENERTZ, *Les Ghisi, Dynastes vénitiens dans l'Archi-
pel: 1207-1390*, Florence, 1975, pp. 97-98.

[17] Date established in R.-J. LOENERTZ, *Menego Schiavo, esclave, corsaire, seigneur
d'Ios: 1296-1310*, in «Studi Veneziani», IX, 1967, pp. 322 n. 30, 336 n. 30.

[18] Cf. M. ANGOLD, *A Byzantine Government in Exile: Government and Society
under the Laskarids of Nicaea, 1204-1261*, Oxford, 1975, pp. 104, 139-140, 230, 249, 266.

[19] Texts in S. CARBONE, *Pietro Pizolo notaio in Candia*, 2 vols., Venice, 1978-1985,
I, pp. 109-110, 263-264.

[20] Texts in G. THOMAS, *Diplomatarium Veneto-Levantinum*, I, Venice, 1880,
pp. 12-19.

[21] Text in R. CESSI-P. SAMBIN, *Le deliberazioni del Consiglio dei Rogati: Senato,
Serie Mixtorum*, I, Venice, 1960, p. 74.

[22] Text in S. CARBONE cit., II, p. 212.

were commercial contacts between Rhodes and Candia[23]. In or just before 1301 some Venetians then on their galleys at Rhodes quarrelled with certain Sicilians there[24]; shortly before April 1303 a group of Venetians at Rhodes detained the galley of the Genoese Percivalle della Turca[25]; and by November 1303 a Venetian galley had in turn been robbed near Rhodes by the Genoese[26]. Before July 1306 the Venetians had been besieging Nisyros, between Kos and Rhodes, with four *ligna*[27]. In January 1309 Andrea Cornaro was granted permission to send grain from Crete to Karpathos which, therefore, he presumably controlled at that time; in the following March the Venetians on Crete were actually considering the acquisition of Rhodes; and by October of that year they were in control of Kos[28].

The granting of Karpathos to Andrea Moresco threatened the Venetian position in that area. Whatever his previous background[29], Moresco emerged from obscurity at a time when Andronikos needed help not only against the Catalans but also to resist the Venetians, with whom the emperor was at war from 1306 to 1310. In March 1303 two Genoese galleys and one from Sicily attacked shipping off Corfu. The Genoese *San Braganzio* was commanded by Andriolo or Andrea Moresco and had a *socio* named *Viguor*, probably Vignolo, de Chiavari; the other, the *Morro da Porto*, carried Samuele Moresco de Chiavari as *socio* and Alvise or Lodovico Moresco as *comito*[30].

---

[23] Texts of 1300 and 1304 *ibidem*, I, pp. 44, 54-55, 132, 150, 166, 315; II, pp. 45, 117.

[24] Texts in R. CESSI-P. SAMBIN cit., I, pp. 41, 62, 81.

[25] ARCHIVIO DI STATO DI VENEZIA, Commemoriali, I, f. 35 r.-v.

[26] Text in E. FAVARO, *Cassiere della Bolla Ducale, Grazie - Novus Liber: 1299-1305*, Venice, 1962, p. 101.

[27] Text in Z. TSIRPANLIS, *He Rhodos kai oi Noties Sporades sta Khronia ton Ioanniton Ippoton (14os-16os ai.)*, Rhodes, 1991, pp. 27-28.

[28] *Infra*, p. 754.

[29] The possibility that Andrea Moresco was on Crete in 1280 seems remote: *supra*, nota 11.

[30] Text in R. PREDELLI, *I libri Commemoriali della Repubblica di Venezia: Regesti*, I, Venice, 1876, pp. 34-35. *Iohaninus de Sancto Anthonio de Ianua, filius quondam Moreschi de Clavaro* was at Famagusta in 1301: text in V. POLONIO, *Notai Genovesi in Oltremare: Atti rogati a Cipro da Lamberto di Sambuceto (3 luglio 1300-3 agosto 1301)*, Genoa, 1982, pp. 328-329; A. FERRETTO cit., pp. 219, 252 n., documents a Loisio Moresco at Chiavari in 1278.

The Moresco family apparently came from Chiavari on the coast to the east of Genoa, as did that of Andrea's uncle Vignolo de Vignoli[31]. In about October 1304 Andrea Moresco entered the emperor's service with his two ships and, after he had defeated a Turkish ship, Andronikos gave him certain honours and the naval title of *vestiarios*; Moresco also attacked the Venetians. In June or July 1305 he captured Tenedos and it was probably then that he and his brother Lodovico inflicted damage on the Venetians there. Soon after that Andrea massacred various Turks, following which Andronikos appointed him Admiral. In July Andrea successfully provisioned the Greeks inside Madytos in the Dardanelles which was under siege by the Catalans. In the same month some of his ships were captured by vessels from Sicily, and only his uncle, presumably Vignolo de Vignoli, was spared. Moresco was not himself captured at that point but he was taken prisoner in a subsequent battle at Halonion in September or October, after which his Catalan or Sicilian captors ransomed him[32]. In July 1306 the Catalans in Gallipoli were unsuccessfully assaulted by eighteen Genoese galleys under Antonio Spinola and by seven imperial galleys commanded by Andrea Moresco, who was wounded there[33]. The honours given Andrea Moresco in 1304 evidently included the lordship of Karpathos, which he held from the emperor *in feudum*[34]; that was in the tradition of Giovanni dello Cavo, the Genoese pirate who in 1278 had also been an impe-

---

[31] ARCHIVIO DI STATO DI GENOVA, Notaio *Vivaldus de Sarzana*, cartolare 107, c. 96 v. (13 June 1308) (kindly supplied by Gillian Moore).

[32] GEORGIUS PACHYMERES, *De Michaele et Andronico Palaeologis*, ed. I. BEKKER, II, Bonn, 1835, pp. 495-496, 556-557, 573, 583-585, with further detail: chronology established in A. FAILLER, *Chronologie et Composition dans l'Histoire de Georges Pachymérès (Livres VII-XIII)*, in «Revue des Études Byzantines», XLVIII, 1990, pp. 62-63, 74-77, 85-86. For Moresco and his brother at Tenedos, see also G. THOMAS cit., p. 156. An undated act shows that one of the Moresco had a Greek wife, Zoe Doukaina Philanthropene Mouriskessa, who was in the vicinity of Patmos and promised that neither her men nor those of her husband's brother would damage the property of the monks of Patmos, who had properties on Kos and Leros: text in F. MIKLOSICH-J. MÜLLER, *Acta et Diplomata Graeca Medii Aevi*, VI, Vienna, 1890, pp. 247-248.

[33] GEORGIUS PACHYMERES cit., II, p. 606, mentioning the wounding; confirmed by RAMON MUNTANER (cit., p. 867 [cap. 227]) who was in charge of the defence: dated in A. FAILLER cit., pp. 78-79, 86, and RAMON MUNTANER cit., p. 985.

[34] *Infra*, p. 755.

rial Admiral and *dominus* of Rhodes. Andrea's uncle Vignolo de Vignoli held from the emperor the islands of Kos and Leros as well as the *casale* of Lardos on Rhodes, for which he claimed to have imperial letters [35].

In addition to Venetian activities, there had repeatedly been Turkish incursions on Rhodes and other islands, including attacks and devastations in 1295 and 1302 [36]. To what extent Moresco and Vignolo exercized any control over the islands they claimed is uncertain. In March 1302 unidentified pirates from Rhodes and Monemvasia, who were probably Greeks but possibly Genoese or some combination of both, arrived in Southern Cyprus with two galleys and a *fusta*; they landed and captured the Count of Jaffa at Episkopi [37]. According to one Cypriot chronicler, many Genoese pirates were caught and hanged on Cyprus in 1303; and it may have been at that time that Vignolo de Vignoli, using Rhodes as his base, caused much trouble to the Cypriots. The king, Henri II, repeatedly sought to catch Vignolo but he retreated to Rhodes or to other Aegean ports and then returned to the attack. In May 1306 Vignolo arrived off Limassol in his galley and sent word that he wished to speak with the Hospitaller Master but that he was reluctant to come ashore since he had caused so much damage in the country [38]. Henri II had been

---

[35] *Infra*, p. 746.

[36] E. Zachariadou cit., pp. 9-10.

[37] Francesco Amadi, in *Chroniques d'Amadi et de Strambaldi*, ed. R. De Mas Latrie, I, Paris, 1891, p. 238, and Florio Bustron, *Chronique de l'île de Chypre*, ed. R. De Mas Latrie, Paris, 1886, p. 134: dated in G. Hill, *A History of Cyprus*, II, Cambridge, 1948, p. 211. P. Edbury, *Cyprus and Genoa: the Origins of the War of 1373-74*, in «Praktika tou Devterou Diethnous Kyprologikou Synedriou», II, Nicosia, 1986, p. 107, interprets these pirates as Genoese. However, Monemvasia was at that moment a flourishing base for Greek shipping: H. Kaligas, *Byzantine Monemvasia: the Sources*, Monemvasia, 1990, pp. 109-112. It was in 1302 that a Venetians force on its way to Kos was attacked by ships from Monemvasia: *supra*, p. 741. Correct A. Luttrell, *The Hospitallers of Rhodes and their Mediterranean World*, Aldershot, 1992, II, p. 83, which describes these pirates as Turks.

[38] Francesco Amadi cit., pp. 239, 254-257; written in the sixteenth century and surviving as an Italian translation from the French, this chronicle used informed earlier sources. Vignolo's arrival evidently preceded the treaty of 27 May 1306. Amadi wrote that before Vignolo's arrival (wrongly placed in June), Andrea Moresco had been captured on his pirate galley and, together with all its crew, been hanged. However, in July 1306 Moresco was at Gallipoli (*supra*, p. 743). Moresco could have attacked Cyprus in 1303 and lost his galley but retained his life and liberty; or he could have been captured in or after 1308 when he was last documented.

involved in a major conflict with the Genoese of Cyprus, and Vignolo probably knew of the royal ordinance of February 1306 commanding all Genoese to leave the coastal towns and live in Nicosia [39].

Vignolo secured an ally in the Hospitallers who were perpetual-
ly hostile to Venice [40] but who had at times, from 1256 to 1258 for
example, been closely allied to the Genoese [41]. The Hospital's Convent or headquarters had been moved to Limassol following the fall
of Acre in 1291. Since then the Order, which could afford only a
small naval force, had been constricted on an island where the government taxed its peasants and limited its activities; the Hospitallers were also embroiled in the crown's dynastic conflicts. The Hospital needed a function which would justify its continued existence
and its enjoyment of its Western wealth and privileges. The acquisition of Rhodes offered it an independent base and a role in opposing
the infidel Turks of Anatolia and in policing the illegal trade in war
materials and slaves to Mamluk Egypt [42]. Who first considered a Hospitaller occupation of Rhodes is uncertain. The contemporary *Gestes des Chiprois* stated that it was the Hospitaller Master, Fr. Foulques de Villaret, who wished to attack Rhodes and so summoned a
leading Genoese, the *grant home* Bonifacio Grimaldi, from Famagusta to discussions at the Hospital's *casale* of Kolossi near Limassol [43];

---

[39] FRANCESCO AMADI cit., p. 241, and *Recueil des Historiens des Croisades: Lois*,
II, Paris, 1843, p. 368; cf. P. EDBURY, *The Kingdom of Cyprus and the Crusades: 1191-
1374*, Cambridge, 1991, p. 111.

[40] A. LUTTRELL, *Hospitallers in Cyprus* cit., VI, pp. 195-212; ID., *The Hospitaller
Priory of Venice in 1331*, in «Militia Sacra: gli Ordini Militari tra Europa e Terrasanta», ed. E. COLI et al., Perugia, 1994, p. 106.

[41] J. RILEY-SMITH, *The Knights of St. John in Jerusalem and Cyprus: c. 1050-1310*,
London, 1967, pp. 183-186.

[42] A. LUTTRELL, *Hospitallers in Cyprus* cit., II, pp. 161-165; see also J. RILEY-
SMITH cit., pp. 198-215.

[43] *Les Gestes des Chiprois*, in «Recueil des Historiens des Croisades: Documents
Arméniens», II, Paris, 1906, p. 863, making no mention of Vignolo at that point. The
Gestes, written by a contemporary between about 1312 and about 1321, seems the
most reliable account. Bonifacio Grimaldi was in Famagusta on 5 April 1307: text in
M. BALARD, *Notai Genovesi in Oltremare. Atti rogati a Cipro: Lamberto di Sambuceto
(31 marzo 1304-19 luglio 1305, 4 gennaio-12 luglio 1307) - Giovanni de Rocha (3 agosto 1308-14 marzo 1310)*, Genoa, 1984, pp. 202-203. The *Gestes* could have confused
Grimaldi and Vignolo; alternatively, there were two meetings, in which case the initiative for the expedition came from the Hospital.

the Amadi chronicle said that Vignolo de Vignoli sailed to Cyprus and asked to discuss an important matter with the Master and Convent, and that he then landed two miles from Limassol to meet the Master and his officers and there promised to give them Kos and Rhodes [44].

By a notarial act drawn up on 27 May 1306 at the church of Saint George of the Greeks near Limassol, Villaret and other leading Hospitallers made a contract, described as a *paragium* or *societas*, with Vignolo de Vignoli, *civis* of Genoa, for the acquisition of various unnamed islands *in Romania*. Specifically excluded from the *paragium*, though its conquest was clearly envisaged, was the island of Rhodes; also excluded were Kos and Leros which Vignolo claimed to hold himself and which he «gave» to the Hospital. Vignolo was to keep the *casale* of Lardos on Rhodes, which he asserted had been granted to him by imperial letters, and he was to have a second Rhodian *casale* of his choice, together with the rights and appurtenances of both. The Master was to have two-thirds and Vignolo one-third of the revenues of all the islands to be acquired, and these incomes were to be collected jointly. Vignolo was to be *vicarius* and *iusticiarius* of all these islands with jurisdictions and powers to impose sentences of mutilation and death over their inhabitants and over any mercenaries or *stipendarii* who might be employed; with the counsel and assent of the Master, Vignolo was to appoint *baylivi*, *servientes* and other officials, and also to create notaries. There were to be rights of appeal to the Master, who was to have other powers of intervention and to exercize jurisdiction over his own *famuli* or household and over brethren of the Hospital [45]. This agreement

---

[44] Francesco Amadi cit., pp. 254-256.

[45] Text in J. Delaville le Roulx, *Les Hospitaliers en Terre Sainte et à Chypre: 1100-1310*, Paris, 1904, pp. 274-276 n. 2. One witness was a Peruzzi, a member of a Florentine bank which made large loans to the Hospital and was subsequently well established on Rhodes: A. Luttrell, *Hospitallers in Cyprus* cit., VIII, pp. 317-320. Another witness was Fr. Sancho de Aragon, then Admiral of the Hospital, apparently the brother of Federigo of Sicily; Sancho had led a Sicilian fleet in the Aegean islands in 1305: A. Rubió I Lluch cit., p. 55 n. 2, and A. Luttrell, *Hospitallers of Rhodes* cit., XV, p. 104. The text in A. Rubió I Lluch cit., pp. 55-56, which seems to show that Sancho was not a Hospitaller in 1310, poses an unresolved problem. There was a church of Saint George at Episkopi near the coast and just west of Kolossi: R. Gunnis, *Historic Cyprus: a Guide to its Towns and Villages, Monasteries and Castles*, Nicosia, 1936, pp. 227-228.

did not create a fief or involve any obligation to military service. Since Vignolo claimed to hold Kos and Leros from the emperor while Karpathos and other islands, none of them named, were held by Andrea Moresco as an imperial vassal, it must have been clear that Vignolo had little right to make any of them over to the Hospital. He would scarcely have organized their conquest if he and his Moresco nephews had effectively controlled them. In reality Rhodes was in the hands of its Greek inhabitants and, in the castle of Phileremos at least, of a Turkish garrison, while the Venetians were predominant on Kos.

The Master left Limassol on 23 June 1306 with a small fleet of two galleys, one *fusta*, one *chutier*, two *panfili*, thirty-five Hospitallers – five from each *langue* according to the chronicler – together with six *turcopuli* and a good number of secular foot soldiers. At Cape Saint Epiphani, the westernmost point of Cyprus, he found the two Genoese galleys of Baldo Spinola and Michele della Volta, both of whom took an oath to join the expedition. Vignolo de Vignoli went ahead, presumably on his own galley, to spy out the situation on Rhodes, while the fleet waited for one month at the island of Kastellorizzo. Vignolo was delayed at Rhodes where he found his nephew Lodovico Moresco, who was an imperial vassal and who initially detained his uncle but later set him free. Perhaps because water and supplies were short on Kastellorizzo, the Hospitaller force had moved to the «island of *Guilla*», which may have been an island or possibly a place on the mainland opposite Rhodes, and Vignolo rejoined the Hospitallers there [46]. The whole expedition then went to the *fiume de Rhodi*, which may also have been on the mainland. The two Genoese, Spinola and della Volta, next sailed to Rhodes in their turn to arrange a surprise attempt on the *castello* whose Greek defenders remained obedient to the emperor. Meanwhile two Hospitaller brethren and fifty foot soldiers were sent to Kos where they captured the castle but failed to guard it, so that the Greeks retook it. At Rhodes, Spinola and della Volta were denounced to the *capitanio*, possibly Lodovico Moresco, by a Greek who had fled from the Hospital's fleet. However, the two Genoese managed to leave Rhodes and return to the Hospitaller force which then sailed to attack the

---

[46] Possibly the late-medieval mainland harbour of *Aguia* or *Guia*, the Turkish Karagatsch-Liman near the classical Ephesus: C. KRETSCHMER, *Die italienische Portolane des Mittelalters*, Berlin, 1909, p. 665.

castello by land and sea, using siege engines. The attackers presumably occupied the suburbs but they failed to take the *castello*. They did capture the castle at Feraklos on 20 September; five days later they unsuccessfully assaulted the *castello* once again and then sent for the rest of the Hospital's Convent, its main force in the East, to come from Cyprus. On 11 November the castle on Mount Phileremos, in which the Greeks had stationed 300 Turks, was taken through the treachery of a Greek defender; the Turks were slaughtered[47].

Even with reinforcements, the Hospitallers' force continued to be too weak to take the main fortified section of Rhodes town or effectively to blockade it[48], and in March 1307 they sent an embassy to Constantinople on ships of the emperor to propose that the Hospital should hold 'Rhodes from Andronikos in return for the service of 300 men against the Turks. The emperor, who had already sent some relief to Rhodes, refused this offer and despatched eight galleys which reached Rhodes in April with further aid for the defenders; meanwhile, eight galleys and a *lignum* came from Cyprus to assist the attackers[49]. In October 1307 there were reported to be twenty imperial ships in the port of Rhodes[50].

There was no sign that Andrea Moresco went to Rhodes with the imperial fleet in 1307 but, following the death of King Hethoum of Armenia on 16 November 1307, Hethoum's brother Sempad, who was at Constantinople, left for Armenia with two imperial galleys and a *fusta* which were captained by Andrea Moresco and his brother Lodovico. They went to Kyrenia on Cyprus where they

---

[47] Francesco Amadi cit., pp. 256-258. However, Florio Bustron cit., p. 141, stated that *Alvise* Moresco joined the Hospitaller force at Kastellorizzo; Bustron also numbered the *fanti* at 500.

[48] Detail on the siege is here omitted: see J. Delaville le Roulx cit., pp. 276-281, A. Luttrell, *Hospitallers in Cyprus* cit., I, pp. 283-285; A. Savvides cit., pp. 223-227, and especially A. Failler, *L'occupation de Rhodes par les Hospitaliers*, in «Revue des Études Byzantines», L, 1992. These accounts, derived largely from chronicle sources, still leave unresolved contradictions and all require revision.

[49] Georgius Pachymeres cit., II, pp. 635-636, and text of 30 April [1308] in H. Finke, *Acta Aragonensia*, III, Berlin, 1923, p. 147; chronology and discussion in A. Failler, *L'occupation* cit., pp. 114-118, 132-135. A. Luttrell, *The Hospitallers in Cyprus* cit., I, p. 284, wrongly places this incident in 1308.

[50] E. Baratier-F. Reynaud, *Histoire du commerce de Marseille*, II, Paris, 1951, pp. 213-214.

stayed a few days and then returned to Constantinople, leaving Sempad on Cyprus; he went to Gastria and was there on 30 April 1308[51]. The Moresco brothers must have passed near the Rhodian islands on these journeys. Their position was ambiguous in that they continued to serve Andronikos II who was attempting to save Rhodes from the Hospitallers and their Genoese collaborators, one of whom was their own uncle. News reached Venice in or shortly before September 1308 that Andrea Moresco with his *lignum* was at sea off Coron as part of a fleet of eleven galleys and two *ligna*, probably in imperial service[52]. After that Andrea disappeared[53]. Lodovico attempted to secure the claims he held to Karpathos as Andrea's brother and as an imperial vassal; he made several attacks on that island until, apparently in 1309, he was captured by the Venetian Andrea Cornaro[54]. Vignolo, who was still with the Hospitaller fleet on the eve of the capitulation of Rhodes, which probably surrendered in August 1309[55], was evidently betraying Andronikos.

During these years the loyalties and attitudes of the Genoese connected with Rhodes varied considerably. Some apparently maintained relations with the besieged Greeks. Thus in July 1308 a Genoese merchant arrived at Famagusta from Rhodes where he had purchased goods *in castro Roddi* only to be robbed three miles out to sea by the Hospitallers[56]. Other Genoese were presumably alongside the Hospitallers in the suburbs outside the main walled town and doing business there. Others perhaps avoided the port. Early in 1307

---

[51] FRANCESCO AMADI cit., pp. 277-278, giving Lodovico as Andrea's nephew *Alvise*. Hethoum died on 16 November 1307: W. RUDT DE COLLENBERG, *The Rupenides, Hethumides and Lusignans: the Structure of the Armeno-Cilician Dynasties*, Paris, 1963, p. 71.

[52] G. GIOMO, *Lettere di Collegio, rectius Minor Consiglio: 1308-1310*, in «Deputazione di Storia Patria per le Venezie: Miscellanea di Storia Patria Veneta», ser. III, I, Venice, 1910, p. 284.

[53] Andrea Moresco was said to have been hanged at Famagusta: *supra*, nota 38. A LAIOU cit., p. 156 n. 101, states that he was alive in 1319/1320 but that text (*infra*, nota 82) shows he was then dead.

[54] *Infra*, p. 755.

[55] *Gestes* cit., p. 864.

[56] MARSEILLES, ARCHIVES DÉPARTEMENTALES DES BOUCHES-DU-RHÔNE, H. 4087 (partly damaged).

Genoese ships from Famagusta were trading in Rhodes. In March 1308 two Genoese at Famagusta were planning a journey to Rhodes but in the same month Manuele Scarlatino of Savona, who was leaving Famagusta to trade somewhere beyond Rhodes, was not to stop there but to go *apud Rodum et per Turchiam, ita tamen quod transsire non debeam Rodum predictum*. In the same month, Edoardo Zaccaria of Genoa agreed in Famagusta to repay a sum of money at Rhodes, since he and another Genoese, Nicola de Magnerri, were sailing there on his galley; this galley had previously belonged to the Hospital which had purchased it from Berthono de Sagona. Two years later, on 19 February 1310, Giovanni Rovereta de Varazze acknowledged receipt in Cyprus from the Hospitaller Treasurer, Fr. Durand, of 7,800 white besants owed him for grain he had recently sold to the Hospitallers at Rhodes; the act was done *in domo Ospitalis sancte domus* at Famagusta [57]. In about May 1308 Baldo Spinola, by then on a mission for King Oshin of Armenia, arrived at Rhodes to find Aitone Doria there with his galley [58]. Doria may have been using Rhodes as a base; by September of that year news had reached Venice that he and his galley had robbed shipping belonging to the Venetian families of Sanudo and Soranzo [59].

The fortified town of Rhodes finally surrendered, on terms, most probably on 25 August 1309 [60]. Andronikos II was at war with

---

[57] Texts in M. BALARD, *Notai Genovesi* cit., pp. 116-117, 134, 144-145, 153-154, 173, 180-181, 185-186, 204, 215-216, 220-221, 375-376. Fr. Durand was already Treasurer in 1306: text in J. DELAVILLE LE ROULX, *Cartulaire général de l'Ordre des Hospitaliers de S. Jean de Jérusalem: 1100-1310*, IV, Paris, 1905, no. 4735.

[58] *Gestes* cit., 867-869; Spinola was to seek the king's brother Sempad who left Cyprus in April or May (*supra*, pp. 748-749).

[59] G. GIOMO cit., p. 284.

[60] J. RILEY-SMITH cit., p. 215 n. 4, establishes the day as 15 August. The year cannot be given with certainty; and all solutions leave unanswered problems, partly because the Western sources, which did not understand events in the Levant, were so confused and contradictory. A. FAILLER, *L'occupation* cit., argues for 1310, but without using all the available evidence; see also ID., *Pachymeriana Alia*, in «Revue des Études Byzantines», LI, 1993, pp. 258-260. In 1315 the Master of the Hospital demanded from the Convent 156,000 florins owing for the «war of Rhodes» which was also said to have cost 50,000 florins a year; since the invasion was launched in June 1306, three times 50,000 florins plus a little more, would give the war as ending in about July 1309: A. LUTTRELL, *Hospitallers of Rhodes* cit., II, p. 110 n. 10. Note also that on 26 June the Grand Commander came from Rhodes with 40 Hospitaller

the Venetians from 1306 until the end of 1310, but his immediate crisis passed when the Catalan company left for Macedonia early in the summer of 1307; the emperor then felt strong enough to make a series of complaints and demands to the government at Genoa, which accepted many of them on 2 March 1308 since the Genoese were themselves under attack from the Mongols in the Black Sea [61]. About a year later followed a renewed appeal for aid from the Greeks on Rhodes, Andronikos despatched arms and supplies for them on a Genoese vessel, but the Hospitallers, who had collected twelve galleys from various Provencals, Genoese and Cypriots to blockade Rhodes, chased away the relief vessel which took refuge in Famagusta; the Hospital's fleet included four galleys from Provence, one of Aitone Doria, one of Vignolo de Vignoli and one, flying the Genoese flag, of Lanfranco Seba. At Famagusta a Cypriot knight named Pierre le Jaune, who had arrived from Rhodes with a small *ligno* armed by the Hospital, captured the Genoese ship and took it to Rhodes, where the Hospitallers pressured the ship's captain into treating with the defenders. The long blockade must have told on their resources and they surrendered on terms [62].

Much of the island of Rhodes had been occupied by November 1306 but the *castello* held out. Meanwhile the centre of action moved to the West. The Hospital's Master, Fr. Foulques de Villaret, had been summoned to France by Pope Clement V and must have

---

brethren and that the Master offered more; it was true that in July the Master was detained on Rhodes by certain *impedimenti*, but on 26 July the Marshal and three Western priors arrived from Rhodes, making a total in Nicosia of 80 *frati cavalieri*, 20 Latin *paggi* (sergeants?) and 200 *fanti*: FRANCESCO AMADI cit., pp. 354, 367-371. That so large a Hospitaller force could be spared from Rhodes might suggest that the war there was over. The present interpretation assumes that a number of sources which gave the Master as present when Rhodes surrendered were mistaken. The whole topic requires yet further discussion.

[61] A. LAIOU cit., pp. 175-177.

[62] *Gestes* cit., pp. 864-865; similarly, FRANCESCO AMADI cit., pp. 258-259, and FLORIO BUSTRON cit., pp. 141-143. On Pierre le Jaune, A. LUTTRELL, *Hospitallers of Rhodes* cit., X, pp. 158-159; for Provencal galleys recruited in the West, E. BARATIER-F. REYNAUD cit., pp. 214-215. The *Gestes* and AMADI said that the surrender was negotiated through the ship's Genoese captain; BUSTRON that it was the Rhodiot envoy sent to the emperor. On 5 November 1309 Ansaldo Grimaldi and other Genoese drew up an act on the mole at Rhodes, but five days later they were at Limassol: texts in M. BALARD, *Notai Genovesi* cit., pp. 309-310, 312.

left the East at about the time of the offer made by the Hospitallers to Andronikos II in April 1307. In France the Master had not only to deal with the problems of concluding the conquest of Rhodes and with the general question of the crusade, but also to confront the dangers to the Hospital which followed the French king's arrest of the Templars, members of a fellow military order, in October 1307. Villaret's solution was to organize a papal crusade which he would lead. It was presented as a project intended to protect the Christians of Cyprus and Armenia, but in reality it enabled him to finance an expedition destined to complete the subjugation of the Rhodian islands; at the same time this scheme, and papal support for it, inhibited Western governments from attacking the Hospital in the way they had the Temple [63]. On 3 June 1307 Andronikos II, who had shown some determination to defend Rhodes against the Hospital, was excommunicated by Clement V, and on 5 September the pope granted Rhodes to the Hospitallers who had, he said, taken it from Greek schismatics and Turkish infidels [64]. In August 1308 the pope issued the letters for the crusading *passagium* [65] and by March 1309 the Hospitallers were even being encouraged from some quarters to direct their expedition against Constantinople itself as part of long-standing schemes to establish the French king's brother, Charles de Valois, as emperor in the East [66].

Meanwhile the Genoese were drawn into participation in the Hospitaller programme in a new and official way. Fr. Foulques de Villaret probably passed through Genoa on more than one occasion, most notably on his journey from Marseilles, where he was in De-

---

[63] J. RILEY-SMITH cit., pp. 220-226; A. LUTTRELL, *Hospitallers of Rhodes* cit., III pp. 70-72; S. SCHEIN cit., pp. 219-230; N. HOUSLEY, *Pope Clement V and the Crusades of 1309-10*, in «Journal of Medieval History», VIII, 1982. R. IRWIN, *How Many Miles to Babylon: the «Devise des Chemins de Babyloine» Redated*, in «The Military Orders: Fighting for the Faith and Caring for the Sick», ed. M. BARBER, Aldershot, 1994, redates another Hospitaller crusade treatise to 1306/7.

[64] Texts in *Regestum Papae Clementis V*, 9 vols., Rome, 1884-1892, II, nos. 1759, 2140.

[65] Text in J. DELAVILLE LE ROULX, *Cartulaire* cit., IV, nos. 4807-4810.

[66] J. HILLGARTH, *Ramon Lull and Lullism in Fourteenth - Century France*, Oxford, 1971, pp. 84-85. Possibly the transfer of the Templars' goods to the Hospital in 1312 was part of an agreement for the Hospital to collaborate in a Valois campaign against Constantinople: A. LUTTRELL, *Hospitallers of Rhodes* cit., III, pp. 73-75.

cember 1308, to Florence and Pisa, which he had reached by late January 1309[67]. One report of January 1309 said that the Master had requested ten or fifteen of the forty galleys he needed at Genoa and that it was being speculated there that they would be used for an attack not in Syria but in Byzantium or Sicily. In March the Aragonese king shrewdly judged that the crusade would be used merely to complete the conquest of Rhodes and the other islands of *Romania* which, the king said, the pope had granted to them[68]. On 27 January Villaret himself announced from Pisa that the Hospital was building twelve galleys at Genoa and was purchasing a *navis magna* there[69]. In October 1309 Hospitaller officials at Marseilles were hiring the ships of Guglielmo Vaca of Finale and Rolando Lameta of Savona[70]. The Genoese probably saw a chance to do business and make gains of some sort. Even before March 1308 Andronikos had complained to the government at Genoa that Benedetto Usodimare and Anicello della Volta were arming galleys at Aigues Mortes in order to attack his empire and its islands[71]. Villaret's departure was so delayed that he was still in the West when the town of Rhodes surrendered, probably in August 1309. He left Genoa on 18 November amid rumours that he might attack not only Rhodes but either Lesbos, Crete or Cyprus, the Venetians being suspicious of what they naturally regarded as a partly Genoese initiative. Villaret was at Brindisi in January 1310 with an estimated twenty-six or twenty-seven galleys, some two or three hundred knights and 3,000 foot, who included the galley crews. Ten of these galleys were Genoese and their captain was Accellino Grillo. By 13 May news had reached Venice that the *passagium* had arrived off Modon and Coron[72].

---

[67] Texts in J. DELAVILLE LE ROULX, *Cartulaire* cit., IV, nos. 4830, 4840-4841.

[68] Texts in H. FINKE cit., III, pp. 191-192, 198-200.

[69] Texts J. DELAVILLE LE ROULX, *Cartulaire* cit., IV, no. 4841.

[70] E. BARATIER - F. REYNAUD cit., p. 215.

[71] Text in L. BELGRANO, *Prima serie di documenti riguardanti la colonia di Pera*, in «Atti della Società Ligure di Storia Patria», XIII, 1877-1884, pp. 110-115.

[72] ARCHIVIO DI STATO DI VENEZIA, Lettere di Collegio, f. 63-64, 69 r.-v., 83 r.-v.; chronicle sources, giving a total of thirty-five galleys, ten Genoese, are collected in A. FAILLER, *L'occupation* cit., pp. 120 n. 19, 121 n. 20. Grillo is named in M.-G. CANALE, *Nuova Istoria della Repubblica di Genova*, III, Florence, 1860, pp. 385, 387.

Whatever objectives this crusade achieved, the Hospital did conquer various islands and, by allying with certain Turks who were
kinsmen of the Emir Masud of Menteshe, it also acquired some territories on the Anatolian mainland[73]. Contemporaries reported that
the Hospital took five islands near Rhodes[74]. In August 1310 the Venetian senate urged its representatives at Constantinople to include
in the truce which they were concluding there a clause guaranteeing
the retention of the «islands acquired in the present war»; these
probably included Karpathos, Amorgos, Siphnos and Ios[75], while
Kos, which had apparently been secured by submission rather than
by conquest, was probably another. Shortly before 31 October 1309
the government of Crete accepted Kos through written pacts and
then sent a hundred mercenaries to defend its two castles. A Hospitaller had arrived on Kos from Rhodes to demand possession of the
island, but in Venice it was agreed on 7 February 1310 to accept the
arrangements proposed by Gioachino Sanudo who had reached
Crete with a request for Venetian protection from the population of
Kos[76]. However, later that year or in the years following Kos was occupied by the Hospitallers[77]. Nisyros, just south of Kos, was apparently taken by two pirates, Giovanni and Bonavita Assanti of Ischia,
who were later rumoured to have secured it as the ransom of a
Turkish lord they had captured and who agreed in 1316 to hold it
in fief from the Hospital[78]. As for Vignolo de Vignoli, on 2 May 1311
he and various merchants had been attacked and robbed while
travelling on Vignolo's *tarida* from Rhodes to Candia; the assailants
were on the Genoese galley of Simone Doria and Antonio Arcanti which was carrying a Genoese ambassador to the Master at
Rhodes[79]. Vignolo was quite probably dead by 1314 and years later,

---

[73] A. LUTTRELL, *Hospitallers of Rhodes* cit., II, pp. 84-86; ID., *Latin Greece, the Hospitallers and the Crusades: 1291-1440*, London, 1982, I, p. 250.

[74] Eg. texts cited in A. FAILLER, *L'occupation* cit., pp. 120 n. 19, 121 n. 20.

[75] R.-J. LOENERTZ, *Menego Schiavo* cit., pp. 321-324.

[76] Text in Z. TSIRPANLIS cit., pp. 32-33 n. 5.

[77] Probably during the 1310 campaign and by 1317 at latest: texts in A. LUT-
TRELL, *Hospitallers of Rhodes* cit., IV pp. 83-86.

[78] A. LUTTRELL, *Hospitallers in Cyprus* cit., III, pp. 759.

[79] ARCHIVIO DI STATO DI VENEZIA, Commemoriali, I, f. 167 v.

in 1325, his *casale* of Lardos was granted in fief to a Fulco de Vignoli, *phisicus* and citizen of Genoa, who had inherited the Vignolo
claims to it according to the agreement of 1306[80].

Another island taken by the Hospitallers was that of Karpathos
which lay between Rhodes and Crete. Karpathos was in the hands of
the Venetian Andrea Cornaro who on 8 January 1309 was granted
permission at Venice to send grain there from Crete[81], but Andrea
and Lodovico Moresco claimed to hold it from the emperor. Perhaps
in about 1309 Lodovico made several armed attempts to acquire
Karpathos by raising a rebellion there; he caused great damage but
was captured by Andrea Cornaro and imprisoned on Crete as a corsair; he was still there in 1319. Andronikos II intervened in about
1314 and again in 1319 to secure his release on the grounds that Lodovico was his vassal and should be treated as a Greek – *computatus
ut Grecus* – rather than as a Latin pirate, and that he had held the
custodia of the islands around Rhodes on behalf of the emperor. Andronikos argued in 1319 that Andrea Moresco, who had been his Admiral and his vassal, had been given these islands *in feudum* and
that the two brothers had owed service for them. For their part, the
Venetians evaded the issue by claiming that in his capacity as lord
of Karpathos Andrea Cornaro was not under Venetian jurisdiction[82].
Karpathos and the small islands of Kassos and Saria nearby were
occupied by the Hospitallers, presumably in 1310 or soon after. This
led to Venetian protests and to the sequestration of Hospitaller
funds at Venice between 1312 and 1314. The Hospital argued that
Andrea Cornaro had no good claim to the islands, which had in earlier times been under the jurisdiction of Rhodes and which had gone
over to the Hospital because the inhabitants considered that Cornaro could not protect them against pirates; these arguments were
rejected by the Venetians. The Hospital made no reference to the

---

[80] A. LUTTRELL, *Hospitallers in Cyprus* cit., III, pp. 757, 763.

[81] Text in S. THEOTOKIS, *Historika kretika eggrapha: Apophaseis meizonos sym-
bouliou Benetias: 1255-1689*, Athens, 1933, p. 56. Andrea Cornaro held Karpathos in
1301: text in R. MOROZZO DELLA ROCCA, *Benvenuto da Brixano: Notaio in Candia 1301-
1302*, Venice, 1950, pp. 93-94.

[82] Texts in R. CESSI-P. SAMBIN cit., I, p. 145, and G. THOMAS cit., I, pp. 131-132,
143-144, 156. Andrea Moresco was not lord of Rhodes, as often asserted, but held *in
feudum* from the emperor the *insule Imperij nostri prope insulam Rhodi*: text *ibidem*,
p. 144.

rights of Andronikos II and the Moresco brothers. In 1314 the Hospitallers agreed to papal arbitration and on 20 June 1316 they announced that they would return the three islands to Andrea Cornaro, which they did[83].

The Venetians had been prevented from acquiring Rhodes, Kos or the surrounding islands, but otherwise the conquest of the islands proved unsatisfactory for the Genoese. The Hospitallers themselves had repeatedly justified the acquisition of Rhodes as providing a base from which they could police the prohibitions on trade with the infidel, but the papal embargo was accepted only half-heartedly by the Genoese authorities[84]. Various forms of economic warfare had been advocated by the majority of the theorists of the crusade, including Fr. Foulques de Villaret[85], and the importance of Rhodes for the blockade had been emphasized by contemporaries such as the author of the *Gestes des Chiprois* who remarked, somewhat unrealistically, that after the conquest of Rhodes «bad merchants» never dared to pass near Rhodes or to take prohibited goods or slaves to or from Turkey and Egypt[86]. The Order faced enormous debts which had been contracted partly to finance the lengthy campaign to conquer Rhodes[87], and the authorization to capture Christian shipping involved in the prohibited trade naturally tempted the Hospitallers. There was correspondence between the Master and the Venetian government on the subject in 1308[88] and again when the

---

[83] J. DELAVILLE LE ROULX, *Les Hospitaliers à Rhodes jusqu'à la mort de Philibert de Naillac: 1310-1421*, Paris, 1913, pp. 3-4; A. LUTTRELL, *Hospitallers in Cyprus* cit., V, pp. 197, 202. The latter (p. 202) was probably wrong to repeat K. Hopf's claim, based only on a modern annotation in a printed work, that Januli de Corogna was a Hospitaller and that he seized Siphnos in the Cyclades in 1307.

[84] E. ASHTOR, *Levant Trade in the Later Middle Ages*, Princeton, 1983, pp. 17-44; see also B. KEDAR, *Segurano-Sakran Salvaygo: un mercante genovese al servizio dei Sultani mamalucchi, c. 1303-1322*, in «Fatti e idee di storia economica nei secoli XII-XX. Studi dedicati a Franco Borlandi», Imola, 1976, and J. RICHARD, *Le Royaume de Chypre et l'Embargo sur le commerce avec l'Égypte (fin XIIIe-début XIVe siècle)*, in «Académie des Inscriptions et Belles-Lettres: Comptes Rendus», 1984.

[85] S. SCHEIN cit., p. 202.

[86] *Gestes* cit., pp. 863, 865; FRANCESCO AMADI cit., p. 259.

[87] A. LUTTRELL, *Hospitallers in Cyprus* cit., VIII, pp. 318-320; ID., *Hospitaller Priory of Venice* cit., p. 107.

[88] Text in R. CESSI - P. SAMBIN cit., I, p. 131.

Venetians wrote on 13 May 1310 expressing approval of the Hospitallers' interventions to enforce the papal embargo[89]. The Hospital's
attacks were, after all, directed chiefly at Venice's rivals from Genoa.

Serious difficulties arose with the Genoese. Since the papal
prohibitions discouraged trade with Egypt and Syria to the advantage of Famagusta, the Cypriot government enforced them actively, to
the annoyance of Genoese merchants who suffered as a result[90]. The
commune of Genoa passed decrees against the trade in war materials in 1305 and 1308, but the Genoese only partially accepted the
papal legislation and their *Officium Robarie* largely nullified their
decrees by permitting merchants whose prohibited merchandise
had been confiscated to claim that they had been attacked by pirates[91]. On 21 December 1309 near Cephalonia the Genoese Andalò,
Raffo and Giuliano Cattaneo della Volta attacked a Sienese merchant returning from Alexandria with pepper and sugar, and he presented claims to the *Officium* at Genoa. Since the della Volta asserted that they had been acting to enforce the papal embargo, the *Officium* raised the question with the archbishop who on 2 June 1310
declared his readiness to produce the papal letters authorizing the
Hospital to act in the *factum passagii*[92]. The Genoese texts did not
state precisely what had happened, but a Venetian complaint to the
Master of the Hospital, made on 14 May 1310 on behalf of Marin
Falier and his partners, claimed that in January of that year Simeo-
ne Giuliano della Volta, described as captain of a Hospitaller galley,
had robbed the Venetians of pepper and sugar which their ship
was taking from Crete to Negroponte[93]. Evidently certain Genoese
were cunningly exploiting the Hospitaller *passagium* as a cover for
piratical operations.

Subsequently, however, the Genoese were themselves to suffer
from the Hospitallers' interpretation of the papal embargo. The cru-

---

[89] G. GIOMO cit., p. 366.

[90] P. EDBURY, *Cyprus and Genoa* cit., pp. 107, 117-120.

[91] E. ASHTOR cit., pp. 19-20.

[92] Texts and discussion in B. KEDAR, *L'«Officium Robarie» di Genova: un tentativo di coesistere con la violenza*, in «Archivio Storico Italiano», CXLIII, 1985, pp. 339-
346, 360-361.

[93] ARCHIVIO DI STATO DI VENEZIA, Lettere del Collegio, f. 84.

sading proposals made in 1311 by Henri II of Cyprus noted that during the winter of 1310 Hospitaller galleys had seized a Genoese galley returning from Alexandria while it was in the waters of Messina and had taken it to Rhodes. Genoa sent envoys to Rhodes where the Master replied that his galleys had been following papal instructions and that he could not release the Genoese ships and goods without the pope's consent. According to Henri II, the envoys themselves accepted this, but two Genoese galleys sailed to Rhodian waters and captured several Hospitaller vessels – *plura vasa* – and their men and goods, inflicting great damage on the Order; the ships attacked included an *userium* of the Master arriving from Brindisi with various Hospitaller brethren, twenty-five horses and many goods, all of which were taken to *Turquia* and in great part sold to the Turks[94]. On 17 July 1311 the pope, apparently referring to a different case, wrote of several Hospitaller galleys and their *stipendiarii* which, while legitimately engaged in controlling the traffic with the infidel, had captured a Genoese galley some way east of Sicily off Crotone and had taken it to Brindisi; the crew confessed and the ship's registers showed their guilt, but the officials of the Neapolitan king had seized the goods and the pope demanded their return to the Hospitallers[95]. On 25 May 1313 the Master at Rhodes imprisoned certain Genoese sailing with two galleys, one *nave* and other vessels from Cyprus to Genoa[96]. Jacobo de Nerono *quondam* Guglielmo Salvaygo, who had been in Syria where he had consigned some cloth to Rainerio de Guisolfo, was among a number of persons detained with their merchandise by the Master at Rhodes in that same month. Some of their goods were returned following a promise by the Master and Convent, probably made on 14 September, to restore everything which had been seized[97].

---

[94] Undated text in R. DE MAS LATRIE, *Histoire de l'île de Chypre sous le règne des Princes de la Maison de Lusignan*, III, Paris, 1855, pp. 118-125.

[95] Text in *Registrum Clementis Papae V* cit., VI, nos. 7118-7119.

[96] FRANCESCO AMADI cit., p. 395.

[97] Text in R. DOEHAERD, *Les relations commerciales entre Gênes, le Belgique et l'Outremont d'après les Archives notariales génoises aux XIIIe et XIVe siècles*, III, Brussels-Rome, 1941, pp. 1106-1107. The text was dated in Genoa on 5 December 1313 and gives the date of the Master's promise made at Rhodes as 14 *decembris* 1313; September seems the most likely emendation.

The conflict had reached crisis point two years earlier in 1311 when Antonio Spinola was sent from Genoa to demand the return of the galley captured off Messina by the Hospitallers, who alleged that they were enforcing the papal prohibitions; the vessel on which Spinola travelled was captained by Simone Doria and Antonio Arcanti, and it was this ship which captured Vignolo de Vignoli and his *tarida*. The Master and council at Rhodes asserted that they had acted legitimately and could not return either the galley or the goods without the pope's assent. According to the pope's letters, they promised Spinola a written reply but when he received no satisfactory answer or letters, he and three Genoese galley captains, Simone Doria, Bernabò de Savignono and Antonio Arcanti, went to the Turkish ruler of Menteshe and, according at least to the Hospitallers, they offered him 50,000 florins to attack Rhodes and various other islands in Byzantine hands. The papal letters also claimed that many merchants and others from Rhodes, who were numbered at about 250 and whose presence suggested some kind of agreement or understanding between Rhodes and Menteshe, were arrested on the mainland where they were seeking food and animals to provision the island of Rhodes. These Turkish collaborations and their consequences may have occurred after Henri II had written his treatise of 1311, which did not mention them. Furthermore, the Genoese captains were said by the papal letters to have captured a number of Hospitallers and their vessels bound for Rhodes, imprisoning and holding to ransom Hospitaller knights and other brethren; they even, it was alleged, threatened to kill and rob the Hospitaller brethren and to expel their Order from Rhodes. The Hospitaller Priors of Rome and Lombardy were sent to Genoa to complain, but after waiting there a month they received no answer and so they went to Clement V at Vienne. On 26 November 1311 the pope protested to Genoa; accepting the Hospital's doubtless onesided version of events, he demanded the liberation of the captive Hospitallers and their goods [98].

The ruler of Menteshe may indeed have taken some action, since by April 1312 news had reached France that the Hospitaller fleet

---

[98] Texts in *Registrum Clementis Papae V* cit., VII, nos. 7631-7632; E. ASHTOR cit., p. 19, regards these papal letters as referring to decrees of the council at Vienne of 1311-1312, but earlier councils were clearly intended.

had pursued twenty-three Turkish ships, whose origin was not reported, to the island of Amorgos. There they burnt the Turks' ships and
destroyed almost their entire force of over 800 men, but they
themselves suffered serious losses amounting to fifty-seven Hospitaller brethren and 300 foot soldiers [99]. The Hospitallers eventually
had to give way to the Genoese and accept arbitration. By March
1315 they had agreed to pay at least 106,956 *libre*, 9 *solidi* and
10 *denarii* for damages done to Genoese ships and goods seized
by the Master before 9 October 1312; this sum was to raised
from the Order's incomes over a number of years [100]. The Hospitallers had taken Rhodes where they successfully established an independent base which ensured their order's continued existence, but
part of the price was paid much later. At Genoa between 27 July and
12 December 1342 the notary Bartolomeo de Bracellis issued at
least forty-nine written quittances to forty-eight named Genoese citizens who were *ex perdentibus et dampnificatis Rodi*, or to their heirs
or successors. The sums recorded varied between 15 and 900 *libbre*;
nineteen of the quittances did not state the amount involved, while
in the others thirty-four individuals received a total of 9,775 *libbre*, 6
soldi, 8 *denarii* [101]. These payments represented part of the damages
for the seizures of 1313 which had brought relations with the
Genoese to a low point.

While Genoa was able eventually to win compensation for its citizens' losses, the Hospital's institutional coherence allowed it to
consolidate a permanent position on Rhodes. Of the piratical Genoese opportunists, Andrea Moresco disappeared, his brother Lodovico was confined to a Cretan prison and their uncle Vignolo de Vi-

---

[99] FRANCESCO AMADI cit., p. 393; cf. A. LUTTRELL, *Hospitallers of Rhodes* cit., II, p.
86. The Turk Sasa seems to have sided with the Latins against his kinsman Masud
Emir of Menteshe: E. ZACHARIADOU cit., pp. 107-109, and N. OIKONOMIDES, *The Turks
in Europe (1305-13) and the Serbs in Asia Minor*, in «The Ottoman Emirate: 1300-
1389», ed. E. ZACHARIADOU, Rethymnon, 1993, pp. 165-168.

[100] MARSEILLES, ARCHIVES DÉPARTEMENTALES DES BOUCHES-DU-RHÔNE, 56 H 4087.
On 12 and 17 September 1319 a Genoese representative issues receipts for 10,000 and
1,000 florins of Florence paid by the Hospital according to an agreement of 1317: VAL-
LETTA, NATIONAL LIBRARY OF MALTA, ARCHIVES OF THE ORDER OF ST. JOHN, Cod. 20 no. 6.

[101] VALLETTA, Cod. 20 nos. 7-55. Recipients included Ambrosio Salvaygo, heir of
Segurano Salvaygo (no. 18) and the Jacobo de Nerono and Rainerio Guisolfo mentioned *supra*, p. 758 (nos. 14, 16).

gnoli was last heard of being captured by fellow citizens. No contemporary source recounted what became of the Genoese galleys
which accompanied the *passagium* of 1310. Collaboration was trans-
formed into conflict. Some Genoese who had served alongside the
Hospital became the victims of Hospitaller attacks. For example,
Giuliano and Raffo della Volta who had captained a galley in Hospitaller service in 1309 had their goods seized on Rhodes in 1313 [102].
The Genoese, whether as individuals or as a commune, had achieved
little more than the exclusion of the Venetians from Rhodes and
Kos. It seemed to some in the West that the Hospitaller expedition
had expended the great sums contributed by the faithful for a crusade merely on the conquest of Rhodes or, worse, for no result at all.
Thus one author remarked *De passagio vero nil sequtum est. Propter
que magnum scandalum in christiano populo sequtum est* [103]. Yet Villaret rescued his Order from its difficulties on Cyprus and he saved
it from any fate such as that of the Temple, which was suppressed in
1312. He pushed back the Turks on the mainland, where the Order
occupied various territories. The conquest of Rhodes acquired for
the Hospitallers a defensible and virtually independent base for their
continued existence as an institution devoted to the struggle against
the Muslims, but in the short term the Hospital's objective of enforcing the embargo on trade with the infidel was frustrated, largely
through Genoese opposition. As Marino Sanudo wrote, the blockade
could succeed only with the co-operation of Venice and of Genoa [104].

---

[102] VALLETTA, Cod. 20 no. 47.

[103] *Quinta Vita Clementis V auctore Paolo Veneto*, in É. BALUZE-G. MOLLAT, *Vitae
Paparum Avenionensium*, I, Paris, 1914, p. 82.

[104] Cited S. SCHEIN cit., p. 233.

II

GLI OSPITALIERI DI SAN GIOVANNI DI GERUSALEMME
DAL CONTINENTE ALLE ISOLE

La caduta di Acri nel 1291 inflisse un colpo serio all'opinione pubblica occidentale, ma non costituì una svolta decisiva nell'evoluzione del suo atteggiamento verso la crociata. Mentre i Latini continuavano ad interessarsi, generalmente in modo solo teorico, al recupero di Gerusalemme, il papato affrontava gravi difficoltà in Occidente. I successivi re di Francia mostravano entusiasmo per una crociata da loro concepita come un quasi monopolio francese nel quale la corona avrebbe dovuto svolgere il ruolo di ispiratore, ma in realtà si preoccupavano soprattutto di raccogliere a spese del clero francese le decime per la crociata e di favorire le pretese dinastiche franco-angioine a Costantinopoli; dopo il 1291 Filippo IV fu sempre meno intenzionato a sprecare soldi per un'effettiva spedizione. I teorici della crociata seguitavano a proporre, con qualche variante, i differenti progetti già discussi al concilio di Lione nel 1274, mentre le città mercantili del Mediterraneo latino mantenevano i loro scambi con i Mammalucchi in Egitto. In fondo la perdita della Siria cambiò poco delle attitudini occidentali[1].

Per i Latini d'Oriente le cose andavano diversamente. Gli ordini militari, avendo perso uomini e risorse, sedi centrali, campo d'azione e ruolo come difensori della Terra Santa, si trovavano a dover fronteggiare una fondamentale crisi materiale e morale. A questi problemi i tre maggiori ordini trovarono soluzioni diverse. Nel 1291 l'Ordine Teutonico si ritirava a Venezia e nel 1309 trasferiva il suo alto comando a Marienburg, dove continuò un'altra guerra santa allargando con grande successo il suo stato continentale, già assai sviluppato, in Prussia ed anche in Livonia. Per i Teutonici fu l'abbandono del Mediterraneo. Il Tempio stabilì il suo convento o quartiere generale a Limassol, cioè a Cipro, dove la sua politica rimaneva quella di continuare la lotta contro i Mammalucchi con assalti alle coste siriane. I Templari si immischiarono nella politica dinastica di Cipro e mantennero, soprattutto in Francia, le loro funzioni di banchieri. Nel 1307, per motivi mai chiariti, Filippo IV di Francia ordinò l'arresto di tutti i Templari nel suo regno e nel 1312, dopo straordinarie accuse, processi e confessioni, il Tempio fu disciolto dal papa. Gli Ospitalieri si stabilirono anch'essi a Limassol nel 1291, e nel 1306 iniziarono un'invasione dell'isola greca di Rodi dove crea-

---

[1] La tesi di S. SCHEIN, *Fideles Crucis: the Papacy, the West and the Recovery of the Holy Land 1274-1314*, Oxford 1991; questo studio è, purtroppo, limitato dal fatto che si ferma all'anno 1314; è assai discutibile la sua interpretazione della politica francese.

rono un *Ordensstaat*, cioè uno Stato diretto da un ordine religioso, evitando così in modo quasi totale le accuse lanciate contro i Templari[2].

Gli Ospitalieri, sia che fossero preti, *milites* o sergenti, erano tutti religiosi professi con voti di povertà, castità e obbedienza, e con una regola approvata dal papato. Inoltre facevano voto di servire i loro «signori infermi», ma il dovere fondamentale degli ordini militari era la guerra perpetua contro gli infedeli. Era loro proibito di prendere il voto della crociata per farsi *crucesignati* o di far guerra ai cristiani, sia Greci sia Latini. Quindi gli Ospitalieri normalmente non partecipavano alle crociate proclamate in Occidente contro i nemici latini del papato. Il quartiere generale dell'ordine, il convento, era in Oriente, ma l'Ospedale contava per uomini, risorse e denaro sui suoi possedimenti, raggruppati in priorati e commende, in Occidente. Fu proprio perché disponevano di questo retroterra, di queste basi in un certo senso coloniali, in Occidente che gli ordini furono capaci di sopravvivere alla perdita dei loro possedimenti orientali in Siria. Tale ricchezza non era, però, intoccabile, come dimostrò la caduta del Tempio[3].

Fino al 1291 l'Ospedale di S. Giovanni era rimasto una potenza continentale. Possedeva varie proprietà e una base di rifornimento sull'isola di Cipro, ma il grosso del suo patrimonio orientale si trovava in Siria, con qualche castello e varie rivendicazioni su beni nella Cilicia armena. Nel XIII secolo il suo carattere militare e la sua componente di *milites* trovarono definizione nel corpo legislativo dell'ordine; in effetti i *milites* appartenevano per la maggior parte alla piccola nobiltà e al patriziato urbano. L'Ospedale fu essenzialmente francese, predominando l'elemento della Francia del sud e della Provenza. Gli Ospitalieri giocarono un ruolo cospicuo nella difesa della Siria, nella sua politica ed anche nelle sue dispute interne. Disponendo in misura consistente di terreni, castelli e forze militari, l'ordine aveva le sue zone di influenza, dove esercitava una libertà considerevole di dominio; tuttavia esso non costituì mai una potenza pienamente indipendente, capace di agire o governare veramente da sola. L'Ospedale era, accanto alla corona, ai baroni, alla Chiesa secolare, agli altri ordini e ai comuni italiani, un elemento fra gli altri con i quali doveva mantenere un rapporto di convivenza. Gli ordini militari costituivano dei gruppi di guerrieri di professione, sperimentati e cauti[4], ma sceglievano istintivamente l'accomodamento con l'infedele. La difficile posizione latina lungo la striscia costiera contribuiva alla formazione di una

---

[2] A. FOREY, *The Military Orders from the Twelfth to the Early Fourteenth Centuries*, London 1992, fornisce l'unico recente trattato comparativo degli ordini militari considerati come categoria; termina però all'anno 1312. N. HOUSLEY, *The Avignon Papacy and the Crusade: 1305-1378*, Oxford 1986, pp. 260-92, contiene uno studio molto interessante sugli ordini militari.

[3] J. RILEY-SMITH, *The Knights of St. John in Jerusalem and Cyprus: c. 1050-1310*, London 1967; questo lavoro si ferma all'anno 1310, come anche la pubblicazione dei testi in *Cartulaire général de l'Ordre des Hospitaliers de Saint-Jean de Jérusalem: 1100-1310*, 1-4, ed. J. DELAVILLE LE ROULX, Paris 1894-1906. Per il periodo successivo, c'è ID., *Les Hospitaliers à Rhodes jusqu'à la mort de Philibert de Naillac: 1310-1421*, Paris 1913, con aggiunte nei lavori di A. Luttrell citati *infra*. Il periodo dopo il 1421 attende uno studio soddisfacente.

[4] M. BENNET, *"La Règle du Temple" as a Military Manual or How to Deliver a Cavalry Charge*, in *Studies in Medieval History presented to R. Allen Brown*, ed. C. HARPER-BILL *et al.*, Woodbridge 1989.

mentalità passiva e difensiva con tendenza alla costruzione di grandi fortificazioni in pietra e a un'economia di difesa con piccole, e quindi relativamente poco costose, guarnigioni. Tale politica e le occasionali rivalità fra gli ordini provocavano critiche in Occidente dove l'opinione era sempre più disposta alla guerra aperta e all'azione diretta per il recupero di Gerusalemme.

In occasione della caduta di Acri i membri degli ordini militari si comportarono con molto coraggio. L'Ospedale aveva già perso 40 *fratres* a Tripoli nel 1289; ad Acri, dove *nous pierdimes a petit peties tout le couvent de no religion*, fu ucciso il suo Maresciallo e ferito gravemente il Maestro[5]. Una parte del suo archivio centrale contenente molti titoli relativi ai possedimenti siriani, fu inviata in salvo in Occidente così come, apparentemente, lo fu il corpo del fondatore, il beato Gerardo. Questi pezzi rappresentavano un elemento di continuità, ma andarono persi il grosso dell'archivio, incluso l'originale della regola con la bolla papale, e tutte le reliquie[6]. L'Ospedale perdette anche i suoi uomini, terreni e introiti siriani, nonché la sua posizione nella società del regno di Gerusalemme; perdette inoltre il contatto con certi elementi caratteristici fondamentali della sua missione, cioè la vicinanza alla città santa di Gerusalemme, la presenza dei pellegrini di passaggio ad Acri, e la possibilità di un confronto continentale permanente con gli infedeli. I suoi membri subirono un grosso trauma morale. Dovettero adattare le loro istituzioni a nuove circostanze difficili, ricostruire un archivio, ristabilire il loro convento e l'ospedale conventuale per poveri e infermi, chiamare nuovi uomini in Oriente, e così via. L'Ospedale diventò molto più dipendente dalle sue risorse in Occidente dove l'opinione pubblica era già da tempo contraria, o almeno critica, nei confronti degli ordini militari e delle loro immunità, e dove il clero secolare protestava contro le sue esenzioni ecclesiastiche; dopo il 1291 gli ordini militari furono, in larga parte ingiustamente, considerati responsabili della perdita della Siria latina. Subito dopo la caduta di Acri il fatto che il Maestro dell'Ospedale si era salvato, anche se gravemente ferito, arrecava più prestigio in Occidente ai Templari, il Maestro dei quali invece era rimasto ucciso ad Acri. In compenso, più tardi l'Ospedale trasse profitto dalla diffusione del *De excidio urbis Acconensis*, racconto molto popolare e conosciuto, che accusava i Templari e lodava il Maresciallo dell'Ospedale, Mathieu de Clermont, come martire coraggioso[7]. In ogni caso, il pubblico considerava tutti gli ordini come responsabili, e nel 1291 il papa incoraggiò questa tendenza invitando una serie di concili ecclesiastici provinciali a dibattere la questione degli ordini nel corso delle loro discussioni sulla crociata[8].

Il soggiorno degli Ospitalieri e dei Templari a Cipro diventò un periodo di incertezza e difficoltà. La corona scoraggiava l'insediamento sull'isola dei due potenti ordini stranieri. Mancavano loro rifornimenti alimentari, cavalli, eccetera, senza contare che essi cercavano un più conveniente campo d'azione. Gli Ospitalieri di S. Giovanni pensavano ad uno sboc-

---

[5] *Cartulaire* (come n. 3), 4050, 4157; RILEY-SMITH (come n. 3), pp. 196-7.

[6] A. LUTTRELL, *The Hospitallers of Rhodes and their Mediterranean World*, Aldershot 1992, XVIII, pp. 7-14, e Addenda et Corrigenda, p. 3.

[7] FOREY (come n. 2), pp. 204-25; H. NICHOLSON, *Templars, Hospitallers and Teutonic Knights: Images of the Military Orders, 1128-1291*, Leicester 1993, pp. 125-8.

[8] SCHEIN (come n. 1), pp. 74-6, 130-1, 136-8.

co nella Cilicia armena, con la quale mantennero contatti di una certa regolarità fino al 1302 o anche dopo[9]. Nel 1291 il papa per aiutare gli Armeni ordinava galee, concedeva indulgenze e otteneva fondi dai Templari e dagli Ospitalieri; nel gennaio 1292 ordinava ai Maestri dei due ordini di intervenire in Cilicia. Nel 1292 i Latini da Cipro attaccavano Alaya in Cilicia, ma poi si ritirarono. Nel 1293 i Templari decisero di armare 6 galee a Venezia, ma due di queste parteciparono ad una battaglia contro i Genovesi[10]. Nella primavera del 1292 i Mammalucchi minacciarono un'invasione della Cilicia, e a un certo momento dopo l'aprile di quell'anno Jean de Villiers, Maestro dell'Ospedale, e Jacques de Molay, Maestro del Tempio, con dei loro *fratres* e con l'inviato inglese, Otto de Grandson, si trasferirono in Cilicia[11]. L'invasione mammalucca fu rinviata al 1293; gli Armeni riuscirono ad evitarla pagando un grosso tributo. Più tardi la Cilicia venne visitata due volte con forze a cavallo e di fanteria da Guillaume de Villaret, Maestro dell'Ospedale, fra il suo arrivo a Cipro, nella seconda metà del 1300, e la sua morte nel 1305[12].

[9] A. LUTTRELL, *Latin Greece, the Hospitallers and the Crusades: 1291-1440*, London 1982, V, pp. 121-5, 134-5.

[10] SCHEIN (come n. 1), pp. 77-9. Il castello templare di Roche Guillaume nella Cilicia fu preso dai Mussulmani nel 1299, ma non è certo che i Templari lo difendessero fino a quell'anno: LUTTRELL (come n. 9), V, p. 122.

[11] Hetoum di Gorighos (in *Recueil des Historiens des Croisades: Documents Arméniens*, 1-2, Paris 1869-1906, 2, pp. 211, 327, 330) narra che il re Thoros III convocò Otto de Grandson e altri in Cilicia e poi rinunciò alla corona, e che lui, Hetoum, dopo due anni trascorsi in Francia (secondo il curatore nel 1299-1301), ritornò in Cilicia e tentò di riprendere il controllo della situazione; citò come testimoni Grandson e i Maestri dei due ordini con i loro *fratres*. Il curatore del testo (*ibid.*, 2, pp. 327, 917) pone la visita di Grandson sia nel 1291/3, sia nel 1299/1302(!). C. KINGSFORD, *Sir Otho de Grandson (1238?-1328)*, in *Transactions of the Royal Historical Society*, 3 ser., 3 (1909), pp. 151-2, e E. CLIFFORD, *A Knight of Great Renown: the Life and Times of Othon de Grandson*, Chicago 1961, pp. 128, 133, seguito da LUTTRELL (come n. 9), V, p. 121, parla erroneamente di una coronazione e pone il ritorno di Grandson nella primavera del 1294. Hetoum di Gorigos, 2, pp. 329-30, colloca il ritorno di Grandson fra l'arrivo in Siria del mongolo Ghazan (1299) e la morte dello stesso (1305). Hetoum sembra aver fatto confusione, dato che il Maestro dell'Ospedale e i suoi *fratres* visitarono due volte la Cilicia fra il 1300 e il 1305: LUTTRELL (come n. 9), V, p. 123. Le fonti citate in C. TYERMAN, *England and the Crusades: 1095-1588*, Chicago 1988, pp. 237-8, non dimostrano che Grandson visitò Gerusalemme dopo il maggio del 1291, anche se tale visita è una possibilità. Nell'aprile 1292 Grandson e il Maestro dell'Ospedale assisterono all'elezione in Cipro di Jacques de Molay: *supra*, p. 87. È possibile che fossero convocati in Cilicia per affrontare la minaccia mammalucca della primavera del 1292. In questo caso fu Molay ad andare in Cilicia: *corrige* M.-L. BULST-THIELE, *Sacrae Domus Militiae Templi Hierosolymitani Magistri*, Göttingen 1974, pp. 293-4. Il Maestro dell'Ospedale era a Limassol in Cipro nell'ottobre 1292 e nell'ottobre 1293: *Cartulaire* (come n. 3), 4194, 4234. Grandson ritornò in Cilicia nel 1293. Il 24 maggio aveva già lasciato l'Inghilterra: testo in *Placita de Quo Warranto temporibus Edwardi I. II. et III.*, ed. W. ILLINGWORTH, London 1818, p. 354. Grandson e Molay erano a Londra nel dicembre 1293: *infra*, n. 56. Grandson non tornò più in Oriente. Molay si trovò in Provenza (forse maggio 1293), era atteso in Aragona (agosto 1293) e fu a Londra (dicembre 1293): BULST-THIELE, pp. 305 n. 50, 306 n. 51, 356-7. Secondo *Les Gestes des Chiprois* (ed. G. RAYNAUD, Genève 1887, p. 279), Grandson si trovava a Corycos, di ritorno dalla corte del re d'Armenia, poco prima della grande battaglia fra Genovesi e Veneziani vicino a Lajazzo; ma questo deve essere un errore, perché la battaglia ebbe luogo il 28 maggio 1294: *Annales Genuenses*, ed. G. PETTI-BALBI, in *Rerum Italicarum Scriptores*, n. ser. 17, 2, Bologna 1975, pp. 34-5.

[12] LUTTRELL (come n. 9), V, p. 123.

Proposte del 1299 e del 1300 per una collaborazione con i Mongoli, che si apprestava-
no a invadere la Siria, portarono solo ad una campagna sulle coste mammalucche, alla quale parteciparono gli Ospitalieri e i Templari. Nel 1300 i Templari occupavano la piccola isola di Ruad, situata molto vicino alla città di Tortosa, che era un vecchio ed importante possedimento templare sulla costa siriana; nel 1301 il papa concesse al Tempio la metà di Ruad,
sebbene non fosse ancora in loro possesso. La bolla papale dichiarò che i Templari stavano
fortificando Ruad e che erano gli unici a difendere l'isola. Probabilmente le alte gerarchie
del Tempio pensavano di trasferire il loro quartiere generale su quell'isola. Una fonte mus-
sulmana asserisce che i Templari stavano fortificando Ruad per controllare le azioni del ne-
mico sulla terraferma e catturare i viaggiatori lungo la costa. In un primo momento gli Ospitalieri parteciparono a questa sfortunata iniziativa, per poi ritirare le loro forze dall'isola, e
nell'ottobre 1302 molti Templari con un gran numero di loro uomini posti a difesa di Ruad,
mancando galee e navi, furono tutti – incluso il loro Maresciallo – presi dai Mammalucchi
e deportati in Egitto[13].

Il Maestro dell'Ospedale si trattenne – a quanto sembra – a Ruad dal novembre 1300 al-
l'aprile 1301 *cum toto passagio suo... et cum gentibus suis Cipri*, mentre il Maestro del Tempio salpò *cum toto conventu suo et pulchris aliis gentibus*; queste forze furono impiegate su
terraferma per più di 25 giorni. Scrivendo da Limassol l'8 aprile 1301, il Maestro del Tempio metteva l'accento sul trasferimento del suo convento a Ruad: *noster conventus cum ga-
leis et teridis nostris totidem*. L'8 novembre, sempre da Limassol, lo stesso Maestro ricor-
dava che *noster conventus stetit cum equis et armis* a Ruad per tutto l'anno, arrecando non
pochi danni agli infedeli[14]. Marino Sanudo, testimone degno di fede, dice che «la maggior
parte del convento» dei Templari era a Ruad, dove essi stavano innalzando edifici; ma, no-
nostante ciò, nel 1302 furono presi prigionieri 120 Templari e uccisi quasi 500 arcieri e 300
altre persone[15]. Secondo Francesco Amadi, i Templari persero 200 *cavaglieri*, 500 arcieri e
400 altre persone, mentre il re di Cipro e i Maestri del Tempio e dell'Ospedale armarono
una flotta a Famagosta per salvare Ruad, ma troppo in ritardo[16]. Le proposte mongole pro-
vocarono disaccordi fra il re e i due ordini[17]. Nel 1306 il re Enrico II fu accusato di aver cer-
cato nel 1301 di bloccare la partenza delle navi che dovevano portare urgentemente vettovaglie alle forze cipriote di Ruad[18], mentre sembra che gli Ospitalieri rifiutassero di ritor-
nare sull'isola perché non si fidavano delle promesse mongole[19]; forse preferivano l'inter-

---

[13] *Ibid.*, V, pp. 122-3, 134-5; Schein (come n. 1), pp. 162-75; P. Edbury, *The Kingdom of Cyprus
and the Crusades: 1191-1374*, Cambridge 1991, pp. 104-6. Vedi i testi in Abou'l Feda, in *Recueil des
historiens des Croisades: Historiens orientaux*, 1-5, Paris 1872-1906, 1, p. 165, e *Les registres de Boniface VIII*, ed. G. Digard *et al.*, 1-4, Paris 1884-1939, n. 4199. Sembra probabile che i Templari non
tenessero Ruad fra il 1291 e il 1300.

[14] Testi in H. Finke, *Papsttum und Untergang des Templerordens*, 1-2, Münster 1907, 2, pp. 3-5;
Id., *Acta Aragonensia*, 1-3, Berlin 1908-1922, 1, p. 79; 3, p. 146; Bulst-Thiele (come n. 11), p. 366.

[15] Marino Sanudo, in *Gesta Dei per Francos*, ed. J. Bongars, 1-3, Hannover 1611, 2, p. 242.

[16] *Chroniques de Chypre d'Amadi et de Strambaldi*, ed. R. de Mas Latrie, Paris 1891, p. 239.

[17] Luttrell (come n. 9), V, p. 122 n. 13.

[18] Testo in C. Köhler, *Documents chypriotes du début du XIV siècle*, in *Revue de l'Orient Latin*,
11 (1905/8), pp. 447-8.

[19] Jean de Paris, in *Recueil des Historiens des Gaules et de la France*, 21, Paris 1855, p. 640.

vento in Cilicia, forse si resero conto dei pericoli della situazione. Il Tempio si impegnò seriamente su Ruad, ma l'isola era piccolissima e indifendibile in mancanza di una flotta: non poteva funzionare come sede di un *Ordensstaat* isolano. Il Tempio pagò caro questo errore del Molay con molti morti e prigionieri. Non mancò, tuttavia, il coraggio, e al Cairo una quarantina di Templari scelse la morte piuttosto che l'apostasia[20]. Nel 1343 l'ex-*miles* del Tempio Gerard de Châtillon si offrì, dopo trentasette anni di carcere, di informare il papa sulla situazione in Oriente[21].

Il trasferimento a Ruad nelle intenzioni dei Templari doveva preludere ad una invasione della terraferma siriana; l'ispirazione era seria e impegnativa, ma fondamentalmente sbagliata. L'isola era troppo vicina al continente e troppo piccola. I due ordini erano alla ricerca di un altro ruolo nella cattura di navi cristiane che commerciavano con gli infedeli in contravvenzione all'embargo papale, provocando così una serie di conflitti con mercanti genovesi e veneziani[22]. Polizia si confondeva facilmente con pirateria. Nel giugno 1306 il papa autorizzava un Templare ad armare varie galee di Marsiglia contro i Mussulmani e contro quei Cristiani che commerciavano illegalmente con loro, con facoltà di trattenere il bottino[23]. Le difficoltà politiche a Cipro culminarono il 26 aprile 1306 con la destituzione del re Enrico II da parte del fratello Amaurie. I Templari, da molto tempo nemici della corona e vittime a Ruad della defezione di Enrico II, appoggiavano il partito di Amaurie, il quale in seguito avrebbe protetto i Templari di Cipro fino al loro arresto nel 1308. In assenza di altri progetti, i Templari pensavano forse a rafforzare la loro posizione a Cipro. Gli Ospitalieri cautamente adottarono una posizione neutrale, e dopo la destituzione del re iniziarono l'invasione di Rodi: cosa che permetteva loro di liberarsi delle limitazioni imposte dalla situazione cipriota. Amaurie prestò qualche aiuto per l'invasione di Rodi, ma nel 1309 si sentì minacciato dal progetto di una crociata in Oriente sotto la direzione degli Ospitalieri; in effetti, dal 1309 in poi l'Ospedale si adoperò attivamente per la restaurazione di Enrico II, avvenuta nel 1310[24].

Nel 1292 uno Statuto dell'Ospedale limitò il numero di *fratres* combattenti a Limassol a soli 40 *milites* e 10 sergenti, ognuno con uno scudiero, un paggio e due cavalli[25]. Nel 1301 e 1302 era già possibile aumentare questa cifra a 70 *milites* con due scudieri e 10 sergenti

---

[20] Testo in K. SCHOTTMÜLLER, *Der Untergang des Templer-Ordens*, 1-2, Berlin 1887, 2, pp. 160-1.

[21] Testo in G. MOYSE, *Les Hospitaliers de Saint-Jean de Jérusalem dans la diocèse de Besançon en 1373*, in *Mélanges de l'Ecole Française de Rome: Moyen âge-Temps modernes*, 85 (1973), pp. 456-8, 514.

[22] SCHEIN (come n. 1), pp. 193-4, 231-3; LUTTRELL (come n. 6), II, pp. 84-5, 110 n. 13.

[23] *Regestum Clementis papae V*, 1-9, Romae 1885-1892, 1, nn. 1034-1036. L'esempio più spettacoloso di un Templare pirata fu Ruggero de Flor: BULST-THIELE (come n. 11), pp. 335-9.

[24] EDBURY (come n. 13), pp. 95-6, 111-3, 121-2; A. LUTTRELL, *The Hospitallers in Cyprus, Rhodes, Greece and the West: 1291-1440*, London 1978, II, pp. 164-9.

[25] Marseilles, Archives départementales des Bouches-du-Rhône, 56 H 4055 (testo mancante in *Cartulaire* [come n. 3], 4194): «Item establi est que doie tenir, au reaume de Chipre .xl. freres cheualiers, et .x. freres sergens d'armes des queaus chascun ait .ij. bestes et .j. escuer et .j. garson». Nel 1309 qualcuno menzionò un capitolo generale dei Templari in Cipro *in quo erant circiter quadringinti fratres*: testo in J. MICHELET, *Procès des Templiers*, 1-2, Paris 1841-1851, 2, p. 139. Probabilmente si tratta di un errore per quaranta. Si parlò di più di 120 Templari a Limassol nel 1304: *ibid.*, 1, p. 562.

con uno scudiero[26], ma tali forze non permettevano grandi azioni continentali. Nel 1306 l'Ospedale, incapace di fornire più di due galee e quattro altre navi per l'invasione di Rodi, fu costretto ad allearsi con certi *patroni* genovesi[27]. Prima del 1291 l'ordine disponeva di varie galee ed altre navi capaci di funzionare come navi da trasporto o da guerra; nel 1246 erano state commissionate a Marsiglia per la prossima crociata un certo numero di navi della larghezza della nave dell'Ospedale chiamata *Comitissa*[28]. Normalmente, però, le navi dell'ordine si limitavano al ruolo di servizio di trasporto di Ospitalieri, di pellegrini, di cavalli e di vettovaglie fra l'Occidente ed Acri[29]. Nel Duecento queste navi erano sottoposte al comando di un *commendator navium*, mentre il Maestro nominava un *comandeor dou frere* per comandare i *fratres* in mare: sembra che quest'ultimo avesse autorità sopra l'altro[30].

Dopo la loro ritirata a Limassol gli Ospitalieri iniziarono il processo di "decontinentalizzazione" con la creazione di una flotta da guerra. Uno Statuto del 1293 trattava della manutenzione di galee ed altre navi sotto un *comandeor*, presumibilmente il *commendator navium*, il responsabile del loro armamento e della ciurma. Nel caso della necessità di imbarcare uomini d'armi, questi dovevano stare sotto il comando del Maresciallo dell'Ospedale e dovevano essere pagati dal Tesoro. Se qualche *frater* dell'ordine doveva salire a bordo delle galee, il Maresciallo poteva nominare un *frater miles* al comando di tutta la flotta; ma in mancanza di un *frater miles* il *comandeor* poteva dare il comando a un *frere de marine* e tutto il bottino doveva andare al Tesoro[31]. Almeno dal 1299 esisteva un nuovo ufficiale, l'Ammiraglio[32]. Nel 1300 fu creato Ammiraglio uno dei *baiulivi* del convento, cioè uno dei grandi ufficiali dell'ordine eletti in capitolo generale, con poteri su tutte le galee e navi armate dall'Ospedale; poteva noleggiare galee, arruolare uomini d'armi e marinai, e farli pagare dal Tesoro. Tutti dovevano essere ai suoi ordini sia nel porto sia in mare, sempre che il Maresciallo non fosse presente. Tutto l'equipaggio doveva essere provvisto del necessario dal Commendatore di Limassol. L'Ammiraglio doveva percepire annualmente 50 misure di

---

[26] *Cartulaire* (come n. 3), 4549 (5), 4574 (14).

[27] Luttrell (come n. 24), II, p. 163 n. 3.

[28] Testo in A. Teulet, *Layettes du Trésor des Chartes*, 1-2, Paris 1863-1866, 2, pp. 632-3.

[29] Riley-Smith (come n. 3), pp. 329-30, 455; J. Pryor, *"In subsidium Terrae Sanctae": Exports of Foodstuffs and war Materials from the Kingdom of Sicily to the Kingdom of Jerusalem: 1265-1284*, in *Asian and African Studies*, 22 (1988), pp. 134-5; cf. M. Barber, *Supplying the Crusader States: the Role of the Templars*, in *The Horns of Hattin*, ed. B. Kedar, Jerusalem 1992, pp. 322-6; M.-L. Favreau-Lilie, *The Military Orders and the Escape of the Christian Population from the Holy Land in 1291*, in *Journal of Medieval History*, 19 (1993).

[30] *Cartulaire* (come n. 3), 2067, 2079, 3317 (6); cf. Riley-Smith (come n. 3), pp. 329-30.

[31] Marseilles, 65 H 4055 (testo mancente in *Cartulaire* [come n. 3], 4234): «Item establi est que quant il couendra faire armement de Galee ou d'autre vassaus, Le comandeor les doie faire aparailler et garnir de ce que besoing sera et de mariners. Et se il couient ametre Gens d'armes que le mareschal les doye retenir, e soient payes au tresor et soient a son comandement. Et si freres uont sur les galees que le mareschal puisse metre un frere cheualier sur tout l'armement. Et si freres d'armes non y uont sur les galees, que le frere de marine que le comandor jmetra soit bailli sur tout l'armement et que le gaaign que les galees au uasseaus feront que le ueigne tout au tresor». Sembra che i *fratres* che facevano bottino lo potessero trattenere, almeno in parte. Il termine *frere de marine* richiede una spiegazione.

[32] Riley-Smith (come n. 3), p. 320.

vino e 100 bisanti saraceni da prelevare dal bottino fatto dalla flotta; qualora il bottino fosse stato insufficiente, il Tesoro avrebbe dovuto pagare la differenza[33]. Vari progetti di crociata assegnarono all'Ospedale il compito di fornire più galee: per esempio Carlo d'Angiò nel 1292/4 ne propose dieci. Ma nel 1300 il re di Cipro, il Tempio e l'Ospedale insieme potevano armarne solo sedici. Il costo delle galee era elevato e la loro capacità operativa assai limitata nello spazio. Nel 1309 Marino Sanudo, esperto di affari orientali, suggeriva la fornitura da parte dell'Ospedale di sole due galee[34].

Dopo il 1291 i teorici della crociata, gli autori dei trattati *De recuperatione* dovettero, per mancanza di altre forze disponibili, assegnare un ruolo importante agli ordini militari[35]. L'unione degli ordini militari, progetto già discusso nel 1274, doveva evitare le rivalità e le dispute fra gli ordini, ma sembra che gli autori francesi e filofrancesi pensassero di assicurare attraverso tale fusione il controllo degli ordini e dei loro beni alla casa di Francia[36]. C'era anche la proposta di installare in una Gerusalemme liberata un *Ordensstaat* governato da un nuovo ordine unito[37]. Questa era un'idea utopica: un monopolio di Gerusalemme sotto il controllo di un ordine militare non sarebbe stato mai realistico. Nel 1306 il Maestro del Tempio, Jacques de Molay, si oppose decisamente alla fusione degli ordini, irritando – come sembra – fortemente il re francese, mentre il Maestro dell'Ospedale, più diplomaticamente, evitò l'argomento; per di più il Molay proponeva come capitano di una crociata un non-francese, Rogerone di Loria, d'origine calabrese[38]. Quanto alla tattica, la maggioranza degli esperti erano per l'embargo sul commercio, combinato con la formazione di una polizia navale e con piccoli attacchi contro le coste e i porti mammalucchi. Tutto doveva precedere un grande *passagium generale* o crociata[39]. Dopo la disastrosa campagna in Egitto di S. Luigi nel 1250, la politica di una grande invasione dell'Egitto era passata di moda, ma fu appoggiata nel 1306 da Jacques de Molay, il quale si opponeva ad una crociata nella Cilicia armena, forse perché l'intervento nell'area faceva parte della politica dell'Ospedale; egli era contrario anche ad una spedizione minore e limitata[40].

---

[33] Testo in *Cartulaire* (come n. 3), 4515 (13). Sul *comandeor dou freres*, RILEY-SMITH (come n. 3), pp. 321, 330. Il testo riporta *maistre*, trasformato in *mareschallus* nella traduzione latina del 1357; *corrige* RILEY-SMITH (come n. 3), pp. 314, 330. Lo stesso (pp. 308, 330, 432) sostiene che il *comandaor de Limason* era il Gran Commendatore conventuale. LUTTRELL (come n. 24), IV, pp. 55-7, riporta ulteriori norme legislative sui poteri dell'Ammiraglio.

[34] RILEY-SMITH (come n. 3), pp. 200-1; LUTTRELL (come n. 24), II, p. 163 n. 3; SCHEIN (come n. 1), pp. 84, 204. RILEY-SMITH (come n. 3), pp. 200, 330, ed EDBURY (come n. 13), p. 103, credono che l'Ospedale disponesse di dieci galee prima del 1300, ma LUTTRELL (come n. 24), II, p. 163 n. 3, respinge questa cifra.

[35] A. FOREY, *The Military Orders in the Crusading Proposals of the Late-Thirteenth and Early-Fourteenth Centuries*, in *Traditio*, 36 (1980).

[36] SCHEIN (come n. 1), pp. 75-7, 197-9.

[37] S. SCHEIN, *The Future "Regnum Hierusalem": a Chapter in Medieval State Planning*, in *Journal of Medieval History*, 10 (1984).

[38] Cf. ID. (come n. 1), pp. 197-9, 202, 241; molti autori dànno come capitano proposto da Molay Ruggero di Loria, già morto nel 1305, invece del figlio Rogerone.

[39] *Ibid.*, pp. 15-9, e *passim*.

[40] *Ibid.*, pp. 50, 201.

Gli Ospitalieri pensavano a progetti ben diversi, volti all'acquisizione di una base in grado di assicurare la loro sopravvivenza. Figura chiave fu il Maestro eletto nel 1305, Foulques de Villaret, personaggio di grande astuzia, come testimonia Marino Sanudo che era stato con lui a Rodi[41]. In due memoriali richiesti dal papa Clemente V, Maestro e convento dichiaravano di non volere una grande, lenta e costosa crociata con lunghi ritardi, dovuti alla necessità di convocare un concilio generale, ma di vedere con favore un *passagium particulare* per portare aiuto immediato ai Cristiani di Cipro e della Cilicia armena. Questa spedizione limitata doveva essere accompagnata dall'embargo economico e da piccoli assalti alle coste per logorare i Mammalucchi; il grande *passagium generale* era rimandato ad un non prossimo futuro. Gli Ospitalieri prevedevano un'efficace preparazione in Occidente del *passagium particulare* e l'esclusione dei crociati dilettanti, inesperti, costosi ed inutili. Volevano inoltre evitare la proclamazione di una crociata formale, con l'attribuzione delle relative decime, per evitare che il re francese potesse accumulare tasse senza poi far nulla. Proposero quindi di presentare il recupero di Gerusalemme come un dovere papale, implicitamente al di fuori del controllo e dell'ostruzione della corona di Francia: *sans le movement de nul des roys*[42].

Per acquisire la propria base ideale a Rodi, gli Ospitalieri dovettero sopravvivere alla crisi degli anni successivi al 1307, nei quali i Teutonici abbandonavano Venezia per la Prussia e dovevano affrontare una grande inchiesta papale, mentre i Templari venivano distrutti da Filippo IV. Per ragioni non tutte comprensibili l'Ospedale non fu oggetto che di poche critiche del tipo di quelle lanciate contro il Tempio. Un Templare dichiarò di essere stato frequentemente canzonato, insieme con altri Templari, da vari Ospitalieri *quod in eorum recepcionibus osculabantur tantum in ano*[43]. Non tutti gli Ospitalieri, però, erano senza macchia. Per esempio, il Priore di Catalogna, Ramon di Ampurias, venne accusato di avere – durante la guerra di Rodi, proprio intorno al 1310 – impedito a due suoi scudieri di ricevere la confessione in punto di morte, allo scopo di occultare così le sue relazioni omosessuali con loro[44]. È probabile che nel regno di Francia, escludendo Provenza, Savoia, Fiandra, Guascogna e Navarra, il Tempio fosse assai più ricco dell'Ospedale; nel nord della Francia nel 1373, per esempio, quasi due terzi delle commende e delle cappelle degli Ospitalieri erano di origine templare[45]. Il Maestro Villaret, abbandonando la politica continentale degli inter-

---

[41] Cit. in LUTTRELL (come n. 6), IV, pp. 79-80.

[42] RILEY-SMITH (come n. 3), pp. 220-1; SCHEIN (come n. 1), pp. 200-4, 219-24. Su un terzo testo, proveniente dal Maestro e convento dell'Ospedale e relativo ad una invasione dell'Egitto, in passato sempre datato 1289/91, ma del 1307 circa: R. IRWIN, *How Many Miles to Babylon? The "Devise des Chemins de Babiloine" Redated*, in *The Military Orders: Fighting for the Faith and Caring for the Sick*, ed. M. BARBER, Aldershot 1994. L'Ospedale accettava il progetto di un *passagium* in Egitto, ma solo nel caso di un'invasione mongola e di un Egitto così lasciato senza difesa. Gli Ospitalieri avevano già approfittato di un'invasione mongola, per attaccare i Mammalucchi nel 1280: R. AMITAI-PREISS, *Mamluk Perceptions of the Mongol-Frankish Rapprochement*, in *Mediterranean Historical Review*, 7 (1992-93), pp. 60, 65.

[43] Testo in MICHELET (come n. 25), 2, p. 153.

[44] Testo in J. MIRET Y SANS, *Sempre han tingut béch les oques: apuntacions per la historia de les costumes privades*, 1-2, Barcelona 1905, 1, pp. 38-46.

[45] Cifre locali in A.-M. LEGRAS, *L'énquête pontificale de 1373 sur l'Ordre de Saint-Jean de Jéru-*

venti in Cilicia, creò un alibi per il suo ordine con l'inizio dell'azione su Rodi, ed evitò di irritare Filippo con un rifiuto troppo esplicito del progetto di unione degli ordini; rimase discretamente lontano dal re, il quale nell'agosto del 1309 protestava per questo fatto. Villaret rimase, invece, vicino al papa Clemente V e attraverso l'organizzazione di una crociata condotta dagli Ospitalieri sotto il proprio comando riuscì a rendersi quasi intoccabile. Con l'aggressione al Tempio Filippo prese una certa iniziativa; con la proclamazione del *passagium* degli Ospitalieri, dal quale il re risultava tagliato fuori, il papa e il Maestro la ripresero almeno in parte. Il sovrano protestò, sostenendo che i francesi erano esclusi dal *passagium*, cercò di imporre persino un inglese come capo della spedizione e rifiutò di versare i 100.000 fiorini promessi per il *passagium*. Come *rex christianissimus* e promotore morale della crociata, faceva assai brutta figura. Villaret aveva promesso la conquista di Gerusalemme o di Antiochia, ma dopo il 1310, senza più denaro e aiuto, non fu in grado di sostenere la costosissima crociata; invece, con risorse fortemente limitate, riuscì almeno a prendere Rodi e certi castelli in Turchia, un'impresa molto significativa per il futuro[46].

Nel 1311 Clemente V riunì un concilio generale a Vienne per dirimere le due questioni della crociata e del Tempio. Nell'aprile 1312 il papa soppresse il Tempio, ma il futuro dei suoi beni, una ricchezza enorme, rimaneva ancora da decidere. Almeno su questo fronte, vinsero ancora una volta il papa e l'Ospedale. Il re francese probabilmente voleva utilizzare i beni templari per un nuovo ordine che fosse sottoposto al controllo francese, e di fatto solo due membri del consiglio della corona si dichiararono favorevoli alla trasmissione dei beni all'Ospedale: Charles de Valois, fratello del re, ed Enguerrand de Marigny, il suo più potente ministro. Marigny era deciso a negoziare un compromesso. Il Maestro Villaret si trovava a Rodi, ma i Priori di Francia e di Alvernia vennero convocati a Vienne; arrivò poi la notizia, presumibilmente esagerata, di una grande vittoria navale degli Ospitalieri contro i Turchi. Nel maggio Clemente V trasferiva i beni del Tempio, ad eccezione di quelli nei regni ispanici, all'Ospedale. Filippo IV dovette accettare ciò, ma in cambio ricevette vari altri vantaggi, incluse le decime per una nuova crociata. Il re insisté, inutilmente, per una riforma dell'Ospedale, il quale di fatto era stato oggetto di varie critiche da parte del concilio: probabilmente l'ordine promise di aiutare Charles de Valois in una futura conquista di Costantinopoli[47]. La tanto discussa fusione degli ordini militari fu così realizzata in modo ina-

---

salem, 1: *L'énquête dans le prieuré de France*, Paris 1987, pp. 93, 100 n. 5. La situazione globale rimane discutibile. BULST-THIELE (come n. 11), p. 350, ha ragione di criticare l'asserzione troppo cruda e soggettiva di LUTTRELL (come n. 24), XI, p. 2, che i Templari erano meno entusiasti per la crociata, più ricchi e corrotti degli Ospitalieri. Secondo una fonte orientale, ma quasi contemporanea e normalmente attendibile, le *Gestes des Chiprois* (come n. 11), pp. 329-30, nel 1307 Molay si era dimostrato molto avaro con il papa e i cardinali, e aveva annullato un enorme prestito promesso a Filippo IV dal Tesoriere del Tempio, espellendo quest'ultimo dall'ordine e rifiutando gli interventi in suo favore del papa e anche del re, che ne fu molto offeso.

[46] SCHEIN (come n. 1), pp. 219-38; LUTTRELL (come n. 6), III, pp. 69-71. Si noti che la lettera di Filippo (testo in *Cartulaire* [come n. 3], 4831) è da datare agosto 1309, perché il latore Pierre de Paray fu inviato presso il papa il 23 agosto 1309: Paris, Archives Nationales, JJ 42A, 64 bis e 68 (gentilmente comunicatomi da Elisabeth Lalou. Cf. A. FAILLER, *L'occupation de Rhodes par les Hospitaliers*, in *Revue des Études Byzantines*, 50 (1992).

[47] SCHEIN (come n. 1), pp. 240-6; LUTTRELL (come n. 6), III, pp. 72-8.

spettato, e l'Ospedale più o meno raddoppiò la sua ricchezza primaria, costituendo così la base economica con la quale mantenere il suo *Ordensstaat* fino al 1798.

Gli Ospitalieri stessi avevano seguito buona parte dei suggerimenti dei teorici della crociata, anche se con certe divergenze. In effetti, organizzarono una specie di *passagium* dell'ordine per completare la sottomissione di Rodi, che era iniziata con un atto di pirateria concepito secondo la tradizione antibizantina della crociata latina di Costantinopoli del 1204. Fecero anche delle conquiste sulla terraferma a spese dei Turchi di Menteshe, e fu quindi possibile presentare la campagna come un attacco a scismatici e infedeli. Successivamente gli Ospitalieri catturavano navi dei Genovesi e dei Veneziani, colpevoli di commerciare in contravvenzione all'embargo papale. La conquista di Rodi durò tre o forse quattro anni e costò molto, contribuendo alla creazione di un grosso debito per l'estinzione del quale occorsero venticinque anni; ma a lunga scadenza divenne un enorme vantaggio il fatto che Rodi fosse un'isola tenuta sotto un teorico dominio papale, sulla quale l'Ospedale poteva installare un regime indipendente, permettendo la creazione di un originale tipo di *Ordensstaat* isolano. Rodi fu relativamente facile da popolare, da proteggere e da sfruttare economicamente: si svilupparono l'economia e il commercio del porto in modo da generare le ricchezze e le truppe capaci di sostenere la difesa dell'isola. Come base di operazioni contro Mammalucchi e Turchi a soli dodici chilometri dalla terraferma turca, l'isola permise la costituzione di una specie di marca marittima. Però, la sola difesa di Rodi non sembrava sufficiente a giustificare l'esistenza dell'ordine. L'opinione pubblica occidentale esigeva anche attività militari in territorio controllato dagli infedeli. L'Ospedale dette in gran parte un nuovo orientamento alla sua guerra santa indirizzandola verso i Turchi nell'Egeo. Così dal 1344 al 1402 gli Ospitalieri mantennero una presenza sulla terraferma con la difesa di Smirne e, perduta la città, iniziarono nel 1407/8 la costruzione a Bodrum di un altro castello nel continente, vicino all'isola di Kos. Per di più, nella seconda metà del Trecento emerse una tendenza favorevole ad un allargamento territoriale dell'*Ordensstaat* e della sua base economica, con ripetuti tentativi di stabilire l'Ospedale in qualche zona della Grecia continentale, sia in Morea, sia in Acaia, sia in Epiro. Approfittando dei suoi uomini e degli introiti occidentali, l'ordine poté creare una solida società capace di difendere Rodi, inaugurando così una tradizione di regime isolano che fu possibile mantenere per quasi cinque secoli[48].

* * *

Il Maestro dell'Ospedale, Folques de Villaret, era senza dubbio molto accorto in fatto di politica[49], mentre quello del Tempio, Jacques de Molay, era meno diplomatico; inoltre, come egli si autodefiniva, era *miles illitteratus*[50]. Questo contrasto non spiega sufficientemente, però, le diverse fortune dei loro ordini. Le divergenze stavano sia nelle personalità, sia nel carattere delle oligarchie dei due ordini. Molay nel 1307 era già Maestro da quindici anni, e presumibilmente gli mancarono durante quel periodo, a causa della loro morte o della lo-

---

[48] *Ibid.*, II, V, VII, XIX, *passim.*; J. SARNOWSKY, *Die Johanniter und Smyrna: 1344-1402*, in *Römische Quartalschrift*, 86-87 (1991-92).

[49] LUTTRELL (come n. 6), IV, *passim.*

[50] Cit. in BULST-THIELE (come n. 11), p. 325.

ro prigionia, molti dei migliori Templari che avrebbero potuto fungere da esperti consiglieri. Sembra che non ci sia stato neppure un tentativo di riforma e che il Tempio non abbia disposto di un'efficace organizzazione costituzionale e di un'élite di dirigenti capaci[51]. Può darsi, per di più, che i Templari si dedicassero troppo alle attività bancarie. La costituzione e le procedure dei Templari erano, grosso modo, poco diverse da quelle dell'Ospedale. Secondo la Regola del Tempio, il suo Maestro non aveva la disponibilità della chiave del Tesoro, mentre negli affari importanti egli doveva agire con il consenso della maggioranza del convento, del consiglio o dei suoi compagni[52]. Inoltre, esisteva una procedura che permetteva al convento di esercitare un controllo su di lui attraverso una limitazione dell'uso della bolla magistrale[53]. Il Tempio tenne tre capitoli generali, tutti in Francia, fra il 1293 e il 1295/6[54], ma successivamente pare che non si riunisse nessun capitolo o adunanza nella quale i Templari potessero limitare o dirigere l'azione del Maestro.

Jacques de Molay, nato prima del 1250, apparteneva alla vecchia generazione; era stato ricevuto *frater* nel 1256 e conosceva la Siria da prima del 1291: sembra che non ricoprisse alcun importante ufficio. Come Maestro, dava l'impressione di essere conservatore, avaro, poco diplomatico, incapace di comprendere gli affari occidentali e con una tendenza a provocare risentimenti fra i suoi *fratres*[55]. Fu eletto Maestro nell'aprile 1292[56]. Il candidato più adatto al magistero nel 1292 sembra essere stato Hugues de Pairaud, un eccellente diplo-

---

[51] Cf. *ibid.*, p. 311. Mancano informazioni e studi sulla politica interna e sulle istituzioni costituzionali del Tempio, forse perché i documenti si sono persi, forse per l'assenza di grandi dissensi nell'ordine.

[52] *La Règle du Temple*, ed. H. DE CURZON, Paris 1886, §§ 81-2, 85-93, 97-8; sul sigillo d'argento, §§ 134, 236. Già nel 1289 un autore presentò un dibattito tra un Templare, ingenuo quanto pessimo oratore, e un Ospitaliere saggio, buon oratore e dalle argomentazioni ben strutturate, che denunciava i Templari come responsabili della crisi della Terra Santa e complici dei Mussulmani: H. NICHOLSON, *Jacquemart Giélée's "Renart le Nouvel": the Image of the Military Orders on the Eve of the Loss of Acre*, in *Monastic Studies*, I: *The Continuity of Tradition*, ed. J. LOADES, Bangor 1990, pp. 182-9.

[53] Secondo Curzon (come n. 52), p. 81, *la boule d'argent* menzionata nella Regola templare (§§ 234, 236) era quella del Maestro; aggiunge, senza citare fonti, che doveva essere custodita sotto tre chiavi tenute dal Maestro e da due altri grandi ufficiali. Una bolla magistrale del 1292 fu utilizzata con la testimonianza di vari grandi ufficiali nominati nella *guarantye de nos prodes homes*, e un'altra del 1306 aveva un *sigillum tumbe plumbee dicti conventus pendens* in cera: testi in A. FOREY, *The Templars in the "Corona de Aragón"*, London 1973, pp. 405-6, 414-5. Nel 1295/6 il Maestro Molay, fuori convento a Parigi, utilizzò il sigillo plumbeo del convento: *Regestum* (come n. 23), 2, 2938.

[54] BULST-THIELE (come n. 11), pp. 305-7. Nel 1310 un Templare testimoniò che Molay aveva partecipato a un capitolo generale *in civitate Nicosiensi* (Nicosia?) con circa [40] *fratres... illo anno quo civitas Aconensis fuit perdita*: testo in MICHELET (come n. 25), 2, p. 139, emendato nella n. 25. Sembra possibile che Molay sia stato eletto a Nicosia da pochi *fratres* il 16/20 aprile 1292 e che un capitolo fu tenuto, sempre a Nicosia, poco dopo, meno di un anno dopo la perdita di Acri del 18 maggio 1291.

[55] BULST-THIELE (come n. 11), pp. 299-301 e *passim*; M. BARBER, *James of Molay, the Last Grand Master of the Order of the Temple*, in *Studia Monastica*, 14 (1972), pp. 91-3, la cui idea – da lui non appoggiata su alcuna fonte – è che Molay probabilmente occupava uno dei grandi uffici prima della sua elezione.

[56] Thibaud Gaudin morì un 16 aprile: BULST-THIELE (come n. 11), p. 294. Molay in veste di Maestro era a Nicosia il 20 aprile 1292 (*nonante et deu*): testo in FOREY (come n. 53), pp. 405-6. A. DEMURGER, *Vie et mort de l'Ordre du Temple: 1118-1314*, Paris ²1989, p. 291, continua, per esempio, a datare la morte di Gaudin al 1293. Da notare che Grandson, come Molay (*supra*, n. 11) si trovava a Londra nel dicembre 1293: *Calendar of Patent Rolls: Edward I A. D. 1292-1301*, London 1895, p. 58.

matico entrato nell'ordine nel 1263, che tuttavia nel 1292 si trovò in Occidente come Maestro di Francia. Più tardi, nel corso del processo contro l'ordine, fu asserito dal Templare Hugues de le Faur, certamente a Cipro all'epoca del fatto, che la maggioranza del convento, gente del Limosino e d'Alvernia, voleva Pairaud come Maestro; che Molay, già sul posto, a Limassol aveva giurato davanti al convento e alla presenza di Otto de Grandson, agente del re d'Inghilterra, e del Maestro dell'Ospedale di non aspirare al magistero e di essere disposto ad accettare Pairaud; così si fece eleggere Gran Commendatore, cioè ufficiale con il controllo sull'elezione magistrale; fu così in grado di organizzare *per impressionem* la propria elezione a Maestro ad opera di un ristretto numero di *fratres* presenti a Cipro. Probabilmente questa storia aveva qualche fondamento. Pairaud era francese, mentre Molay era con molta probabilità della Franca-Contea, regione fuori del regno di Francia, dove in quel momento la nobiltà si trovava in conflitto con Filippo IV di Francia. Ad Otto de Grandson, un savoiardo al servizio di Edoardo I d'Inghilterra, nel 1295 o 1296 fu assegnata dal Molay una pensione annua di 2.000 *livres tournois*. In qualche modo, forse attraverso un intervento antifrancese di Grandson, un'elezione poco soddisfacente ebbe l'effetto di procurare al Tempio un Maestro poco soddisfacente[57].

A differenza del Tempio, l'Ospedale, pur sperimentando parecchie difficoltà e scandali, si sviluppò costituzionalmente in modo significativo negli anni dopo il 1291. Il suo Maestro doveva sentire il consiglio dei *prud'hommes*, cioè dei *fratres* saggi e capaci di offrire buoni consigli, e poi seguire il parere della maggioranza. Il Maestro era eletto in convento e i *fratres* potevano far *esgart de freres*, appellare in capitolo contro di lui. Le decisioni più importanti potevano essere convalidate soltanto con il sigillo comune del Maestro e del convento. L'ordine si presentava pertanto come un'oligarchia. Chi governava poteva mantenere il suo prestigio e un potere di comando, sempre che non esagerasse; ma l'oligarchia era assai sensibile e pronta a reagire in caso di mal governo. Nel 1295 i dirigenti occidentali dell'Ospedale, incluso il Priore provenzale Guillaume de Villaret, protestavano vigorosamente contro gli eccessi del Maestro Eudes de Pins, proponendo che l'ordine fosse governato da sette *diffinitores*, uno per ciascuna lingua o nazione, con decisioni prese a maggioranza. Dal 1297 al 1300 i *prud'hommes* litigarono a lungo con il Maestro Guillaume de Villaret, che era deciso a rimanere in Occidente, a convocare capitoli generali in Provenza e a spostare il centro del comando fuori dell'Oriente. Questo costrinse il convento ad una decisa opposizione, basata sul proprio diritto di controllo sul Maestro attraverso il sigillo comune. Alla fine il Maestro dovette trasferirsi a Cipro contro la sua volontà. Il capitolo generale del 1302 introdusse un nuovo Statuto per rafforzare il controllo del Maestro mediante il vecchio meccanismo del sigillo comune, mentre Guglielmo di Santo Stefano raccoglieva una quantità di *esgarts* e altri documenti per poi comporre un trattato sulle questioni costituzionali e sui limiti formali del potere magistrale. Accadde anche che il capitolo generale fosse riunito ogni anno dal 1300 al 1306[58].

---

[57] BULST-THIELE (come n. 11), pp. 295-303, 307 n. 57, 357; sulla funzione elettorale del Gran Commendatore, *Règle* (come n. 52), §§ 198-223. Per Barber (come n. 55), pp. 93, 108, l'«Odo of Grandisson» del 1291/2 era un Templare, e diverso da «one Othon of Granson» beneficiario della pensione templare.

[58] RILEY-SMITH (come n. 3), pp. 290-303; A. FOREY, *Constitutional Conflict and Change in the Ho-*

Il caso di Villaret fu esemplare. Nel 1317 questo Maestro, salvatore dell'ordine con le conquiste di Rodi e in Turchia, con la crociata del 1309/10 e con l'acquisizione dell'eredità dei Templari, fu deposto da un colpo di stato eseguito all'unanimità dai *fratres* del convento, i quali elessero un nuovo Maestro, Maurice de Pagnac. Villaret era accusato di vari eccessi e di comportamento tirannico, di aver trattato con gli infedeli e di aver agito contro la costituzione dell'ordine. Dietro tali accuse c'era, con tutta probabilità, il fatto che Villaret, avendo contratto enormi debiti, cercava di farsi pagare dal convento la grossa somma di 154.000 fiorini, da lui spesa durante i tre anni della guerra di Rodi. Nel 1319, dopo un lungo dibattito giuridico presso la curia papale ad Avignone, dove il legista Olrado de Ponte dimostrò in un dettagliato *consilium* che il Maestro era stato sempre subordinato al convento e al capitolo generale, il papa Giovanni XXII, agendo di concerto con alcuni tra i maggiori ufficiali dell'Ospedale, nominò al magistero Hélion de Villeneuve[59]. In conseguenza dell'affare Villaret, il capitolo generale del 1320 introdusse o confermò molti, dettagliati provvedimenti costituzionali. Il Maestro doveva giurare di rispettare gli Statuti; i suoi atti dovevano essere ritenuti privi di validità, se non fatti d'accordo con un consiglio di sette *fratres*, che dovevano essere eletti dalle singole *langues*. E fu proprio il Consiglio dei Sette – di fatto i sette *diffinitores* proposti nel 1295 – ad essere costretto a denunciare e a mettere in stato di accusa un Maestro che agiva in modo improprio. Il sigillo conventuale doveva essere conservato nel Tesoro sotto la custodia del Gran Precettore, del Maresciallo, del Priore del Convento e dell'Ospedaliere. Sembra, però, che questi Statuti riformatori del 1320 non fossero mai entrati in vigore: scomparvero prima del 1330[60].

La continua, quasi feroce resistenza da parte di un gruppo di uomini d'esperienza ed abituati ad una certa tradizione corporativa di buon governo era fondata su uno spirito costituzionale. Il gruppo di responsabili nell'oligarchia conventuale si mostrava determinato ad esercitare un controllo sulla politica magistrale. C'era fra loro qualche superstite del periodo siriano, come il teorico Guglielmo di Santo Stefano, divenuto Commendatore di Cipro, e forse il Maestro Hélion de Villeneuve, il quale aveva lottato contro gli infedeli: *in partibus Terre Sancte... contra barbaras nationes*. Una parte dell'opposizione del 1295 si trovava in Occidente, inclusi il Priore di Provenza e Bonifacio di Calamandrana, già Gran Commendatore in Siria. Il Maestro Guillaume de Villaret era stato per lungo tempo rettore papale della contea di Venaissin, e fra i suoi oppositori dopo il 1296 c'era il proprio nipote Foulques de Villaret, nel 1299 Ammiraglio dell'Ospedale[61].

Altro fattore positivo era la composizione cosmopolita dell'oligarchia conventuale. Filippo IV protestò nel 1309 per la riduzione della componente francese nel convento[62]. Nel

---

spital of St John during the Twelfth and Thirteenth Centuries, in *Journal of Ecclesiastical History*, 33 (1982). Questi due studi si fermano al 1310 senza prendere in considerazione la deposizione del Maestro Villaret nel 1317/9.

[59] LUTTRELL (come n. 6), II, p. 110 n. 10; IV, *passim*.

[60] Paris, Bibliothèque Nationale, Ms. franç. 13531, ff. 59v-65r.

[61] RILEY-SMITH (come n. 3), pp. 205-7, 272-3, 330; per Villeneuve, vedi il testo del 1319 in S. PAOLI, *Codice diplomatico del sacro militare ordine Gerosolimitano, oggi di Malta*, 1-2, Lucca 1733-1737, 2, pp. 399-401.

[62] *Cartulaire* (come n. 3), 4831.

1306 l'Ammiraglio, Sancho de Aragón, e il Priore del Convento, Joan de Laodicea, erano catalano-aragonesi; il Maresciallo, Albrecht von Schwarzburg, era tedesco; il Drappiere, William of Henley, inglese. Nel novembre dello stesso anno Richard of Pavely, inglese, era Drappiere e Vasques Martins, portoghese, Ospitaliere; nel 1309 l'Ammiraglio era Ramon de Ampurias, catalano. A parte il Maestro, che era originario della Linguadoca, francesi furono Gautelme de Tournel, Gran Commendatore nel 1308 e nel 1310, Simon le Rat, Maresciallo dal 1306 al 1310, e Durand de la Prevoté, Tesoriere nel 1306[63]. Non tutti i francesi provenivano dal regno di Francia: per esempio, Hélion de Villeneuve era provenzale[64]. Gran Commendatore da molti anni, vincitore di battaglie navali contro i Turchi, era il nobile tedesco Albrecht von Schwarzburg[65]. Molti di questi ufficiali del convento diventarono anche titolari di priorati occidentali[66], e questo scambio fra i dirigenti occidentali e ufficiali conventuali, ugualmente occidentali, fu importante per assicurare la coerenza nella direzione dell'ordine.

Stabilitosi a Rodi, l'Ospedale doveva contribuire allo sviluppo dell'isola, creando una società greco-latina capace di sostenere il convento, portando avanti la lotta antiturca e partecipando a varie azioni di crociata. Eccellente amministratore, il nuovo Maestro estinse i colossali debiti dell'ordine, e poi nel 1332 passò a Rodi, dove fece migliorare la difesa dell'isola. Importante inoltre fu il mantenimento dell'appoggio papale, necessario per conservare le risorse occidentali[67]. Una resistenza contro gli infedeli era essenziale per mantenere appoggi in Europa, e dopo il 1345 circa bisognò affrontare le disastrose conseguenze di decenni di guerre occidentali, di grandi pestilenze e dell'universale crollo economico e demografico, che incise fortemente sul numero dei *fratres* e sui loro redditi. Dopo il 1378 l'Ospedale fu parzialmente diviso dallo scisma papale e dal conseguente scisma interno all'ordine. Anche in tale circostanza gli Ospitalieri mostrarono una compattezza straordinaria, un *ésprit de corps* che limitò gli effetti dello scisma. Il convento a Rodi appoggiava il papa di Avignone, ma il pontefice romano, Urbano V, nominò un "antimaestro", il napoletano Riccardo Caracciolo. Costui non otteneva nemmeno l'obbedienza di tutti gli Ospitalieri italiani, mentre quelli d'Inghilterra, regno formalmente di obbedienza romana, continuavano a inviare i loro uomini e denari a Rodi. Nessuna parte portò l'ostilità alle estreme conseguenze, e lo scisma nell'Ospedale effettivamente era già concluso nel 1409, qualche anno prima di quello del papato[68].

---

[63] J. DELAVILLE LE ROULX, *Les Hospitaliers en Terre Sainte et à Chypre: 1100-1310*, Paris 1904, pp. 274-6 n. 2, 410-3 (per «Panelli» leggi «Pavely»); per Henley, vedi TYERMAN (come n. 11), p. 237. Per Ramon de Ampurias, vedi E. BARATIER, *Histoire du commerce de Marseille*, 2: *de 1291 à 1423*, Paris 1951, p. 215 n. 1. Le origini di Sanzolius Grassie, Ammiraglio nel 1307 (*Cartulaire* [come n. 3], 4756), sono incerte.

[64] DELAVILLE LE ROULX (come n. 3), p. 52.

[65] *Ibid.*, pp. 7-9, 24.

[66] Vedi i numerosi appunti prosopografici in DELAVILLE LE ROULX (come n. 3), *passim*. FOREY (come n. 2), p. 28, fornisce l'esempio di Girardo de Gragnana, Ospitaliere e poi Maresciallo del Convento, divenuto Priore di Pisa e poi di Venezia.

[67] Cf. HOUSLEY (come n. 2), pp. 260-92, che sottolinea il contrasto con la politica papale verso i Teutonici.

[68] LUTTRELL (come n. 24), XXIII, *passim*; ID. (come n. 9), I, pp. 258-60; ID. (come n. 6), XI, *passim*.

La creazione dello stato degli Ospitalieri a Rodi fu possibile soltanto su un'isola piccola e difendibile. Il fabbisogno di effettivi era ridotto al punto che ogni tanto l'ordine rimandava vari *fratres* in Occidente, per risparmiare le spese che il loro soggiorno a Rodi comportava[69]; mentre l'afflusso di denaro dalle commende occidentali rimase sempre di importanza vitale. Al contrario, l'*Ordensstaat* dei Teutonici in Prussia, contando una popolazione di forse 300.000 o 350.000 abitanti, non aveva necessità di esigere denaro dai suoi baliati tedeschi, ma richiedeva invece un buon numero di *fratres* per poter amministrare il suo territorio e difendere i suoi estesi confini. Il Ricevitore generale dell'Ospedale in Occidente era ufficiale del Tesoro a Rodi, con il compito di riscuotere denari per conto del convento. Ogni tanto si nominava in convento un Gran Precettore in Occidente; si trattava, tuttavia, di un ufficio transitorio con poteri vaghi e mal determinati[70].

I Teutonici si confrontavano con un'esperienza militare in Prussia molto più brutale e con condizioni molto più aspre di quelle che riservava la vita relativamente pacifica e comoda di Rodi. Essi entravano spesso in contesa con i propri sudditi ed effettuavano troppe spedizioni militari contro i vicini pagani e cristiani; per questo dovevano assoldare troppi mercenari. La conversione dei Lituani dopo il 1389 privò l'Ordine Teutonico della giustificazione per le sue guerre. Inoltre la grande sconfitta a Tannenberg nel 1410 doveva dimostrare la sua debolezza, e poco dopo gli attacchi di natura giuridica nel concilio di Costanza rivelarono una sua crisi morale. L'Ordine Teutonico divenne solo un'oligarchia conservatrice di se stessa, superficialmente efficiente, ma incapace di dirigere il proprio *Ordensstaat*. Il suo declino continuò durante il Quattrocento e la Riforma protestante dette il colpo finale al suo stato in Prussia[71]. Anche nei regni ispanici i vari ordini militari nazionali finirono per perdere la loro ultima ragion d'essere. La centralizzatrice monarchia castigliana si intrometteva ripetutamente per limitare o controllare l'eccessivo potere politico ed economico degli ordini, i quali persero la loro indipendenza quando i re, agendo spesso in connivenza con il papa, imponevano candidati inadatti come Maestri attraverso la manipolazione delle elezioni e il meccanismo dell'omaggio dovuto alla corona[72]. Dopo la fine della Riconquista nel 1492 gli ordini militari vennero nazionalizzati formalmente e in modo perpetuo. Da quel momento sopravvissero come enormi corporazioni esenti, fonti di ricchezza e di uffici da distribuire per la corona, ma sempre meno militari[73].

L'espansione ottomana del Quattrocento rese Rodi sempre più tagliata fuori e, quindi, sempre più utile ai Latini come base commerciale e militare. Così la città divenne ricca e cosmopolita sotto due Maestri catalani, due italiani e sei francesi fra il 1421 e il 1522. La flotta dell'ordine rimase con due o tre galee di guardia e con la possibilità, come nell'asse-

---

[69] ID. (come n. 24), I, pp. 296, 304; XXIII, pp. 36-7.

[70] RILEY-SMITH (come n. 3), pp. 365-71.

[71] La bibliografia è molto estesa; sommario conveniente in M. BURLEIGH, *Prussian Society and the German Order – an Aristocratic Corporation in Crisis: c. 1410-1466*, Cambridge 1984. Molto materiale è contenuto in *800 Jahre Deutsche Orden*, ed. U. ARNOLD et al., München 1990.

[72] Cf. S. MENACHE, *A Juridical Chapter in the History of the Order of Calatrava – the Mastership of Don Alonso de Aragón: 1443-1444*, in *Tijdschrift voor Rechtsgeschiednis*, 55 (1987).

[73] L. WRIGHT, *The Military Orders in Sixteenth and Seventeenth Century Spanish Society: the Institutional Embodiment of a Historical Tradition*, in *Past and Present*, 43 (1969).

dio mammalucco del 1440, di ingaggiare altre navi genovesi e catalane, per attività di commercio o di pirateria[74]. Già nel 1413 esisteva un sistema ufficiale di corsa autorizzata dall'ordine, con una divisione del bottino tra i *fratres* partecipanti[75]. La tendenza però fu sempre più verso l'attività difensiva, soprattutto dopo la caduta di Costantinopoli nel 1453. Negli assedi del 1480 e del 1522 gli Ospitalieri si difesero dietro le poderose mura di pietra che essi continuamente costruivano, tanto che nel 1522 la città dovette arrendersi più che altro per mancanza di polvere da sparo.

Con la perdita di Rodi doveva manifestarsi la natura dell'*Ordensstaat*. Come corporazione l'Ospedale di S. Giovanni non fu posto in discussione in nessuna sede; poteva mutare la posizione geografica del suo convento senza cambiare la struttura essenziale dell'organizzazione dell'ordine e senza perdere la sua base economica in Occidente, ma di fatto poteva spostarsi solo su un'altra isola. L'esperienza del 1291 con il suo trauma morale, lo sforzo di conservare archivi, tradizioni ed altri elementi di continuità si ripete dopo il 1522. Dopo sette anni di trattative, durante le quali il convento vagabondò attraverso l'Italia, l'imperatore Carlo V, dovendo sistemare un'istituzione prevalentemente francese dentro un impero spagnolo, infeudò all'Ospedale l'isola di Malta e costrinse l'ordine ad accettare una base sulla terraferma infedele, a Tripoli d'Africa[76]. La difesa di Malta contro gli Ottomani nel 1565 dimostrò la sopravvivenza della tradizione degli assedi, mentre la costruzione della nuova città di La Valletta ripeteva la politica delle enormi fortificazioni di pietra[77]. Anche la guerra di corsa fu mantenuta fino al Settecento[78]. L'Ospedale sopravvisse come ordine militare fino al 1798, perché seppe trasformare la sua vocazione continentale in una specie di *Ordensstaat* isolano, che permise al suo convento di mantenere una missione di guerra santa, di difendere una base con impegni limitati e di vivere delle sue rendite occidentali. La svolta decisiva in questo prolungato sviluppo risale agli anni successivi alla caduta di Acri del 1291.

[74] LUTTRELL (come n. 6), VII, p. 321 e n. 23.

[75] *Ibid.*, II, pp. 103-4.

[76] R. VALENTINI, *I Cavalieri di S. Giovanni da Rodi a Malta: trattative diplomatiche*, in *Archivum Melitense*, 9 (1933-35).

[77] Per queste continuità, LUTTRELL (come n. 6), XVIII, *passim*, e ID., *Malta and Rhodes: Hospitallers and Islanders*, in *Hospitaller Malta 1530-1798: Studies in Early Modern Malta and the Order of St. John of Jerusalem*, ed. V. MALLIA-MILANES, Malta 1993. W.-D. BARZ, *Der Malteserorden als Landesherr auf Rhodos und Malta im Licht seiner strafrechtlichen Quellen aus dem 14. und 16. Jahrhundert*, Berlin 1990, utilizza le fonti in modo poco soddisfacente: cf. LUTTRELL (come n. 6), VI, *passim*.

[78] M. FONTENAY, *Les Chevaliers de Malte dans le "Corso" méditerranéen au XVIIe siècle*, in *Las Ordenes Militares en el Mediterràneo Occidental (s. XII-XVIII), Madrid 1989*; ID., *Les missions des galères de Malte: 1530-1789*, in *Guerre et commerce en Méditerranée: IXe-XXe siècles*, ed. M. VERGÉ-FRANCESCHINI, Paris 1991; cf. ID., *De Rhodes à Malte: l'évolution de la flotte des Hospitaliers au XVIe siècle*, in *Atti del V Congresso internazionale di Studi Colombiani*, Genova 1990; A. LUTTRELL, *Eighteenth-Century Malta: Prosperity and Problems*, in *Hyphen* (Malta), 3 (1982); V. MALLIA-MILANES, *Venice and Hospitaller Malta 1530-1798: Aspects of a Relationship*, Malta 1992.

III

THE GREEKS OF RHODES
UNDER HOSPITALLER RULE: 1306-1421 *

Western expansion into the Eastern Mediterranean naturally led to new relationships and confrontations between Latins and Greeks who had differing languages, religious traditions and historical backgrounds (¹). The island of Rhodes largely escaped Western occupation after the Latin conquest of Constantinople in 1204 and it thus enjoyed a degree of independence which preserved it from Latinization, allowing it to retain predominantly Greek governmental forms and institutions on the fringe of the surviving Byzantine world. A variety of Latin merchants and corsairs had temporarily established themselves in the port, but the comparative isolation of Rhodian society persisted until its invasion by the Order of the Hospital in 1306 (²). By that time

---

* This article revises a brief paper on a wider theme first given at the Dumbarton Oaks Center for Byzantine Studies, Washington, in 1980 and published, without correction of proofs, in A. LUTTRELL, *Greeks, Latins and Turks on Late-Medieval Rhodes*, in *Byzantinische Forschungen* 11 (1987); the five documents published there are summarized, with two others and certain amendments, below. The earlier paper covered the period 1306 to 1522, but the subsequent appearance of major works by Z. Tsirpanlis and E. Kollias render the reproduction of the post-1421 material superfluous; for pre-1421 relations with the Turks, A. LUTTRELL, *The Hospitallers of Rhodes and their Mediterranean World*, London 1992, II *passim*. The essential bibliography for Rhodes is given in works by Tsirpanlis, Kollias, Luttrell and others here cited. A much fuller study of the Greeks on Rhodes from 1306 to 1522, based on the surviving parts of the Hospitallers' rich central archives now in Malta, is in preparation by Julian Chrysostomides, Kara Hattersley-Smith and the present author. Meanwhile only a small sampling of the available material is utilized below. On Rhodes Elias Kollias, Anna Maria Kasdagli and Vassilis Karabatsos provided generous collaboration, as also has Joanna Christoforaki.

(¹) Recent surveys and bibliography in D. JACOBY, *Social Evolution in Latin Greece*, and H.E. MAYER – J. McLELLAN, *Select Bibliography of the Crusades*, both in *A History of the Crusades*, ed. K. SETTON, VI, Madison 1989.

(²) A. SAVVIDES, *Βυζαντινὰ στασιαστικὰ καὶ αὐτονομιστικὰ κινήματα στὰ Δωδεκάνησα καὶ στὴ Μικρὰ Ἀσία: 1189-1240*, Athens 1987; IDEM, *Rhodes from the End*

194

Rhodes had apparently been seriously depopulated, partly as a result of repeated devastations by Turks from the mainland; some of these may even have settled on the island (³), though the three hundred Turks who in 1306 garrisoned the castle at Phileremos against the Hospitallers had come to Rhodes from the mainland (⁴). It was probably in 1309 that the main harbour town of Rhodes finally surrendered to the Hospitallers on terms which were subsequently to condition the nature of the island's settlement (⁵). To the Greek inhabitants the Hospitallers must have appeared as Western pirates seizing yet one more outpost of Byzantium; from the Latin viewpoint they were liberating and defending schismatic fellow-Christians from the infidel Turk. Under Hospitaller government Rhodes became a cosmopolitan town, a busy seaport and pilgrim station harbouring Latin settlers, residents and visitors of many types, and minority groups including Syrians, Jews, Cypriots and many Greeks from outside Rhodes (⁶). The Syrians, probably Maronites, were often entrusted by the Hospital with minor military commands in the countryside (⁷).

The Hospitallers who served on Rhodes were members of a military-religious order whose collective experience in Syria before 1291 and in Cyprus before 1306 had accustomed them to the administration of a subordinate foreign peasantry. They were not Western nobles grabbing lands and castles, but a few hundred brethren, many of knightly or urban patrician origin, who managed their Rhodian regime in paternalistic fashion, and though they doubtless appeared authoritar-

---

of the Gabalas Rule to the Conquest by the Hospitallers: A.D. c. 1250-1309, in Βυζαντινὸς Δόμος 2 (1988); E. MALAMUT, *Les îles de l'Empire Byzantin*, 2 vols., Paris 1988; E. PAPAVASSILIOU – T. ARCHONTOPOULOS, *Nouveaux Élements historiques et archéologiques de Rhodes à travers des Fouilles dans la Ville médiévale*, in *XXXVIII Corso di Cultura sull'Arte Ravennate e Bizantina*, Ravenna 1991.

(³) SAVVIDES, *Rhodes* cit., pp. 212-220; LUTTRELL, *Hospitallers of Rhodes* cit., II p. 83; IDEM, *Latin Greece, the Hospitallers and the Crusades: 1291-1440*, London 1982, I p. 250 and n. 57, VI p. 81 and n. 2.

(⁴) *Les Gestes des Chiprois*, ed G. RAYNAUD, Geneva 1887, pp. 320-321.

(⁵) For the date, LUTTRELL, *Hospitallers of Rhodes* cit., II p. 110 n. 10; SAVVIDES, *Rhodes* cit., pp. 223-230; A. FAILLER, *L'Occupation de Rhodes par les Hospitaliers*, in *Revue des Études Byzantines* 50 (1992), arguing for 1310.

(⁶) LUTTRELL, *Latin Greece* cit., VI *passim*; IDEM, *Hospitallers of Rhodes* cit., XIX *passim*; IDEM, *The Hospitallers in Cyprus, Rhodes, Greece and the West: 1291-1440*, London 1978, IV pp. 57-58.

(⁷) IDEM, *Hospitallers of Rhodes* cit., XIX pp. 137-138, 149 n. 25.

ian and militaristic to many Greek inhabitants, their despotism was a comparatively benevolent one. The Hospital provided security and employment while it invested on Rhodes considerable funds derived from its European properties. A community of Latins grew up in the main town and a few lived in the countryside and on the Hospital's lesser islands northwest of Rhodes. In 1391 the Order was supposed to maintain on Kos twenty-one Hospitallers, ten Latin men-at-arms, a hundred Levantine *turcopoli*, a doctor and an apothecary [8]; but in 1433 Nisyros was to have only two Hospitaller *milites* and a Hospitaller priest [9]. Conditions on the smaller islands could be extremely harsh for all concerned; to the east of Rhodes a visitor to Kastellorizzo in 1396 mentioned a Hospitaller castellan and sixty Greeks working the salt there [10].

There was a continual influx of Westerners into Rhodes, but most of these did not remain permanently in the East and it is doubtful whether more than a minority brought womenfolk with them to establish any genuinely Latin family settlement. It was important that Hospitaller brethren took oaths of poverty and chastity and could therefore have no dynastic stake on the island. Many spent only a few years at Rhodes, and any lands or properties they held there temporarily would revert to the Order on their death; they had no perpetual proprietary interest in their estates. Furthermore, Levantine Latin nobles were refused entry to the Order. Thus in 1373 the pope requested the Master of the Order to receive as a *miles* of the Hospital the *nobilis* Giorgio de Lippo *domicellus* of Rhodes, notwithstanding the Hospital's statute which stated *quod nullus de ultramarinis partibus oriundus possit in praefato Ordine recipi sicut miles* [11]. Giorgio's family was well established on Rhodes; in 1383 Pope Clement VII pro-

---

[8] J. DELAVILLE LE ROULX, *Les Hospitaliers à Rhodes jusqu'à la mort de Philibert de Naillac: 1310-1421*, Paris 1913, pp. 230-231. Ruy Gonçalez de Clavijo was presumably confused when reporting 100 Hospitaller *frayres* on Kos in 1403: *Embajada a Tamorlán*, ed. F. LÓPEZ ESTRADA, Madrid 1943, p. 23.

[9] Valletta, National Library of Malta, Archives of the Order of Saint John, Cod. 350, f. 242v-243.

[10] A. LUTTRELL, *The Latins and the Smaller Aegean Islands: 1204-1453*, in *Mediterranean Historical Review* 4 (1989), p. 153.

[11] Text in *Pontificia Commissio ad Redigendum Codicem Iuris Canonici Orientalis: Fontes*, ser. 3, 15 vols., Rome 1943-1990, XII, pp. 112-113; the text of the statute does not survive. Giorgio de Lippo never appears as a Hospitaller.

vided Manuele de Lippo, already a canon of Rhodes, as archbishop of the island ([12]) and in 1391 Niccolino de Lippo, *civis* of Rhodes, was granted the Rhodian fief of Lardos ([13]). No class of *archontes* or Greek nobles survived, and since initial attempts to create a group of Latin fief-holders were, with a few exceptions, unsuccessful, there was never any significant class of individuals with a permanent, heritable lordship over the land and people ([14]).

The inhabitants of Rhodes were conceivably fewer than 10,000 in 1310 ([15]), rising to perhaps 20,000 or more by 1522 ([16]). The population in the countryside and on the other islands was periodically reduced by Turkish and other razzias ([17]). Many properties and vineyards on Rhodes were leased by the Hospital in emphyteusis at an annual census to both Greeks and Latins ([18]). Most Greeks outside the town were either free peasants sometimes called *francomati*, or they were *parichi*, or serfs, or slaves; on the island of Nisyros there were *rustici* who dug the volcanic sulphur for wages ([19]). Slaves when manumitted became wholly free or *franci* ([20]). *Francomati* and *marinarii*, the latter with hereditary obligations to serve at sea, were legally free

---

([12]) *Ibid.*, XIII part 2, p. 58.

([13]) LUTTRELL, *Hospitallers in Cyprus* cit., III p. 764.

([14]) Cf. *ibid.*, III *passim*.

([15]) This figure is largely guesswork: *ibid.*, III p. 755 n. 8.

([16]) An Ottoman *defter* datable between 1523 and 1535, that is following the final siege and the consequent deaths and emigrations, listed 1,121 Muslim and 5,191 Christian households on Rhodes: Ö. L. BARKAN, *Osmanli Impararatorlu-ǧunda Bir Iskan ve Kolonizasyon Metodu Olarak Sürgünler*, in *I. U. Iktisat Fakül-tesi Mecumuasi* 5 (1953-1954), p. 237 [information kindly provided by Heath Lowry].

([17]) A magistral letter of 8 July 1457 stated that there were *xijm animarum incirca* on Kos: text in Z. TSIRPANLIS, Ἡ Ῥόδος καὶ οἱ Νότιες Σποράδες στὰ χρόνια τῶν Ἰωαννίτων ἱπποτῶν (14ος-16ος αι.): Συλλογὴ ἱστορικῶν μελετῶν, Rhodes 1991, pp. 122-124. J. KODER, *Topographie und Bevölkerung der Agäis-Inseln in spätby-zantinischer Zeit: Probleme der Quellen*, in *Byzantinische Forschungen* 5 (1977), p. 231 n. 20, gives figures from Giacomo Rizzardo for 1470: 20 *anime* on Leros; 400 on Astypalia; 400 for Kalymnos and Patmos together, and 1500 for Kos and "Chexenia"(?).

([18]) A. LUTTRELL, *Hospitallers of Rhodes* cit., V *passim*; IDEM, *Emphyteutic Grants in Rhodes Town: 1347-1348*, in *Papers in European Legal History: Traba-jos de Derecho Histórico Europeo en Homenaje a Ferran Vals i Taberner*, V, Bar-celona 1992.

([19]) IDEM, *Hospitallers in Cyprus* cit., III pp. 762-763.

([20]) IDEM, *Latin Greece* cit., VI pp. 93-96, 100.

but if they married *servi* or *parichi* then their children would be *servi* or *parichi* ([21]). A *paricho* inherited not a bondage to the soil but a subjection to a lord or to an institution; in the tradition of the Byzantine *paroikos* he was in some ways free and could hold land and transmit it to his heirs, but if he had no heirs it would revert to his lord ([22]).

The distinction between the free and the unfree was often ambiguous. The town statutes, the *Capitula Rodi* which were probably established early in the fourteenth century, laid down that children of either sex born of a father who was *francus*, which in that context meant Latin, and of a Greek mother were legally to be *franchi* or Latins, a rule presumably applying only to the Latins of the town: *Item quod omnes tam masculi, quam femine, tam nati, quam nascituri de franco, et Greca, habeantur, et teneantur pro franchis.* However a later amendment decreed that they should be *marinarii* and should reside in the *borgo* where they were needed, evidently so that they could board ship rapidly: *Additio. qui scilicet marinarij fuerint, et morabuntur in burgo Rodi.* Presumably it was decided that children of mixed parentage had increased and that they were not to be considered as entirely Latin but should, after all, be compelled to galley service ([23]). There could also be complications in the countryside if the mother was a serf. Thus in 1352 a Greek named Maria Maistrisse, who was the daughter of a *papas* or priest and of a *serva* or serf of the Hospital, was manumitted when her father gave the Hospital a female slave in her place; she was then licensed "to make a will, to stand in justice and to do those other things permitted to a *mulier franca et libera*", and freely to dispose of her goods ([24]). In 1366 the four sons and two daughters of a free Latin, a *francus homo* from Provence, had to seek their freedom from serfdom. Their father had settled on a

---

([21]) As declared in 1448 in Malta, Cod. 361, f. 281-281v; cf. IDEM, *Hospitallers in Cyprus* cit, IV pp. 61-63.

([22]) The Rhodian peasantry awaits detailed examination.

([23]) Text in IDEM, *Hospitallers of Rhodes* cit., VI p. 210 [but revise *ibid.*, p. 206 n. 8]. W.-D. BARZ, *Der Malteserorden als Landsheer auf Rhodes und Malta im Licht seiner strafrechtlichen Quellen aus dem 14. und 16. Jahrhundert*, Berlin 1990, requires considerable caution. BARZ, *ibid.*, pp. 66-68, 169-170, claims, unconvincingly, that the *marinarii* constrained by the *Capitula* to residence in the *borgo* were sailors rather than men and women obliged to the *servitudo marina*.

([24]) Malta, Cod. 318, f. 221.

Rhodian *casale* as a *sargentus* and had married a Greek *serva* belonging to the Hospital; the father had received a licence which established that his children were to be free *more franchorum*, that is to be Latins in status, and they were baptized as Roman, not Greek, Christians (²⁵).

A contemporary Latin chronicler recounted how the late-Byzantine town held out for several years after 1306 and finally surrendered on terms or *covenanses devizees* of which he gave no details except to say that the Hospitallers respected the agreements; the Hospitallers then moved the Greek inhabitants from the *forteresse dou chastiau* to the less strongly defended *bourc*, strengthened the defences of the *chastiau* and brought in settlers (²⁶). The internal late-Byzantine wall with large square projecting towers which divided the castle or *castrum* from the *borgo* had a gate leading into the *borgo* (²⁷). Within this wall the *castrum* constituted an area which was known as the *collachium* and included the *kastron* or fortress which became the Master's palace. Technically the *collachium* may have been reserved to Hospitallers (²⁸), but eventually the towers of the *collachium* wall came to be used as houses and the wall must have lost much of its defensive, anti-Greek function (²⁹). In fact, there were other Latins inside the *collachium*, including the mercenary garrison, those attached to the cathedral and to the arsenal, and the staff and inmates of the Order's great hospital. In 1357 a statute of the Hospital decreed that thenceforth no Turkish slaves should be kept within the *castrum*, except that each

---

(²⁵) Malta, Cod. 319, f. 272.

(²⁶) *Gestes des Chiprois* cit., pp. 320-322.

(²⁷) Current excavation is establishing the Byzantine foundations of Hospitaller Rhodes: details and references in PAPAVASSILIOU – ARCHONTOPOULOS, *Nouveaux Élements* cit. The precise history of the *collachium* wall is still uncertain: interim detail *ibid.*, pp. 337-345; E. KOLLIAS, *The City of Rhodes and the Palace of the Grand Master*, Athens 1989, pp. 61-63, plans I-II, figs. 1, 21, 23, 72; IDEM, *The Knights of Rhodes: the Palace and the City*, Athens 1991, pp. 62-63 (plan), figs. 45, 66-67.

(²⁸) A. GABRIEL, *La Cité de Rhodes: MCCCX - MDXXII*, 2 vols., Paris 1921-1923, I, pp. 6-7. Cf. B. WALDSTEIN – WARTENBERG, *Mittelalterlichen Bauten von Rhodos auf der Grundlage von Beschreibungen zeitgenössischer Riesender*, in *Annales de l'Ordre Souverain Militaire de Malte* 35 (1977). The Hospitallers' own documents were most inconsistent in their use of such terms as *castrum*, *civitas*, *burgum* and *collachium*.

(²⁹) PAPAVASSILIOU – ARCHONTOPOULOS, *Nouveaux Élements* cit., p. 339.

Hospitaller *auberge* might keep one as a servant ([30]). There were also properties within the *castrum* which belonged to Greeks, who presumably lived in them. In 1351 a house there which had once been the property of the *presbiter* Georgios stood between the church of Saint Demetrius and the *hospitium* of *magister* Nicola Coquirasserij ([31]). In 1358 a two-storeyed *hospicium* within the *castrum* which had belonged to Sophia the daughter of Johannes Diastrique stood next to the houses of Anna widow of Petroto, of Marossa de Stranofodilo and of Margocia sister of Leonardello's widow; the very same text also described a single-storeyed house *in civitate* ([32]). A later statute establishing hours in which Hospitaller brethren were to stay within the walls and gates of the *castrum* ([33]) suggests that the notion of a *collachium* was as much concerned with enclosing the brethren as with excluding others ([34]).

In the *borgo* Latins and Greeks lived side by side. In about 1420 Cristoforo Buondelmonti wrote of a quarter "inhabited by the merchants together with the Greeks" ([35]). In addition to the Hospitaller brethren, Western merchants, sailors, pilgrims, lawyers, clerics, artisans and others established themselves in the town and conducted business which brought them into contact with the Greeks. Arrangements in town government reflected an element of equality at certain levels. Thus in 1385 the Latin and the Greek *habitatores* of Rhodes town complained of excessive taxes, and it was decided that the officials who controlled the importation of foodstuffs were to act only in the presence of two Latin and two Greek *burgenses* ([36]). When in 1429 a *commerchium* of eight percent had to be raised to pay for peace

---

([30]) Text in Luttrell, *Latin Greece* cit., VI pp. 86-87.

([31]) Malta, Cod. 318, f. 204v.

([32]) Malta, Cod. 316, f. 316v; *Diast*[...] is unclear.

([33]) Text in *Prohemium in Volumen Stabilimentorum Rhodiorum Militum...*, ed G. Caoursin, Ulm 1496, *De fratribus*, lij.

([34]) However, those not Hospitallers were sent out of the *colachio* and the gates closed during the magistral election of 1437: *Andanças é Viajes de Pero Tafur por diversas partes del Mundo: 1435-1439*, ed. M. Jiménez de la Espada, Madrid 1874, p. 127.

([35]) *Cristophori Buondelmontii, Florentini, Librum Insularum Archipelagi*, ed L. von Sinner, Leipzig – Berlin 1824, p. 73, discussed in Gabriel, *Rhodes* cit., I, pp. 6-7; numerous documents concerning properties describe the adjoining properties in terms of their owners or occupants.

([36]) Malta, Cod. 323, f. 216-216v/218-218v.

embassies to the Turks, the consent of both Greek and Latin *cives* and *subditi* was required according it was said to the *antiqua consuetudo* of earlier Masters, and one Greek and one Latin were to be elected annually by the *giurati* to supervise its collection. The agreement was for ten years only and it was reconsidered in 1439 ([37]). Except for the clause concerning children of mixed marriages which was an addition, the early fourteenth-century *Capitula Rodi* contained no overt discrimination between Latins and Greeks ([38]); the same was true of the much lengthier recodification of 1590/10 which continued to recognize the Latins and Greeks of the *borgo* as separate but still ensured them equal representation ([39]).

Developments in the town were conditioned by the emergence of a Greek bourgeoisie. There must always have been some short-range shipping in local Greek hands operating from Rhodes. There were Greeks and local Latins who were running small-scale, short-distance trade or cabotage within the Aegean on ships from Rhodes by the mid-fourteenth century ([40]), but before that there was apparently no substantial class of Greeks who were merchants and shippers. Greek merchants at Rhodes were not necessarily natives of the island. In 1360 Georgios Caligopulos of Constantinople, *nunc habitator* of Rhodes, was empowered at Famagusta to act on behalf of a Sicilian lending money there, and also in Famagusta in 1362 Antonio de Sacha of Sicily empowered Dimitri *de Rhodo* to act on his behalf in Venice or elsewhere ([41]). In 1381 Johannes Susomeni, a *burgensis* of Rhodes, employed a factor in Cyprus named Michalli Conderato who was transferring monies to Rhodes from Cyprus on behalf of the Hospital; and in the same year Nicholas of Corinth, a *burgensis* of the town of Kos, was licensed to send to Rhodes grain grown on his lands in

---

([37]) Malta, Cod. 354, f. 258-259.

([38]) Text in LUTTRELL, *Hospitallers of Rhodes* cit., VI pp. 207-211.

([39]) Modern copies in Valletta, National Library of Malta, Biblioteca, Ms. 153, Ms. 617 and Ms. 740, f. 1-94. This extensive text, fundamental to any study of the *borgo*, is inexplicably ignored in BARZ, *Malteserorden* cit.

([40]) LUTTRELL, *Hospitallers in Cyprus* cit., V pp. 200-201, VI pp. 169-172; merchants and ships from Rhodes are seldom demonstrably Rhodian.

([41]) Texts in *Nicola de Boateriis Notaio in Famagusta e Venezia: 1355-1365*, ed. A. LOMBARDO, Venice 1973, pp. 32-33, 192.

Kos (⁴²). A fragmentary page of accounts from Rhodes, datable to the end of the fourteenth century, showed local lendings and a range of business within an area stretching from Ephesus to Kastellorizzo and Cyprus (⁴³). By then merchants and shipping from Rhodes were active in the Adriatic. Costa Somian of Rhodes was captain of a *cocha* which arrived at Dubrovnik from somewhere in Anatolia in 1390, and in the following year two captains of a ship belonging to a citizen of Rhodes were leaving Dubrovnik for Alexandria. In 1397 a Greek from Negroponte, inhabitant of Rhodes, was at Constantinople. There were at least five Rhodian merchants at Dubrovnik in 1409. Above all Manuel de Costabilibus or Comestabilibus of Rhodes was, at least from 1404 to 1414, a leading businessman at Dubrovnik, dealing in oil and grain, buying and hiring ships, and trading in the Adriatic, Byzantium and Egypt (⁴⁴). Merchants from Rhodes, some of them Greek, continued to trade between Dalmatia, Anatolia and Egypt. At Alexandria, Antonius Myverbeti, *burgensis* and inhabitant of Rhodes, became Rhodian consul in 1413; in 1419 and 1420 a Rhodian Greek named Archondizi de Assarino had two or more ships, one of which was seized at Beirut; and a ship captained by Stamati de Rodo was at Alexandria in 1422 (⁴⁵). When some time before 1412 Angelina, daughter of Costa Megulusiane, *burgensis* of Rhodes and probably a Greek, married Andrea Janni, *burgensis* of Venice, her dowry amounted to no less than 4000 ducats (⁴⁶).

In the Rhodian countryside and on the lesser islands the leading Greeks of the villages met together as a *universitas grecorum* to settle local matters or protest to the government. Thus in 1351 six Greeks, including four *pappates* and a *protopapas*, and the *universitas habitancium* of the island of Symi complained that the *mortuaria* or death

---

(⁴²) Malta, Cod. 321, f. 214v, 231; that these men were Greeks rather than Latins or Syrians remains an assumption.

(⁴³) Text in P. Schreiner, *Texte zur spätbizantinischen Finanz- und Wirtschaftsgeschichte in Handschriften der Biblioteca Vaticana*, Vatican 1991, pp. 68-70.

(⁴⁴) B. Krekić, *Dubrovnik (Raguse) et le Levant au Moyen Âge*, Paris – The Hague 1961, pp. 129-130, 229-230, 232, 243, 245-247, 249, 253, 257, 263.

(⁴⁵) Luttrell, *Hospitallers of Rhodes* cit., X p. 199, XIX p. 140; E. Ashtor, *Levant Trade in the Later Middle Ages*, Princeton 1983, pp. 245 n. 223, 365 and n. 566, 536, 540-541.

(⁴⁶) Malta, Cod. 339, f. 241.

duties the Greek islanders had long had to pay were insupportable; the Hospital accepted their suggestion that the *universitas* pay the Order 500 *asperi* a year in place of the death duties, but with the condition that the possessions of deceased *calogeri* and *calogere*, that is of Greek monks and nuns, and of those dying without heirs should revert to the Order (⁴⁷). In 1386 the goods of a deceased nun on Rhodes did devolve to the Hospital (⁴⁸), and the point emerged in 1422 when the Master made a concession to the *protos* of the *castellania* of Katagro by which the movable and immovable goods, but not monies, jewels or plate, belonging to deceased monks in the *monasterium* of Saint Michael *Camberidj*, which the *protos* had founded, should remain in that monastery, notwithstanding existing custom to the contrary; their bodies were to be buried in the monastery, and its rector or abbot was to inform the castellan and the *protos* on the same day (⁴⁹). In 1460, following a damaging Turkish razzia, Symi's annual *census* or *jus dominij* was temporarily reduced from 750 to 400 florins (⁵⁰). In the absence of a Greek nobility on Rhodes, village affairs were often handled by a *protos* or head man who might be a priest; in 1347 *papas* Janni Macrigerij was *protos* of Appollakia and Michaellj Culichi was *protos* of Archangelos (⁵¹). Especially where matters of fortification and defence were involved, the Hospitallers sought to accommodate or protect their subjects. When the small islands of Khalkia and Piskopia were granted out in 1366 the Hospital stipulated that no new services

---

(⁴⁷) Malta, Cod. 318, f. 205v-206; TSIRPANLIS, *Ρόδος* cit., p. 130, uses a defective summary of this text in G. BOSIO, *Dell'Istoria della Sacra Religione et Illustrissima Militia di San Giovanni Gerosolimitano...*, 2nd ed., II, Rome 1630, p. 82. TSIRPANLIS, cit., pp. 130 n. 1, 191 n. 1, 239 n. 1, 422, considers Bosio's *mortuario* to be the Byzantine *mourti*, which was a tax of a fourth on agrarian produce. LUTTRELL, *Hospitallers of Rhodes* cit., VII pp. 322-323, considered the *morti* paid at Lindos to be a customary death duty, citing also the Symi *mortuaria* of 1351 and monies due on Leros *ratione mortuariorum*, in 1436: Malta, Cod. 352, f. 141v. LUTTRELL, *ibid.*, XIX p. 150 n. 56, stated that the *mortuaria* was really the *morte*, a tithe or tenth, but clearly it was a duty, payable at Symi in 1351, on the goods of deceased monks and nuns and of those without heirs, and is to be distinguished from the *mourti*.

(⁴⁸) Malta, Cod. 323, f. 213-213v.

(⁴⁹) Malta, Cod. 346, f. 167v.

(⁵⁰) Text in TSIRPANLIS, *Ρόδος* cit., pp. 133-135.

(⁵¹) Malta, Cod. 317, f. 235, 236.

were to be imposed on their inhabitants (⁵²). In 1445 the *plebs* and *populus* of the island of Kalymnos produced a *sacramentale* of uncertain antiquity written in Greek claiming that they were *liberi ab omnibus servitutibus* and not bound to work on the castle. Legal debate followed at Rhodes where it was decided that the population did owe castle service but was free of all other *servitia* (⁵³).

Arrangements for military service, watch towers, road and castle building, the fortification of villages and the system by which the islanders were to retreat to safe castles in time of danger were all of benefit to the Rhodians (⁵⁴). The exemption from military service granted to the men of Lindos in 1314 in return for the *xili*, the carting of timber for ship-building, was a case in point (⁵⁵). Communities were given a degree of autonomy and local leadership was recognized while what were probably ancient Byzantine institutions were preserved or adapted; the Hospital's officials were occasionally censured or restrained when their behaviour was oppressive, the Hospital being prepared to accept legal process and to ratify privileges in the interests of all parties (⁵⁶). This was another reason for the absence of major revolts such as the Venetians experienced on Crete. There were occasional uprisings but they were not necessarily the result of bad or tyrannical government. The revolt on Leros in 1319 saw more than 1900 rebel Greeks slaughter the Hospitallers and their garrison and go over to the emperor at Constantinople (⁵⁷), while that on Nisyros in 1347 occurred on an enfeoffed island not under direct Hospitaller rule (⁵⁸).

The Hospital generated employment for the population in wall

(⁵²) LUTTRELL, *Hospitallers in Cyprus* cit., III p. 761.

(⁵³) Text in TSIRPANLIS, *Ρόδος* cit., III pp. 167-171.

(⁵⁴) LUTTRELL, *Hospitallers of Rhodes* cit., XIX pp. 136-140 *et passim*; J.-C. POUTIERS, *Rhodes et ses Chevaliers 1306-1523: Approche historique et archéologique*, Brussels 1989, pp. 28-34, 192, 251-298, 301-314, with plans of villages and enceintes.

(⁵⁵) LUTTRELL, *Hospitallers of Rhodes* cit., VII pp. 323-324, 330-332.

(⁵⁶) Texts and discussion in TSIRPANLIS, *Ρόδος* cit., pp. 190-192, 208-209 *et passim*. Most of the documents used by Tsirpanlis date after 1440 circa. Where an institution is not otherwise explained, and especially when the privilege was presented in Greek, TSIRPANLIS cit., pp. 246-249, 419-422 *et passim*, plausibly seeks Byzantine origins.

(⁵⁷) Text in DELAVILLE, *Hospitaliers à Rhodes* cit., pp. 365-367.

(⁵⁸) LUTTRELL, *Hospitallers in Cyprus* cit., III p. 761.

and castle building, in providing supplies and services, in running the port and the great hospital, and so forth. For example, in 1347 the Master had a Greek cook and there was a Greek *serviens* in the *curia* [59]. Some Rhodian Greeks found employment as oarsmen on Western galleys [60]. The number of Greek slaves diminished during the fourteenth century, and as manumissions freed many slaves and serfs and with land available on emphyteutic leases, the class of largely independent Greek peasants was strengthened. Their holdings were often rather small. The Latin Antonio Contarelli, who was granted a large property, the *monasterium* and *domus* of Artamitis, in the centre of the island in 1359, held about 31 square kilometres at an annual census of 55 florins, while in 1347 the Greek *protos* of Archangelos held seven modiates, perhaps 0.75 square kilometres, there [61]. These non-urban Greeks paid a variety of dues including a tax on their animals, the *mourti* of a quarter on agricultural produce and a sales tax, while they owed castle building and other corvées or services. Those who held land in emphiteusis owed an annual *census* and other payments [62]. On Kos there was a *testagium* or poll tax [63]. Greek priests could be lowly in status; in about 1375 *papas* Costa Chrimeli of the *casale* of Archangelos, who was a *servus* of the Hospital, was freed by the Master, and this manumission was confirmed in 1427 when his children were being impressed for marine service [64].

The status in law of the Rhodian Greeks was a complicated matter. The agreement of 1309 circa guaranteed them – *a la fiance de l'Ospitau* – their property and such personal freedom as they had enjoyed in Byzantine times – *si come il esteent de l'emperour de Costantinople*; the Order was said soon after 1309 to be respecting this agree-

---

[59] Malta, Cod. 317, f. 239v, 239v-240.

[60] IDEM, *Hospitallers of Rhodes* cit., XIX p. 139.

[61] K. HATTERSLEY – SMITH, *Documentary and Archaeological Evidence for Greek Settlement in the Countryside of Rhodes in the Fourteenth and Early Fifteenth Centuries*, in *The Military Orders: Fighting for the Faith and Caring for the Sick*, London forthcoming.

[62] The condition of the peasantry awaits detailed study, but in addition to TSIRPANLIS, *Ρόδος* cit., see LUTTRELL, *Hospitallers in Cyprus* cit., III pp. 768-769, IV pp. 60-63; IDEM, *Latin Greece* cit., VI pp. 81-91; IDEM, *Hospitallers of Rhodes* cit., V pp. 275-277, VII pp. 319, 322-324, XIX pp. 136-138.

[63] Text of 1441 and discussion TSIRPANLIS, *Ρόδος* cit., pp. 240, 246-249.

[64] Malta, Cod. 347, f. 200.

ment ([65]). The Hospitallers, virtually independent rulers in the islands, had their Rule and statutes which regulated their own affairs; they also enjoyed a general lordship over the islands which allowed them to free slaves and serfs ([66]), to pardon those exiled for murder ([67]) and other crimes ([68]), to compel the inhabitants of a *casale* to construct a castle ([69]) and so forth. Disputes over such matters sometimes came before Hospitaller officials sitting with the council of the Order, and with professional lawyers in attendance, as a court in which Greeks could present certain classes of appeals, act as witnesses and take oaths made in the Greek metropolitan church according to the Greek custom, probably by touching an ikon rather than the bible. Some such cases concerned personal status, manumissions, corvées, exemptions for village communities and various problems of the smaller islands. The Order sometimes dealt with such matters according to its own decrees which seem never to have been codified into a legal corpus ([70]). In 1420 a statute laid down that the Master or his lieutenant, together with the Conventual *baiulivi* and the Vice Chancellor, should hold a weekly public audience every Friday to hear quarrels and complaints, to each according to his own law: *et cuique ius suum tribuat* ([71]). Grants of property, churches and monasteries were made or confirmed by the Master. Property throughout the island was largely held through standard leases involving the Roman law of emphyteusis with the *maior dominium*, the *jus praelationis*, the *laudimium* and so on ([72]).

In the town of Rhodes affairs were regulated by the *Capitula Rodi* which were probably applied in primitive form early in the fourteenth century and were recodified, for the last time, in 1509/10 ([73]). Juris-

---

([65]) *Gestes des Chiprois* cit., p. 322.

([66]) Eg. LUTTRELL, *Hospitallers in Cyprus* cit., IV pp. 61-62; IDEM, *Latin Greece* cit., VI pp. 92-100.

([67]) Eg. Malta, Cod. 319, f. 272v (1366).

([68]) Text in IDEM, *Hospitallers of Rhodes* cit., VI pp. 208, 210.

([69]) Eg. Malta, Cod. 330, f. 121 (1400).

([70]) Eg. IDEM, *Hospitallers in Cyprus* cit., IV pp. 57-59.

([71]) Text in *Prohemium in volumen Stabilimentorum* cit., De consilio, iij.

([72]) LUTTRELL, *Hospitallers in Cyprus* cit., III pp. 773-774; IDEM, *Hospitallers of Rhodes* cit., V pp. 275, 277.

([73]) Text and discussion *ibid.*, VI and BARZ, *Malteserorden* cit.; the *statutum municipale terre nostre Rodi* existed by 1381 at latest (*infra* Doc. II) but the

diction lay with the *curia* which was under the overall control of a Hospitaller acting as Castellan of Rhodes and of judges ordinary, criminal and appeal; these were always Latins, usually with Italian degrees (⁷⁴), and evidently they applied Western civil law. When an Italian *legum professor* was confirmed as judge of appeals in the *civitas* of Rhodes in 1390, he was to exercize his post *secundum jura et statuta dicte terre* (⁷⁵). A possible exception was Nicholaus Gorgostari of Rhodes, son of Georgios Gorgostari of Rhodes who may have been wholly or partly Greek; he was a *legum doctor* who had graduated at Padua and in 1453 he was a judge in the *maleficiorum curia* at Rhodes (⁷⁶).

Cases under Byzantine law and custom were presumably decided in Greek ecclesiastical courts. The Greeks could do business in the Greek metropolitan church, as in the case of the evidence taken there in 1401 (⁷⁷). These arrangements must have evolved across the years. By 1509/10 there had long been a *tabulario*, a notary or scribe appointed by the Master, who was available in the metropolitan church to write letters, dowries, testaments and legacies in Greek and to record copies in bound registers to be kept under lock in a notarial archive in the *Castellania* (⁷⁸). An act drawn up in Greek in 1336 by Johannes Kalliandres, who was a priest and *nomikos* and also chartophylax or archivist of the metropolitan church, recorded a declaration made before four ecclesiastical officers, the grand *oikonomos*, the *skeuophylax*, the *sakellarios* and the *protopsaltes*, and three worthy men, Iohannes Akyndinos, Joseph Markapha and Georgios Calokyres. Another Greek act of 1337 concerning a financial transaction between Leon Ligeros and his son was done before the clergy and *kritai* or judges of the metropolitan church and before Nikolaos Ieraki, Konstantinos Zenarites and Kristianos *servente tes cortes*, that is sergeant

---

Capitula probably dated to the first half of the century (BARZ, *Malteserorden* cit., pp. 79-80, 84-86, 173).

(⁷⁴) Eg. LUTTRELL, *Hospitallers in Cyprus* cit., III pp. 765-766, IV p. 57, XVI pp. 452, 454.

(⁷⁵) Malta, Cod. 324, f. 148.

(⁷⁶) Text and discussion in TSIRPANLIS, *Ρόδος* cit., pp. 282-284, 344-347.

(⁷⁷) LUTTRELL, *Hospitallers in Cyprus* cit., IV p. 59.

(⁷⁸) Malta, Biblioteca, Ms. 740 part 1, f. 10-10v.

of the *curia* ([79]). In 1358 Georgios Calokyres, *notarius publicus*, drew up in Rhodes an act by which one *papas* donated a Rhodian *ecclesia patrimoniale* to another ([80]). Greek notarial offices were variously described from 1381 onwards as a *scribania* held by a *scriba* or *notarius* or by a *scribus grecus* or sometimes as the notarial office of the *condillus grecorum*. The offices served both the city and island of Rhodes; appointments were in the power of the Master; and the notaries issued and preserved legally valid acts. The office could be granted to a Latin who appointed a Greek-speaking lieutenant to exercize them ([81]). In 1427 an *officium scribanatus* concerned with drawing up acts and codicils between Greeks on Kos was known as *lo condilj* ([82]).

Greeks were on occasion drawn into the working of Latin justice. An example was the experience of the brothers Nicholas and Nikephoros Crossocopolo, who lost a case over a vineyard brought against them by Anna Stratigissa before *magister* Amellenus de Tricaris, judge ordinary in the *curia*; his sentence was later confirmed by Buchio de Muto, judge of appeals. Anna's rights seem to have passed to Johannes Falconeri, apparently a Latin, and the brothers Crossocopolo then brought an unsuccessful case against him before *magister* Bartholomeus, also a judge ordinary. After that Nicholas appealed to the Master, then at Avignon, who handed over the acts to various *professores* in civil and canon law. These found the judgements of Amellenus and Buchio to be defective, and on 20 September 1391 the Master instructed the Lieutenant Master on Rhodes that the case against Anna was to be retried entirely and that Nicholas was to be given back the vineyard. Nicholas had also taken his case to the Latin archbishop, but the papers relevant to the latter's decision were not sent to Avignon ([83]).

One major reason for the largely peaceful Latin occupation of Rhodes was an acceptable religious accommodation. Relations be-

---

([79]) Texts in I. SAKKELION, *Πατμιακὴ Βιβλιοθήκη*, Athens 1890, pp. 115-116; these two private acts in Greek seem to be unique survivals from Rhodes.

([80]) Malta, Cod. 316, f. 301-301v.

([81]) *Infra*, Docs. II-IV, VI-VII.

([82]) Malta, Cod. 347, f. 161v.

([83]) Malta, Cod. 325, f. 142v-143: this case happens to survive because the appeal went to the Master at a time when both he and his register were at Avignon. In 1390 Amellenus de Tricaris *iurisperitus* was *iudex curie nostre Rodi ciuilium et criminalium*: Cod. 324, f. 147-147v.

tween Latins and Greeks had for centuries been entangled in a complex heritage of linguistic incomprehension, religious dispute and other perennial hatreds and divisions. On Rhodes, arrangements concerning religion formed part of the general *covenanses devizees* of 1309 circa according to a *sacramentale* or agreement made at the time of the surrender on terms. The Rhodians evidently retained the Greek rite and at least some ecclesiastical property, but they had formally to acknowledge papal supremacy and the overall control of ecclesiastical matters and appointments by the Master and Convent of the Hospital [84]. Relations between the Greek and Latin churches on Rhodes were revised after the decree of union at the Council of Florence in 1439 [85]. There was a Latin Archbishop of Rhodes with subordinate bishops of Kos and Nisyros, and the pope interfered to make provisions in a way which became normal throughout the Latin Church [86]; in 1324, for example, he translated the Bishop of Kos to the Archbishopric of Rhodes [87].

Some Greek churches and incomes passed to the Latins, which led the Hospital and the Latin archbishop to quarrel over properties, churches, monasteries, *servi, rustici, villani*, tenths and services due to the archbishop from the Hospital and from other Latins on Rhodes. Two cardinals held lengthy negotiations at Avignon and produced an agreement confirmed by the pope on 1 March 1322. The archbishop was to be assigned sufficient goods and rents to provide him with 8000 besants of Rhodes, equivalent to 1231 florins, yearly. He was to have

---

[84] The *sacramentale* was mentioned in 1366: *infra*, Doc. 1.

[85] The discussions in TSIRPANLIS, *Ρόδος* cit., are largely based on post-1439 materials and seem not to apply entirely to the earlier period.

[86] G. FEDALTO, *La Chiesa Latina in Oriente*, I, 2nd ed., Verona 1981, pp. 449-451; II, 1st ed., Verona 1976, pp. 88-89, 137, 181-182. The frequent claim (eg. in GABRIEL, *Rhodes* cit., II, p. 159) that just before the conquest Pope Clement V gave the Hospital the right to appoint the archbishop derives from E. FURSE, *Mémoires numismatiques de l'Ordre de Saint-Jean de Jérusalem*, Rome 1889, p. 27, without source. In 1433 the pope agreed that only Hospitaller priests who could speak Greek should be appointed to the sees of Rhodes and Nisyros: texts in *Pontificia Commissio* cit., XV, pp. 137-139. In July 1436 the Master and Convent elected Fr. Matthieu de Chaselles, Commander of Chanonat, to Nisyros following the agreement that they could appoint suitable Hospitaller brethren *in ydiomato greco simul, et moribus gencium dictarum ecclesiarum dyocesanarum experti*: Malta, Cod. 325, f. 141.

[87] Archivio Vaticano, Reg. Aven. 23, f. 549v-550.

"half" of all Rhodian churches with their goods and incomes: *habeatis medietatem omnium ecclesiarum consistentium in civitate et insula Rodi cum universis et singulis bonis redditibus et rebus earum*. The archbishop was to have: the canonical portion, probably a fourth, of the fees of all who chose burial in the Hospital's churches; the *iurisdictio libera* over all Greeks, lay and clerical, both in visiting them and in receiving procuration payments when doing so; all other rights enjoyed over the Greek subjects of their churches by Latin prelates in Cyprus; the cathedral church within the *castrum*, the Greek archbishop's former house with both its upper and lower floors, its oven and baths, and the *hospitia* or houses on either side of the cathedral *usque ad muros civitatis seu castri*; and other advantages not detailed in the bull ([88]). The *medietas* apparently involved a half of the churches' incomes. In 1383 Pope Clement VII not only maintained as rector of the parish in the *borgo* a man whom he had provided despite protests from the archbishop and chapter that the parish was subordinate to them by ancient custom, but he also exempted the rector from paying them the *medietas* of all his incomes; furthermore Clement abolished the custom by which the archdeacon received five *solidi* for every marriage conducted in the parish church ([89]).

The Hospital had no wish to provoke ideological resistance. The Cypriot settlement of 1260 had established that a Latin metropolitan should supervise subordinate Greek bishops, confirming their election and receiving an oath of obedience. Greeks were to be free to use their own courts, unless Latins were involved, and to appeal from them to the Latin bishop or to the pope. On Cyprus, Latin bishops could visit Greek churches, but without interfering or exacting procuration payments, and the Latin clergy were to receive tithes ([90]). On

---

([88]) Reg. Aven. 16, f. 326-327, partially and inaccurately published in *Dépouillement des Tomes XXI-XXII de l'"Orbis Christianus" de Henri de Suarez*, in *Archives de l'Orient Latin* I (1881), p. 269. The Augustinians in the *borgo* were exempted from paying the canonical portion in 1435: text in *Pontificia Commissio* cit., XV, pp. 178-179.

([89]) Texts *ibid.*, XIII part 2, pp. 54-57.

([90]) Text in *Pontificia Commissio* cit., IV part 2, pp. 91-121; cf. G. Hill, *History of Cyprus*, III, Cambridge 1948, pp. 1059-1061, with later references in J. Gill, *The Tribulations of the Greek Church in Cyprus: 1196-ca. 1280*, in *Byzantinische Forschungen* 5 (1977); J. Darrouzès, *Textes Synodaux Chypriotes*, in *Revue des Études Byzantines* 37 (1979); J. Richard, *The Institutions of the King-*

Rhodes, the Latins took over the Greek cathedral and any other churches they may have found within the *collachium*, and Latin churches were established in the *borgo* and outside the city walls (⁹¹). The Hospitallers also annexed Byzantine churches existing within various castles, as for example at Lindos (⁹²). However, the Greeks retained many churches and monasteries (⁹³) and presumably they taxed their own laity and clergy, as on Cyprus.

There was little sign of any attempt at conversion, and indeed proselytization would have been difficult. As late as 1436 the Latin archbishop Andreas Chrysoberges, who was a Greek from Constantinople, was licensed by the pope to preach and celebrate mass in Greek for the sake of the Rhodian Uniates who could not understand Latin and for the conversion of other Greeks who were technically *infideles* (⁹⁴). The missionary orders were slow to be installed, though an abortive scheme for the transfer of the hospice of Santa Caterina in the *borgo* to the Franciscans was proposed in 1411 (⁹⁵). The Augustinians had a church in the *civitas* by 1388 (⁹⁶), but apparently no other Latin religious order established a house on Rhodes before the arrival of the Franciscans some time before 1457 (⁹⁷). There was probably no Latin parochial system outside the main town, though Latins did occasionally found chapels in some of the larger centres. Thus shortly before 22 January 1412 Fr. Juan de Mur, the Prior of Aragon and *Baiullivus* of Rhodes, founded a *capellania beati Antonij latinorum* outside the cas-

---

dom of Cyprus, in *A History of the Crusades*, ed. K. SETTON, VI, Madison 1989, pp. 168-174.

(⁹¹) Incomplete list in GABRIEL, *Rhodes* cit., II, pp. 167-177, 179-182, 211-212. The Latin parish church of Santa Maria existed in the *borgo* by 1363: text in *Pontificia Commissio* cit., XI, p. 36.

(⁹²) L. SØRENSEN – P. PENTZ, *Excavations and Surveys in Southern Rhodes: the Post-Mycenaean Period until Roman Times and the Medieval Period = Lindos*, IV part 2, Copenhagen 1992 pp. 209-216.

(⁹³) Lists in PAPAVASSILIOU – ARCHONTOPOULOS, *Nouveaux Élements* cit., passim.

(⁹⁴) Text in *Pontificia Commissio* cit., XV, pp. 248-250.

(⁹⁵) LUTTRELL, *Hospitallers of Rhodes* cit., X pp. 199-200.

(⁹⁶) Text in L. BELGRANO, *Seconda Serie di Documenti riguardanti la Colonia di Pera*, in *Atti della Società Ligure di Storia Patria* 13 (1877-1884), pp. 953-965; cf. E. GAMURRINI, *Istoria genealogica delle Famiglie nobili toscane et vmbre*, III, Florence 1673, p. 154.

(⁹⁷) GABRIEL, *Rhodes* cit., II, p. 206; LUTTRELL, *Hospitallers of Rhodes* cit., X p. 200 n. 44.

trum at Kattavia, endowing it with 220 goats or sheep to support a
Hospitaller chaplain (⁹⁸). In 1390 a Latin inhabitant of Rhodes was
permitted to build a church of Saint Honophrius in the *contrata* of
Eleimonitria which was *extra suburbia* (⁹⁹). There may have been outlying parts where isolated Latins worshipped in Greek churches. In a
rather special case at the shrine on Mount Phileremos, a visitor
reported in 1396 that the ikon of the Virgin in a small church there,
which had two Greek hermits or priests, performed miracles and was
revered by "Hospitallers and Greeks and other merchants" (¹⁰⁰). The
Latins intervened there as well; thus in September 1404 the priory or
chaplaincy of Saint Mary of Phileremos was granted to the Hospitaller
Fr. Johannes Tensar (¹⁰¹).

The Rhodian Greeks reacted to the Latins in a variety of ways,
some maintaining an allegiance to the patriarch at Constantinople who
naturally refused to recognize new arrangements and who therefore
continued to nominate titular absentee metropolitans. The Hospitallers evidently banned or discouraged these Greek bishops from the
islands. The Bishopric of Chios, deprived of its pastor, was detached
from Rhodes and confided to Smyrna in 1318/9. Gerasimos, apparently Archbishop of Kos, was in Constantinople in 1330, but following
the Hospitaller occupation of that island in about 1336 its archbishopric was transferred to the metropolis of Corinth in 1343. Joannes
Syropoulos, Metropolitan of Rhodes, was at Constantinople in 1350.
In April 1357 the patriarch wrote to the clergy and faithful of Rhodes
announcing the appointment of a new metropolitan and stating that
Rhodes had been without a bishop since he was prohibited from residence; that someone on Crete or elsewhere had made ordinations and
consecrations for Rhodes without synodal mandate; that the new
bishop would come to Rhodes; that he was empowered to ordain dea-
cons and priests and to consecrate churches; and that any other pre-
tender would be excommunicated. In fact from 1369 onwards the
titular see of Rhodes was regularly given to Orthodox metropolitans

---

(⁹⁸) Malta, Cod. 339, f. 53v-54.

(⁹⁹) Malta, Cod. 324, f. 147; other examples in *Pontificia Commissio* cit.,
XV, pp. 211, 226.

(¹⁰⁰) *Le Saint Voyage de Jherusalem du Seigneur d'Anglure*, ed F. BONNARDOT
– A. LONGNON, Paris 1878, p. 93; cf. G. FERRARIS DI CELLE, *La Madonna di Fileremo*, Verona 1988, pp. 26-27, 97, 148-151 *et passim*.

(¹⁰¹) Malta, Cod. 333, f. 122.

elsewhere; in 1401 this was the Metropolitan of Stauropolis who was in trouble for ordaining as deacon a Rhodian monk named Moisis who lived in Constantinople (¹⁰²). None of these titular metropolitans ever functioned on Rhodes (¹⁰³).

On Rhodes, the metropolitan's cathedral was moved from the *castrum* to the *burgum* (¹⁰⁴), where a number of other churches also served the Greeks (¹⁰⁵). The Rhodians largely accepted the theoretical religious supremacy of the Roman pope, of the Hospitaller Master and of the Latin archbishop. Apparently they did not choose a Uniate metropolitan before 1439 but were ruled by a dean or vicar known as the *dicheus* (¹⁰⁶); in fact, the church in the *borgo* called *metropoli* was

(¹⁰²) *Les Régestes des Actes du Patriarchat de Constantinople*, i: *Les Actes des Patriarches*, ed. J. DARROUZÈS, V-VI, Paris 1977-1979, V, pp. 68, 116-117, 189, 258-260, 271, 277, 282-283, 289-290, 292-293, 316, 329-331, 474-475, 509, 516-517; VI, pp. 76, 110-112, 124-125, 218-219, 417-418; J. GOUILLARD, *Le Synodikon de l'Orthodoxie: Édition et Commentaire*, in *Travaux et Mémoires: Centre de Recherche d'Histoire et Civilisation byzantines*, II, Paris 1967, pp. 26-27, 113, 278-279. This subject remains obscure and controversial.

(¹⁰³) A possible exception was Neilos Diasorenos who may have visited Rhodes; TSIRPANLIS, *Ρόδος* cit., pp. 335-337, proposed that he exercized a cultural influence over the Master Fr. Juan Fernández de Heredia.

(¹⁰⁴) By 1348 there was a *contrata* and a *domus* of the Greek metropolitan church: text in LUTTRELL, *Emphyteutic Grants* cit., pp. 1415-1416. It was probably the fourteenth-century church at the Demirli Djami: GABRIEL, *Rhodes* cit., II, pp. 185-188; KOLLIAS, *City* cit., p. 85; PAPAVASSILIOU – ARCHONTOPOULOS, *Nouveaux Élements* cit., pp. 333-337.

(¹⁰⁵) GABRIEL, *Rhodes* cit., II, pp. 182-211; PAPAVASSILIOU – ARCHONTOPOULOS, *Nouveaux Élements* cit., pp. 325-326, 332-333.

(¹⁰⁶) *Papas* Georgios Kalliandres was *diquio* until his death in about 1380: *infra* Doc. II. On 21 October 1399 the Master confirmed for life the grant of the office of *dicheios* on Kos (Lango) to *Papa cartofilaca Agonelli diquius Langon[ensis]* made *per olim politi de Rodo Langon[ense] et Scarpento*, and this was done by licence of Fr. Roger de Loubaut, Commander of Kos, as shown by letters of that commander and of the *metro politj*: he was to have the powers and incomes enjoyed *per ipsum metro politj insule Langon[ensis]*: Malta, Cod. 330, f. 119v. Note that the Latin Bishop of Kos disappeared after 1349: FEDALTO, *Chiesa Latina* cit., II, p. 137. A Filippo Bishop of Kos, possibly a titular bishop named during the papal schism, was on Andros in 1384/5: R.-J. LOENERTZ, *De quelques Îles grecques et de leurs Seigneurs vénitiens au XIVᵉ et XVᵉ siècles*, in *Studi Veneziani* 14 (1972), pp. 5, 28. On 20 September 1399 *papas* Janni de Sinapigue (?) was *diqueus* of Hospitaller Smyrna: Cod. 330, f. 119v. In 1428 *presbiter Costa diquio* held a house in the *borgo* on Rhodes: Cod. 347, f. 162. On 17 March 1435 the Master appointed *papas Michali sachellari*, the *sakellarios*, to

held until his death in about 1380 by *papas* Georgios Kolliandres, *diquius*, and it was then granted to two of his nephews who were priests ([107]). Many Greeks must have been confused. Some perhaps welcomed the exclusion of patriarchal interference from Constantinople. Others, immigrant exiles perhaps, followed the doctrines of Gregorios Palamas concerning the divine essence. Between 1343 and 1347 Palamas sent his work to the Master of the Hospital in order to explain his allegedly heretical ideas ([108]), but in 1347 the Greeks of Rhodes were among those who wrote to Constantinople anathematizing Palamas and all his followers ([109]). There remained a party of "schismatics", probably Orthodox supporters of the patriarch, and on 16 February 1376 Pope Gregory XI ordained that "Greeks and schismatics" were no longer to exercize the *officium tabellationis*, that is to act as notaries, at Rhodes; that schismatics there claiming to be vicars of the patriarch were to be stopped from granting dispensations for marriages of persons within the prohibited degrees of kinship and from conducting such marriages; and that, except in the case of *servi* and *scismatici* of the Hospital, schismatics of the *ritus grecorum* who were refusing to pay the *decime* or tithes due to the Latin church on Rhodes on the grounds that by custom they never had paid them, were to be compelled to do so ([110]).

The Master and Convent controlled the Greek church on Rhodes

---

be *dichio seu decanus* for the Metropolitanate of Kos in the same way as there was a *dichio* on Rhodes – *cum in insula nostra langonensi sit presentialiter mitropolita constitutus, et iuxta consuetudinem ciuitatis nostre Rhodi apud metropolitanum quemlibet dichio esse debeat, prout est consuetum in omnibus grecorum ecclesijs*, and the *Mitropolite* and all Greek priests and clergy on Kos were to obey this nomination: Cod. 351, f. 156. In 1511 the *dicheus* was the senior Greek cleric on Rhodes after the metropolitan: text in Tsirpanlis, *Ρόδος* cit., pp. 323-326. In 1453 the *dicheus* was named by the Master and took an oath to him in the metropolitan church: text *ibid.*, pp. 285-286. On Chios, the δικαῖος administered the church as the metropolitan's lieutenant: *ibid.*, p. 267 n. 3.

([107]) Malta, Cod. 322, f. 291v; cf. *infra*, p. 222.

([108]) Cited in J. Meyendorff, *A Study of Gregory Palamas*, London 1964, p. 81.

([109]) Nicephorus Gregoras, *Byzantina Historia*, edd. L. Schopen – I. Bekker, 3 vols., Bonn 1829-1855, II, p. 787.

([110]) Texts in *Pontificia Commissio* cit., XII, pp. 381-383.

somewhat as if they had taken the place of the Greek emperor ([111]). A statute of 1428 decreed that any secular Rhodian *civis* or *subditus* should on his marriage take an oath of homage and fidelity to the Master and recognize the superiority of the Master and Convent ([112]). The latter could appoint abbots and priests within the Greek church in the islands and grant out its properties. They could license a man to become a deacon or priest ([113]) and permit a monk to bequeath goods by will, as in the case of Athanasios de Saloniqui in 1347 ([114]). The Master could suspend a priest from celebrating mass and grant his church to another *papas* ([115]). The Master and Convent could grant a monastic house together with its appurtenances, for example a flock of goats, to a *papas* and his heirs to be held in perpetual emphyteusis in return for an annual payment or tithe, the *decatia* ([116]), or they could provide a *monasterium*, usually a minor institution often without monks, to the Greek layman who had founded it and to his heirs in perpetuity ([117]). One magistral bull of 1389 granted two churches to a *papas* with the succession to one of his sons. Greek laymen, or even laywomen, might enjoy offices and benefices or the incomes of churches they had founded or repaired, but they had obligations to maintain their churches, to ensure divine service, and so on ([118]). In 1358 the Master confirmed the donation by one Greek priest to another of the *ecclesia patrimonali* of Ayia Maria *Calisteni* ([119]).

Hospitaller interference must often have irritated the Greeks of Rhodes but their position was probably rather favourable compared with that of Greeks in many other parts of the Latin East. The Rhodians were at least able to maintain their liturgical life and to manage

---

([111]) The best published documentation, in TSIRPANLIS, *Ρόδος* cit., pp. 269-286 *et passim*, largely concerns the changed situation after 1439.

([112]) Text in *Prohemium in Volumen Stabilimentorum* cit., De magistro, viiij.

([113]) Eg. Malta, Cod. 321, f. 216v (1382); Cod. 322, f. 330 (1383).

([114]) Malta, Cod. 317, f. 234 (1348).

([115]) Malta, Cod. 319, f. 306v (1366). Ayios Ipatios was twice mentioned on the late fourteenth-century account sheet in SCHREINER, *Finanz- und Wirtschaftsgeschichte* cit., pp. 68-69.

([116]) Malta, Cod. 317, f. 235 (1347).

([117]) *Infra*, Doc. 1.

([118]) Malta, Cod. 324, f. 140v (1389), later texts of 1452 in TSIRPANLIS, *Ρόδος* cit., pp. 269-278.

([119]) Malta, Cod. 316, f. 301-301v.

their own church, and their enthusiasm for doing so was demonstrated in a continual succession of numerous if minor foundations and endowments in town, village and country which were granted, confirmed or revoked, often according to documents copied into the Hospital's registers. The Rhodian beneficiaries were acquiring confirmation of what was virtually perpetual tenure, while the Hospital was assuring for itself an element of security and a source of income. Families were enabled to establish a secure title to a property with an income which was often hereditable by their children or heirs, who might be priests. The Hospital was in effect amalgamating the Latin form of endowment which a family could hold in *jus patronatus* with the old Byzantine practice of *charistike* which had possibly survived on Rhodes during the period of isolation between 1204 and 1306 ([120]).

There was a series of ecclesiastical posts attached to the metropolitan church ([121]). One family in particular stood out. In 1292 the priest Symeon Kalliandrès was both *nomikos* and *prodekdikos* or judge of the Rhodian church and was copying monkish writings, and in 1336 *papas* Johannes Kalliandres was *nomikos*, priest and *chartophylax* or archivist in the metropolitan church ([122]). *Papas* Georgios Kalliandres, who was *dicheios* and who held the church called *metropoli* in Rhodes town died in about 1380, and on his death the Master granted this church to Georgios' nephews, *papas* Agaconicho Paula and *papas* Johannes Kalliandres, inhabitants of Rhodes ([123]). *Papas* Georgios had also held a notarial office ([124]). In 1381 the Master granted for his lifetime to *Papas* Johannes Kalliandres the church of Ayios *Pati* or Hypatios in the *borgo* which an earlier Master had granted to a woman ([125]).

Many Greek clerics were prepared to accept a Uniate position as long as their own liturgy and language were not threatened. The Rhodians' religion, probably sustained by a lower clergy to which

---

([120]) Cf. J. THOMAS, *Private Religious Foundations in the Byzantine Empire*, Washington 1987, pp. 246-249 *et passim*.

([121]) Listed in a text of 1511 in TSIRPANLIS, *Ρόδος* cit., pp. 323-326.

([122]) *Supra*, p. 206; P. GÉHIN, *Un Copiste de Rhodes de la fin du XIII siècle: le Prêtre Syméon Kalliandrès*, in *Scriptorium* 40 (1986), pp. 172, 175, 177-178, 183.

([123]) Malta, Cod. 322, f. 291v; cf. *infra* Doc. II.

([124]) *Infra* Doc. III.

([125]) Malta, Cod. 321, f. 213v.

political leadership passed by default, evidently reinforced their awareness of their Greek identity. In the town, co-existence and a community of interests naturally led to a degree of collaboration on the part of Greeks in Latin service [126]. Merchants, notaries and priests displayed their relative wealth in the foundation and patronage of churches and monasteries. The connection between business and culture was exemplified in the manuscript of the Aristotelian treatise in Greek which contained both a late fourteenth-century merchant's accounts in Greek and, in the same hand and language, a list of classical Greek books presumably in a Rhodian library [127]. A prosperous urban group sought social prestige from churches, chapels and tombs in town and country which they decorated with ikons and frescoes containing their patron's portraits and personal inscriptions [128]; some even aspired to forms of nobility by adopting a Latin-style system of heraldic family arms [129]. A Hospitaller document referred to certain Greeks of the city as *greci nobiles* as early as 1347 [130]. When the ground outside the town walls was cleared before the 1480 siege some twenty churches, mostly Greek, had to be destroyed [131]. In addition to the Latin architecture and sculpture, Western paintings decorated buildings, most notably the early fourteenth-century Tuscan-style frescoes in the Latin cathedral [132] and the frescoes in a vaulted room above the sea wall of the *collachium* not far from the Sea Gate which were probably painted at the end of the fourteenth century [133]. The Greeks continued to build churches in the Byzantine style [134] and to decorate them in the older Palaeologan manner. The frescoes of

---

[126] KOLLIAS, *City* cit., p. 49, speaks of such a movement in the 1430's; to what extent it may earlier have had an ideological base is uncertain.

[127] SCHREINER, *Finanz- und Wirtschaftsgeschichte* cit., p. 66.

[128] KOLLIAS, *City* cit., and IDEM, *Knights* cit.; PAPAVASSILIOU – ARCHONTOPOU-LOS, *Nouveaux Éléments* cit., pp. 324-328, 332-336, 342; part of this work is datable pre-1421.

[129] KOLLIAS, *Knights* cit., Figs. 31-32, 37; A.-M. KASDAGLI, Εἰσαγωγὴ στὴν Ἐραλδικὴ τῆς Ρόδου, in Δελτίον Ἐραλδικῆς καὶ Γενεαλογικῆς Ἑταιρίας Ἑλλάδος 7 (1988), pp. 44-45; fig. 22.

[130] LUTTRELL, *Hospitallers in Cyprus* cit., IV p. 60.

[131] They are named in Malta, Cod. 76, f. 47-48v.

[132] KOLLIAS, *City* cit., p. 92 (Fig. 30); IDEM, *Knights* cit., p. 37 (Fig. 35).

[133] B. DE BELARBE, *Rhodes of the Knights*, Oxford 1908, pp. 89-93, figs. 74-76; GABRIEL, *Rhodes* cit., I, p. 67.

[134] KOLLIAS, *City* cit., pp. 78-85.

1335/6 in Ayios Phanourios in the *borgo* included portraits of the founders, and there was other fourteenth-century painting in Ayia Ekater-
ini, in the frescoes of 1407/8 in the Holy Trinity church at Psinthos,
and elsewhere (¹³⁵). More original, perhaps the fruit of evolving attitudes among elements of the bourgeoisie, were those eclectic paintings
in a mixed Latin-Byzantine style which appeared mainly in the town
late in the fourteenth century (¹³⁶).

There were educated Rhodian Greeks, some of them found in exile
or residence at Constantinople (¹³⁷). Other cultured Greeks visited or
settled on Rhodes. A certain Georgios Kydones Gabrielopoulos known
as "the philospher", a correspondent and doctor of the distinguished
Dimitrios Kydones, visited Rhodes in about 1362 (¹³⁸). At some point
between 1382 and 1402 Niketas Myrsiniotes, a priest at Rhodes, wrote
an anti-Latin treatise on the procession of the holy spirit and consulted
the theologian Josephos Bryennios on fourteen theological questions (¹³⁹). Early in the fifteenth century Johannes Marmoras was
active on Rhodes as a scribe and book collector (¹⁴⁰). Other writers
may have been involved in the development on Rhodes of a secular
poetic literature in Greek (¹⁴¹). From 1405 at the latest, some Rhodians
were studying civil law in the university at Padua but none of them
was clearly Greek (¹⁴²). Latins with Greek wives and Rhodians of

---

(¹³⁵) *Ibid.*, pp. 94-97 (Figs. 45, 46, 49); IDEM, *Knights* cit., p. 38; PAPAVASSI-
LIOU – ARCHONTOPOULOS, *Nouveaux Élements* cit., pp. 324-328. There is no datable pre-1421 Byzantine sculpture, while the provenance of pre-1421 ikons cannot be established.

(¹³⁶) KOLLIAS, *City* cit., pp. 97-101; IDEM, *Knights* cit., pp. 38-39; PAPAVASSIL-
IOU – ARCHONTOPOULOS, *Nouveaux Élements* cit., p. 326. For "eclectic" sculptures, all post-1421, GABRIEL, *Rhodes* cit., I, pp. 97-98 (Plates XXVIII 1, 4; XXIX
1-3): G. JACOPI, *Monumenti di Scultura del Museo Archeologico di Rodi: II*, in *Clara Rhodos* 5 part 2 (1932), pp. 48-58 (Figs. 31-35).

(¹³⁷) Eg. *supra*, p. 212.

(¹³⁸) *Prosopographisches Lexikon der Palaiologenzeit*, II, Vienna 1977,
p. 137.

(¹³⁹) R.-J. LOENERTZ, *Pour la Chronologie des Oeuvres de Joseph Bryennios*,
in *Revue des Études Byzantines* 7 (1949), pp. 14-15.

(¹⁴⁰) TSIRPANLIS, *Ρόδος* cit., p. 365.

(¹⁴¹) However, no Rhodian poetry is datable pre-1421: G. SPADARO, *Problemi
di Poesia greca medievale rodia*, in *Studi di Filologia Bizantina*, III = *Quaderni
del Siculorum Gymnasium*, XV, Catania 1985.

(¹⁴²) TSIRPANLIS, *Ρόδος* cit., pp. 91, 344-347.

mixed descent may also have been culturally and politically active [143].

The church provided leaders for the Greek community, and it was sometimes their cultural qualities which raised Greek churchmen to relatively influential positions, especially through the attainment of notarial and secretarial offices. Some such Greeks played a part in translations and cultural transmissions from the Greek. An early example was the first Plutarch to be translated into a Romance language. The Greek manuscript was apparently discovered on Rhodes where, at the command of the Master Fr. Juan Fernández de Heredia, it was turned from classical into demotic Greek by a *philosopho greco* named Dimitri Calodiqui de Saloniqui, possibly an immigrant from Thessalonika, who was a scribe but not a priest and who in 1381 was granted a *scrivania* or notarial office; his wife was a Rhodian *serva marina*, that is to say her male children would owe galley-service. The Plutarch in demotic Greek was then translated into some Western language by a Dominican named Nicholas who was titular Bishop of Adrianopolis and, in 1384, vicar of the Latin Archbishop of Rhodes; in 1369 this Nicholas had acted in Rome as interpreter to the Emperor John V Palaeologus, but evidently he could not read classical Greek. Dimitri Calodiqui was dead by 1 October 1389, having previously acquired a *scribania* or notarial office known as the *condillus grecorum* [144]. Greek texts do not seem to have been copied into the chan-

---

(143) It is not possible to document such developments at an early date. TSIRPANLIS, *Ρόδος* cit., pp. 331-335, claims Dragonetto Clavelli as a Rhodian Greek, though no document indicates his origins. For some thirty years until his death in January 1415 *circa* he grew wealthy as the Master's proctor on Rhodes and in 1413 was described as "almost lord" of the island; he married Agnese Crispo, possibly a daughter of Francesco I Duke of the Archipelago: LUTTRELL, *Hospitallers in Cyprus* cit., III pp. 764-765. By 1412 he was Lord of Nisyros and of Lardos on Rhodes, and titular Marshal of the Roman Curia: Cod. 339, f. 350. His arms of three nails (*clavelli*) appear with those of the Master, Fr. Philibert de Naillac, on a silver processional cross, on other such crosses, and on towers at Rhodes and Bodrum: IDEM, *Hospitallers of Rhodes* cit., XVIII pp. 11-12. He built and was buried in a chapel in the Augustinian church in Rhodes: texts in Malta, Cod. 347, f. 163, and *Pontificia Commissio* cit., XIV part 2, pp. 1139-1140. Clavelli's does not sound like a Greek career, though he could have had a Greek mother.

(144) LUTTRELL, *Hospitallers in Cyprus* cit., XX-XXI *passim; infra*, Docs. II-VII; on the *condillus grecorum*, TSIRPANLIS, *Ρόδος* cit., pp. 267 n. 1, 284, 390.

cery registers at Rhodes before 1440 ([145]). As the Byzantine world of *Romania* contracted during the fifteenth century, Rhodes became more important as a minor centre of Greek studies ([146]). The humanist Guarino Guarini of Verona found an almost illegible copy of the *Lexicon* of Suidas there in about 1408 ([147]), and Rhodes was the chief residence of the Florentine Cristoforo Buondelmonti who, apparently just before 1420, wrote there his *Liber Insularum Archipelagi* which recorded classical remains on Rhodes, Kos and many other islands ([148]). Some of the ancient sites on Rhodes were visited in about 1351 by the historian Nikephoros Gregoras, whose description made reference to Homer and who noticed that there was no surviving vestige of the Colossus of Rhodes ([149]). In about 1427 the antiquarian Ciriaco d'Ancona was inspecting classical remains there, and he had Buondelmonti's book with him; later he corresponded with the learned Vice-Chancellor of the Hospital, Fr. Melchiore Bandini, about ancient coins ([150]). None of these scholars realized that the site opposite Kos on the mainland at Bodrum where the Hospitallers constructed a castle in about 1407 was actually the classical Halikarnassos ([151]).

Cultural contacts inevitably depended on men understanding each other's languages. There were problems among the Latins themselves, with the English and German brethren in particular having to

---

([145]) Written in a crude demotic Greek to summon the Greeks of Lindos to resist a Mamluk attack: text in LUTTRELL, *Hospitallers of Rhodes* cit., VII pp. 325-326. A Greek text of 1453 concerning Nisyros is in TSIRPANLIS, *Ρόδος* cit., pp. 195-200.

([146]) V. FLYNN, *The Intellectual Life of Fifteenth-Century Rhodes*, in *Traditio* 2 (1944); see also G. SOMMI-PICENARDI, *Itinéraire d'un Chevalier de Saint-Jean de Jérusalem dans l'Île de Rhodes*, Lille 1900, pp. 127-128.

([147]) R. SABBADINI, *Le scoperte dei codici latini e greci ne' secoli XIV e XV*, Florence 1905, p. 45 n. 14.

([148]) BUONDELMONTI, *Librum Insularum* cit., pp. 71-74, 104-105 *et passim*, dated in H. TURNER, *Cristoforo Buondelmonti and the "Isolario"*, in *Terrae Incognitae* 19 (1987). At least 59 Mss. survive to indicate its popularity: A. LUTTRELL, *The Later History of the Maussolleion and its Utilization in the Hospitaller Castle at Bodrum* = *The Maussolleion at Halikarnassos*, II, Aarhus 1986, pp. 189-194.

([149]) Nicephorus Gregoras, *Historia* cit., III, pp. 11-12.

([150]) Texts in C. COLUCCI, *Delle Antichità Picene*, XV, Fermo 1792, pp. lxxx-lxxxi, and C. MITCHELL, *Ex Libris Kiriaci Anconitani*, in *Italia Medioevale e Umanistica* 5 (1962), pp. 288-289; on Bandini, LUTTRELL, *Hospitallers in Cyprus* cit., II pp. 146, 150; III pp. 67-68.

([151]) LUTTRELL, *Maussolleion* cit., pp. 163-166.

rely on French or even Latin. A few Westerners would have spoken some demotic Greek but their ability to write it must have been rare, at least in the fourteenth century. Greeks or half-Greeks probably knew some French, Italian or Catalan, or spoke a Levantine lingua franca. Much later, in 1521, a visitor observed that on Rhodes there were people from so many lands that each corrupted the other with the result that no language was spoken properly[152]. Contacts with Turks were limited by the recurrent hostilities with the infidel. The Turkish coast is only a short distance from Rhodes town, and commercial contacts with the mainland were often close; horses, grain and other supplies were imported from Ephesus, Miletus and elsewhere. Some trade was possible, though in 1393 the Hospitallers rejected proposals from the Ottoman sultan Bayezid, who had recently annexed Aidin and Menteshe, for a treaty permitting Turkish merchants to bring Christian and other slaves to sell in Rhodes[153]. Despite the Hospitallers' tendency to slaughter Turks taken in battle, there were some Turkish slaves on Rhodes[154]. There were occasional Latins who spoke Turkish[155], but there is no evidence for Turkish-speaking Hospitallers in the period before 1421[156]. For dealings with the Turks the Hospital apparently relied on Greeks such as the Georgios Calokyres who in 1348 was acting as notary for the Hospital and who knew some Latin since he then composed the Latin text, presumably a translation from the Greek, of a treaty between the pope and the Emir of Ephesus[157], and in 1358 he drew up a public instrument in Greek for two Greek *pappates* at Rhodes[158].

The Latins introduced to Rhodes various more material forms of

---

(152) Text in R. RÖHRICHT - H. MEISNER, *Deutsche Pilgerreisen nach dem Heilige Lande*, Berlin 1880, p. 370.

(153) LUTTRELL, *Hospitallers of Rhodes* cit., II pp. 96-97.

(154) IDEM, *Latin Greece* cit., VI pp. 86-87.

(155) An early example was Ancelin de Toucy who was born at Constantinople in the first half of the thirteenth century: *Libro de los Fechos et Conquistas del Principado de la Morea*, ed. A. MOREL-FATIO, Geneva 1885, p. 81.

(156) After 1471 the Hospitaller Fr. Laudivio Zacchia knew Turkish and also owned Greek books, including a Lexicon written in 1310 which he purchased on Rhodes: *Memorie Melitensi nelle Collezioni della Biblioteca Apostolica Vaticana*, ed. G. MORELLO, Rome 1987, pp. 32-33.

(157) E. ZACHARIADOU, *Trade and Crusade: Venetian Crete and the Emirates of Menteshe and Aydin (1300-1415)*, Venice 1983, pp. 184, 210.

(158) Malta, Cod. 316, f. 301-301v.

culture; modern fortifications and building techniques, Gothic palaces, tapestries, illuminated missals, liturgical articles and numerous domestic items ([159]). The Hospitallers were not for the most part intellectual men but they did make Rhodes a place where Latins and Greeks could mix in reasonable freedom and friendship. Rhodes was not a colony in the true sense; Hospitaller rule provoked no major revolts such as those the Venetians occasionally faced on Crete, and race relations on Rhodes seem to have been comparatively good. The Greek historian Nikephoros Gregoras noted in about 1351 that old men bewailed the loss of their independence, but the Rhodians also told him that they were effectively defended and well governed under good laws and judges, while they benefited from the fine harbour and from the imports and plentiful food supplies which freed them from material hardship. Gregoras remarked that the people were not greedy and that both rich and poor had an easy life ([160]).

APPENDIX

I Rhodes, 1 April 1366. Fr. Raymond Bérenguer, Master of the Hospital, and the Convent of Rhodes, confirm in perpetuity to Vestiariti Mirodi, *burgensis* of Rhodes, and to his heirs and successors the *monasterium* of Santa Maura in the Castellany of Rhodes and the *contrata* of *Kyparrisi*, with the church of Ayios Soulas, with two *curtes* situated between the monastery and the church, *ac cum hospicijs altis et bassis domuncullis siue cellis* (with details of contiguous *hospicia, jardina* and public roads); Mirodi has founded and built the monastery; also confirmed are the *jardinum*, vineyards and *hospicium altum et bassum* in the *platea* of Santa Maria in the *burgum* of Rhodes (all with much detail of contiguous properties) with which Mirodi has endowed them; the above are to pay the Hospital ten *asperi* of Rhodes every year from these endowments, and to maintain and repair the monastery and

---

([159]) Examples in *The Order's Early Legacy in Malta*, ed. J. AZZOPARDI, Malta 1989.
([160]) Nicephorus Gregoras, *Historia* cit., III, pp. 12-13; cf. A. LUTTRELL, *Malta and Rhodes: Hospitallers and Islanders*, in *Hospitaller Malta 1530-1798: Studies on Early Modern Malta and the Order of St John of Jerusalem*, ed. V. MALLIA-MILANES, Malta 1993.

church, and to provide a chaplain *et alium ministrum* for them; the Hospital is not to take away any or all of the above *Non obstante eo quod canetur in sacramentalj facto in captione Insule nostre Rodj, quod donaciones Monasteriorium et ecclesiarum uacancium in Ciuitate et Insula nostra Rodj ad Magistrum nostre dicte domus debeant pertinere.*

Malta, Cod. 319, f. 296v-297 = LUTTRELL, *Greeks, Latins and Turks* cit., pp. 370-372, where read *Rodj; Michaelis; Burgarj; successores; reperare; necessarijs; succesorum.* Xeno *Uistiarity Mirodi* was freed *ab omni nexu seruilj marino et terestry* on 10 July 1347: Malta, Cod. 317, f. 222v.

II Rhodes, 17 April 1381. Fr. Juan Fernández de Heredia, Master of the Hospital, and the Convent of Rhodes, grant Dimitri Calodiqui *phylosopha*, in recognition of his literary virtues and of his services, the *scribania* or notarial office held by the late *papas* Georgios, *diquio*, to be held for life *iuxta statutum municipale terre nostre Rodi*; acts issued by Calodiqui or in his name were to be regarded as fully valid.

Malta, Cod. 321, f. 210v = LUTTRELL, *Greeks, Latins and Turks* cit., p. 372, where read *vigentia* (Ms. *vigentiam*); *peribetur* (Ms. *sic*); *premissis* (Ms. *permissis*). In about 1380 the *dicheios* was Giorgios Kalliandres: *supra*, p. 212-213.

III Rhodes, 6 March 1382. Fr. Juan Fernández de Heredia, Master of the Hospital, licences Dimitri Calodiqui *phylosophus scriba seu notarius* to name *papas* Janni and *papa* Nichita Muntanioti his lieutenants in the *scribania* or notarial office *in ciuitate et insula* on Rhodes which had formerly been held by *papas* Georgios *Coliandri* and to which Calodiqui had recently been appointed by the Master and Convent.

Malta, Cod. 321, f. 217 = LUTTRELL, *Greeks, Latins and Turks* cit., p. 373, where read *vniuersis; dimicti; poss[e]*. On earlier members of the Kalliandres family on Rhodes, *supra*, p. 215. Note that in this and the following documents the form *etc* in the registered copy leaves it unclear whether the Master was acting alone or, as in Docs. II and III, was acting with the Convent and using the Conventual seal.

IV Rhodes, 12 March 1382. Fr. Juan Fernández de Heredia, Master of the Hospital, authorizes Dimitri Calodiqui, *phylosophus ac scribus grecus scribanie ciuitatis et Insule nostrarum Rodi*, to acquire, retain, copy and have himself or others publish *in publicam formam*, the *cartularia* which had belonged to the late *papa* Cacilli, a former *nomikos* or lawyer, and which are held by Cacilli's brother Gavidotti; the latter or anyone else holding the *cartularia* was to hand them over to Dimitri without imposing any condition.

Malta, Cod. 321, f. 217v = LUTTRELL, *Greeks, Latins and Turks* cit., p. 373, where read *nomici* and *jre* (Ms. *gre*). The *cartularia* were evidently notarial registers; there is no proof that the text involved was the Plutarch translated by Calodiqui.

V Avignon, 26 May 1383.   Fr. Juan Fernández de Heredia, Master of the Hospital, at the request of Dimitri Calodiqui de Saloniqui and in recognition of his services, frees in perpetuity his children, male and female, by his wife Maria Auemina, who is bound to marine service, from that service; they are to be obliged to serve with their arms by land and sea in defence of the island of Rhodes whenever necessary.

Malta, Cod. 322, f. 330 = LUTTRELL, *Greeks, Latins and Turks* cit., p. 374, where read *gratuita seruitia per te; astricte; obedientie*.   On the *servitudo marina*, IDEM, *Hospitallers in Cyprus* cit., IV *passim*.

VI Avignon, 1 October 1389.   Fr. Juan Fernández de Heredia, Master of the Hospital, grants to his *familiaris*, Nicholaus Trasmontanie, the *scribania seu officium notarie quam et quod quondam Dimitrius Calodichi philosofus tenebat et exercebat per eius obitum vacans* to be exercized by him, or by some competent lieutenant, for his lifetime.

Malta, Cod. 324, f. 140.

VII Rhodes, 16 February 1403.   Fr. Philibert de Naillac, Master of the Hospital, grants to his *familiaris*, Franciscus Monerij, the *Scribania seu officium nottar[iatus] vocatum be* [sic] *condillj grecorum in ciuitate et Insula Rodj, quam et quod quondam Dimitrius Calodichi philosophus grecus tenuit et exercuit*; he is empowered to have someone else exercize the office *iuxta statutum municipale terre nostre Rodj*.

Malta, Cod. 332, f. 146v; Monerij was evidently a Latin.

IV

SUGAR AND SCHISM:
THE HOSPITALLERS IN CYPRUS FROM 1378 TO 1386

The military order of the Hospital of Saint John of Jerusalem held estates on Cyprus before its surviving brethren retreated to Limassol following the fall of Acre in 1291. The Convent or headquarters moved from Cyprus to Rhodes in about 1310 but the Hospitallers retained their extensive Cypriot holdings, which were augmented in 1313 by the transfer of the possessions of the recently suppressed Order of the Temple. After 1310 the number of Hospitallers resident on Cyprus was very small, but the Order's agrarian incomes, especially those from its sugar plantations, were considerable.[1] Rhodes and Cyprus maintained a special relationship. On both islands a Greek population had come under Western rule in consequence of Latin expansion in Syria. Hospitallers participated in Cypriot crusading expeditions, such as that against Alexandria which sailed from Rhodes in 1365, and they intervened in Cypriot affairs at moments of crisis, as in 1374 when the Master of the Hospital went to Nicosia and died there. The Hospitallers of Rhodes and the Lusignan rulers of Cyprus shared their French speech, and they both governed their islands as a metropolis rather than as the colonial possession of a Western power; it was only after 1373 that the Genoese began the process of converting Famagusta into an Aegean-style commercial outpost.

Together with the secular clergy and the other religious orders, both monastic and mendicant, the Hospital formed part of the Latin establishment on Cyprus. Down to 1378 a strong French element was predominant among the island's higher Latin clergy.[2] Few, if any, Hospitaller brethren were indigenous Cypriots, since the Hospital's statutes prevented local families from securing any interest or control within the Order by prohibiting the reception as a knight or *miles* of any noble born in the East.[3] There were Hospitaller houses at Limassol, Nicosia and Famagusta, while the Order's great estates were con-

1. A. Luttrell, *The Hospitallers in Cyprus after 1291*, in *Acts of the First International Congress of Cypriot Studies*, II, Nicosia, 1972; idem, *The Hospitallers in Cyprus: 1310-1378*, in Κυπριακαί Σπουδαί, 50, 1986. A number of errors in the 1986 article will be corrected in a forthcoming publication. These works indicate the essential bibliography. P. Edbury, *The Kingdom of Cyprus and the Crusades: 1191-1374*, Cambridge, 1991, contains further information and bibliography.

2. W. Rudt de Collenberg, *État et origine du haut Clergé de Chypre avant le Grand Schisme d'après les Registres des Papes du XIIIe et XIVe siècle*, in *Mélanges de l'École française de Rome: Moyen Âge - Temps Modernes*, XC, 1979.

3. Luttrell, *Cyprus*, 1986, *op. cit.*, p. 155 and n. 4.

centrated in the south of the island. There was a small tower at Kolossi near Limassol,[4] and there the Hospital's lucrative sugar production and refinery were centred.[5] The knowledgeable Venetian Marino Sanudo claimed in 1329 that the Hospital's Cypriot incomes were 20,000 florins a year, one ninth of his estimate of the Order's total incomes in West and East which included those from Rhodes and Cyprus. Part of this Cypriot wealth, due from the commander as *responsiones* payable to the Treasury at Rhodes, was fixed in 1365 at 12,000 florins a year; that sum was greater than the *responsiones* of any single Western priory and it would, if paid, have exceeded a quarter of the total Western *responsiones* received at Avignon in 1373/4 and 1374/5.[6] The rest of the Hospital's Cypriot incomes went to support the commandery and its brethren, with the balance being retained by the commander. The sugar and other crops represented a useful security, since the Hospital could borrow from Western merchants in Rhodes and promise repayment in Famagusta out of the commandery's future income.[7]

Such wealth provided a benefice for a senior Hospitaller at Rhodes who did not normally reside on Cyprus in person. Between 1319 and 1365 the commandery was, with the possible brief exception of the unidentified Fr. Bernardus Malavicina, granted only to Southern French brethren. Alternatively, the Master might make no appointment, naming a lieutenant to govern the commandery and keeping the profits for himself. In 1357 a Hospitaller statute declared that the Master was not to appropriate the commandery to the brethren of the *langue* of Provence but that it should be common to all *langues*. A later statute of 1379 decreed that the commandery be divided into seven parts to be shared, in a complicated way, among the seven *langues*. Such reforms could,

---

4. The Kolossi tower requires further investigation: Luttrell, 1972, pp. 170-171, and E. Aristidou, *Kolossi Castle through the Centuries*, Nicosia, 1983. The house at Kolossi was in a poor state in 1450 since the King had refused to allow the commander to restore it: G. Grivaud, *Excerpta Cypria Nova*, I, Nicosia, 1990, p. 67. It appears highly likely that the existing structure was built in the time of Fr. Louis de Magnac, circa 1454/6: cf. G. Hill, *A History of Cyprus*, II-III, Cambridge, 1948, II, p.22 n. 3; III, pp. 1132-1133, and C. Enlart, *Gothic Art and the Renaissance in Cyprus*, trans. London, 1987, pp. 69, 376, 383-384, 494-502.

5. On sugar at Kolossi, possibly first documented in 1343, Luttrell, *Cyprus*, 1986, pp. 165-166, 184 *et passim*. Sugar manufacturing there was described in 1450: Grivaud, *op. cit.*, p. 67. Any eventual excavations at Kolossi should be preceded by a study of the materials in Valletta, National Library of Malta, Archives of the Order of Saint John. On 1 May 1379 184 cases of sugar powder weighing 100 quintals of Rhodes and worth 6,457 florins were loaded at Rhodes for Clarenza, Avignon and Bruges (Malta, Cod. 48, f. 11) and in 1382 *circa* sugar shipped from Rhodes was sold in Provence for 8,803 florins (Cod. 322, f. 52v); it is not, however, certain that this sugar came from Cyprus.

6. Luttrell, *Cyprus*, 1986, *op. cit.*, pp. 164, 173; cf. *idem, The Hospitallers' Western Accounts: 1373/4 and 1374/5*, in *Camden Miscellany*, XXX, London, 1990, pp. 8-9.

7. Eg. text of 1351 in Luttrell, *Cyprus*, 1986, *op. cit.*, pp. 178-179.

however, be frustrated by the papacy. Between 1366 circa and 1374 first Urban V and then Gregory XI persistently demanded that Cyprus be given to Fr. Daniele del Carretto who was serving the pope in Italy as rector of various papal provinces. For years the Hospitallers at Rhodes refused this papal demand, but they had to give way in 1374 when Gregory XI invoked his apostolic powers to provide Carretto to the commandery; Gregory had already in 1373 instructed Fr. Giorgio de Ceva, Prior of Messina, to go to Cyprus to govern the commandery on Carretto's behalf and to pay the *responsiones* of 12,000 florins to Rhodes; in March 1378 Ceva was in Nicosia with the king. The brethren on Rhodes had lost control of the patronage of an appointment which had previously provided one of their own number with a useful income.[8]

Gregory XI left Avignon for Rome and he died there in 1378; the cardinals elected first an Italian as Urban VI, and then, amid much controversy, a Frenchman who became Clement VII and soon returned to Avignon. The results were most confusing for it was not at first recognized how definite the split was to become. Not all governments took sides along evident diplomatic lines. For example, the Aragonese king adopted a policy of *indiferència*, declaring that he could not determine which was the true pope and that in the meanwhile the crown would take all monies normally due to the papacy; the King of England supported the Roman obedience but allowed the English Hospitallers and their monies to go to Avignonist Rhodes.[9] Initial reactions in Cyprus were ambiguous and fluctuating; some contemporaries stated that King Pierre II declared for Avignon or that he remained neutral, while the Genoese controlled Famagusta and seem to have insisted on neutrality there. Clement VII continued to nominate bishops and to issue bulls for Cyprus for many years; in June 1382 he approved supplications submitted by Pierre II,[10]

8. Details *ibid.*, pp. 162-163, 172-174, 177 *et passim;* cf. *idem, Carretto, Daniele del,* in *Dizionario Biografico degli Italiani,* XXXVI, Rome, 1983, pp. 394-397.

9. A. Luttrell, 'Intrigue, Schism and Violence among the Hospitallers of Rhodes: 1377-1384', in *Speculum,* XLI, 1966; *idem, Le Schisme dans les Prieurés de l'Hôpital en Catalunya et Aragón,* in *Jornades sobre el Cisma d'Occident a Catalunya, les Illes i el País valencià,* I, Barcelona, 1986, pp. 107-110.

10. N. Valois, *La France et le Grand Schisme d'Occident,* I-11, Paris, 1896, I, p. 197 n, 1; II, p. 219-221. The only extended treatment of the earlier period of the schism in Cyprus is W. Rudt de Collenberg, *Le Royaume et l'Église de Chypre face au Grand Schisme: 1378-1417,* in *Mélanges de L'École française de Rome: Moyen Âge - Temps Modernes,* XCIV, 1982 (the secondary remarks concerning the Hospital at p. 662, require amendment); see also J. Richard, *Le Royaume de Chypre et le Grand Schism: à propos d'un Document récemment découvert,* in *Academie des Inscriptions: Comptes Rendus,* 1965. An apparently unlocated *capella* of Saint Catherine *in suburbis* at Famagusta in 1390 had been founded by an unidentified Johannes de Ripparia: Rudt, 1982, *op.cit.,* pp. 680, 685. Catherine was the patron saint of the Italian Hospital. This hospital was conceivably connected with the unidentified Hospitaller church at Famagusta described in Enlart, pp. 290-293. Fr. Giovanni de Rivara, Commander of Casal Monferrato, was made a proctor to rule the Cypriot commandery in 1358: Luttrell, 1987, *op.cit.,* p. 163.

and by July 1382 the papal collector in Cyprus had paid 3,100 florins to Clement VII.[11] Meanwhile on 10 March 1382 Clement instructed that 2,000 florins which were owed to the papacy in Cyprus should be transferred to the Hospital for the defence of Smyrna against the Turks;[12] in the same month the Hospitallers at Avignon paid for papal bulls declaring that, notwithstanding appeals made from Cyprus by the Archbishop of Nicosia and the Cypriot clergy, these should pay the Hospital the 'two parts of the tenth' for Smyrna along with 2,000 ducats to be taken from the Cypriot goods of the late Patriarch of Jerusalem.[13] In such ways Cyprus remained within the Avignonese orbit.

By 1381, however, the Urbanists were gaining some ground in Cyprus. From 1382 onwards the incomes of the Cypriot clergy assigned to the Hospital for the defence of Smyrna were no longer paid.[14] On 8 May 1382 Clement VII instructed the Archbishop of Nicosia to act against Urbanists, secular and religious, on Cyprus; he was to imprison the Urbanist Bishop of Cerenza, a Cypriot Dominican named Jean Fardin.[15] Confusion increased when King Pierre II died on 3 October 1382 leaving his successor Jacques a prisoner in Genoa who was unable finally to return to Cyprus until April 1385. In Cyprus a council of regency and the bulk of the Cypriot church avoided recognition of either papal obedience.[16] In 1385 King Jacques also evaded the question by having himself crowned at Nicosia by an unscrupulous Greek impostor, Paulus Palaeologus Tagaris the Latin Patriarch of Constantinople, who received 30,000 gold pieces and even dared to create new bishoprics on Cyprus.[17] Meanwhile the Clementist Archbishop of Nicosia, the Venetian Andrea Michiel who had been appointed in 1383, was never able to take possession of his see.[18] The Bishop of Limassol was resident in France from December 1384 onwards, while on 20 May 1385 Clement VII instructed Michiel, who was then being sent to Cyprus, to act against Urbanists there and to recover lands and monies held by others who may also have been supporting Urban.[19] Neither obedience secured much support or money in Cyprus. Jacques declared for neither side, appropriating the revenues of the Latin church and continuing to exclude bishops and legates until 1395/6 when he recognized Clement VII's successor, Benedict XIII. After 1378 ecclesiastical links with the West, and especially with France,

11. Rudt, 1982, op.cit., p. 681.

12. Valois, II, op.cit., p. 224 n. 1.

13. Malta, Cod. 48, f. 68.

14. Richard, 1965, op.cit., p. 504.

15. Partial text ibid., pp. 502-503.

16. Rudt, 1982, op.cit., p. 669.

17. R.-J. Loenertz, Byzantina et Franco-Graeca, Rome, 1970, pp. 579.

18. Rudt, 1982, op.cit., pp. 681-682.

19. Valois, II, op.cit., p. 220.

were weakened and the Latin clergy was reduced in strength and numbers.[20]

The situation of the Hospital on Cyprus after 1378 did not follow this general pattern. The Commander of Cyprus, Fr. Daniele del Carretto, died shortly before 29 December 1378,[21] and the chapter general which met at Rhodes in February 1379 replaced him with another Italian, Fr. Domenico de Alamania.[22] For some reason this appointment lapsed and for several years neither Clement VII nor the Master of the Hospital ratified or recognized it.[23] The 1379 chapter general did pass a statute dividing the Commandery of Cyprus into seven parts[24] and it sent all its statutes for confirmation at Avignon, thus implicitly recognizing Clement VII who confirmed the new statutes, with certain reservations, on 6 August 1379.[25] On 22 April 1381 Clement named Fr. Bertrand Flotte, Grand Preceptor of Rhodes, to hold for his lifetime the Commandery of Cyprus which was said to be vacant following Carretto's death.[26] Clement also appointed Flotte as papal receiver empowered to deal with or destitute Urbanists in many Eastern parts, including Cyprus.[27] Flotte died in about March 1382,[28] and on 12 March 1383 the next Hospitaller chapter general confirmed Alamania as Commander of Cyprus, this confirmation itself being confirmed by Clement VII on 5 September 1383.[29]

The Commandery of Cyprus had been sub-divided in various ways. The lesser Commandery of Anoyira and Phinikas, held in 1365 by Fr. Bertrand de Orsanis, was sometimes given to lieutenants governing the main commandery. Brethren could also hold individual casals, as Fr. Giorgio de Ceva held the casal of Apsiou north of Limassol in 1365.[30] On 20 September 1381 Fr. Giovanni de Pozzo was rented Apsiou for ten years at an annual *responsiones* of 4,500 white besants of Cyprus, worth some 1,125 florins, to be paid yearly to Ceva; on the expiry of the ten years he would be repaid 2,000 gold ducats he had advanced to the Master and Convent. With Apsiou he was also to hold the Hospital's estates at Yeras, *Marameno,* Paramytha, Yermasoyia and Mathikolomi,

20. Rudt, 1982, *op.cit.*, pp. 629-630, 670.

21. Luttrell, *Cyprus*, 1986, *op.cit.*, p. 174.

22. Archivio Vaticano, Reg. Vat. 294, f. 149v-151.

23. Alamania was not entitled Commander of Cyprus in magistral bulls dating at least between 28 February 1379 and 23 March 1382: eg. Reg. Vat. 294, f. 150-152v, 152v; Malta, Cod. 321, f. 225, 234.

24. Luttrell, *Cyprus*, 1986, *op.cit.*, p. 174.

25. Luttrell, 1966, *op.cit*, p. 34.

26. Archivio Vaticano, Reg. Aven. 226, f. 32.

27. Reg. Aven. 227, f. 4v-5v.

28. Luttrell, 1966, *op.cit.*, p. 34.

29. Reg. Vat. 294, f. 149v-151v.

30. Details in Luttrell, *Cyprus*, 1986 *op.cit.*, pp. 161, 163, 171-174 *et passim*.

while he was to maintain the various houses, stables, cellars, granaries, animals, wheat and barley of the casal. Pozzo was licensed to leave Rhodes on 24 January 1382 and on 2 February Ceva was instructed to pay him 250 ducats lent to the Treasury at Rhodes by a Genoese merchant whom Pozzo was to repay.[31]

During 1381 and early 1382 the government of the Hospital at Rhodes maintained control of the Cypriot commandery and its various affairs. Fr. Giorgio de Ceva was still there.[32] On 11 May 1381 Ceva, as *arrendatarius*, was ordered to pay 200 besants of Cyprus to Pozzo, and on 18 July he was instructed to make to the factor of a Rhodian merchant another payment out of 7,000 florins he was due to pay in August for the *apaltum* or farm of the commandery.[33] On 13 May 1381 Fr. Giovanni de Pozzo and Fr. Foulques de Montaigu were commanded to inquire into the activities of Fr. Bertrin de Gagnac, a recalcitrant Hospitaller soon to attempt the assassination of the Master at Rhodes; he had caused much damage to the men of the Cypriot commandery and had left the island without licence.[34] On 17 July Fr. Federigo Malaspina was licensed to leave Rhodes for Cyprus and to reside there under obedience to the *arrentor;* on 2 February 1382 Fr. *Pontius Iuven* was expelled from Rhodes for his sins and sent to Cyprus where Ceva was to maintain him in the way customary for sergeant-brethren; on 22 February Fr. Niccolò de Cipriano was sent to Cyprus in order to reduce expenses at Rhodes and to reside there under obedience to Ceva.[35] During November 1381 Fr. Antonio Sellarii, chaplain of the chapel of Saint Mary in the Conventual church at Rhodes, exchanged that post for the chapel of Saint Mary of the Temple at Nicosia held by Fr. Johan Faber, while Fr. Antonio Xeno was removed from the chaplaincy of Saint John at Nicosia and Fr. Niccolò Michele was sent to serve it until the arrival of Fr. Jean Morin, Prior of Saint John at Nicosia; the Master issued the relevant travel licences and instructed Ceva to make the necessary inductions to office.[36]

The papal schism did after several years eventually divide the Hospital. The legitimate Master, Fr. Juan Fernández de Heredia, and the governing oligarchy at Rhodes supported Clement VII at Avignon. Urban VI opened a formal inquiry into disobedience within the Hospital on 2 May 1381 and he convoked an assembly of Italian and German brethren to Bologna for 29 September of that year, but not until 15 December 1382 did the Roman pope

31. Malta, Cod. 321, f. 213v, 214, 216v, 232; place names identified in J. Richard, *Documents chypriotes des Archives du Vatican (XIVe et XVe siècles)*, Paris, 1962, pp. 68 n. 5, 112, 118.

32. A lieutenant was named to govern Ceva's Sicilian priory on 9 May 1381: Malta, Cod. 321, f. 200. The Master's registers for the six years previous to 1381 do not survive.

33. Malta, Cod. 321, f. 230v, 231.

34. Malta, Cod. 321, f. 212; for Gagnac, Luttrell, 1966, *op.cit.*, pp. 37-40.

35. Malta, Cod. 321, f. 213v, 216v.

36. Malta, Cod. 321, f. 214v-215v.

'depose' Fernández de Heredia, by then resident at Avignon; only in March 1383 did Urban provide an 'anti-Master', the Neapolitan Fr. Riccardo Caracciolo, who remained in Italy and held a Romanist chapter general at Naples during March and April 1384 which was attended by a considerable number of Italian brethren. Some German, Bohemian, Flemish, Gascon and English brethren supported the Romanist Master. There was a good deal of confusion on all sides, and especially in Italy, with much chopping and changing of allegiances. Some Hospitallers sought confirmation of their offices from both obediences; some paid their *responsiones* to neither.[37]

These events had repercussions in Cyprus where Fr. Giorgio de Ceva was involved in a plot conducted by an Urbanist agent, the Piedmontese Fr. Ribaldo Vagnone, to win Rhodes to Caracciolo's obedience. Shortly before October 1383 Vagnone went from Rhodes to Cyprus to plot with Ceva who had held the Hospital's Cypriot casal of Apsiou in 1365 and had governed the Commandery of Cyprus from about 1373 onwards as its *arrendatarius*.[38] In March 1383 Ceva's rule on Cyprus was formally terminated by the Avignonist chapter general at Valence; he was to hand the government of the commandery to the proctor of Fr. Domenico de Alamania who was named, or confirmed, as commander for ten years on 12 March at annual *responsiones* of 5,000 florins, while the *responsiones* of Anoyira and Phinikas were to be paid to him by Fr. Bertrand de Orsanis; the magistral bull declared the office vacant *quovismodo* without any reference either to Fr. Daniele del Carretto or to Fr. Bertrand Flotte.[39] Further magistral bulls of 12 April 1383 made it clear that Alamania would not go to Cyprus and that Fr. Giovanni de Pozzo was to rule it for him; the Hospital's brethren and vassals were to do homage and fealty to Pozzo to whom Ceva was to hand over possession of the commandery when his three-year lease on it expired on 1 September 1383.[40]

Fr. Domenico de Alamania was a Neapolitan who remained faithful to the Rhodian Convent and the Avignon allegiance, eventually ruling Rhodes in the Master's absence.[41] Urban VI, Caracciolo and many of their proteges were also

37. To Luttrell, 1966, *op.cit.*, add *idem, Le Schisme*, 1986, *op.cit.*, pp. 107-110; for Caracciolo, J. Delaville le Roulx, *Les Hospitaliers à Rhodes jusqu'à la mort de Philibert de Naillac; 1310-1421*, Paris, 1913, pp. 248-264. Urban's bull was dated 2 March: Biblioteca Vaticana, Vat. Lat., 6772, f. 37-37v. The coming September assembly is mentioned in Marseilles, Archives départementales du Bouche-du-Rhône, 56 H 4086 (undated paper roll).

38. Luttrell, 1966, *op.cit.*, pp. 42-46; *idem, Cyprus*, 1986, *op.cit.*, p. 173.

39. Malta, Cod. 322, f. 283 = Reg. Vat. 294, f. 150v.

40. Malta, Cod. 322, f. 283v. Rudt, 1982, *op.cit.*, p. 662, seems incorrectly to imply that Alamania was in Cyprus, but he was in Italy and went to Flanders in 1382/3: Luttrell, 1966, *op.cit.*, p. 41 n. 49.

41. Delaville, *op.cit.*, pp. 190/1 n. 3, 305; Alamania was a Neapolitan and belonged to the *langue* of Italy, but his Provençal commanderies may suggest connections with Provence.

Neapolitans. Another Neapolitan, Fr. Bartolomeo Carafa, was named regent in the Priory of Rome by the Master Fernández de Heredia on 13 April 1383; [42] possibly about the same time Urban VI may have nominated Carafa Commander of Cyprus,[43] and the latter was Prior of Rome in March 1384 when his proctor attended Caracciolo's chapter general at Naples.[44] However, it was especially the Genoese who were under suspicion at Rhodes;[45] Fr. Ribaldo Vagnone was a Piedmontese and Fr. Giorgio de Ceva, whose family were Marchesi of Ceva in Piedmont, was losing his lucrative position in Cyprus where his appointment dated in fact from 1373, the year of the Genoese intervention on the island. By some point in mid-1383 Ceva had changed or was changing sides, having been appointed administrator of the Cypriot commandery by Urban VI. The plan was that Ceva and Vagnone were to win Rhodes over to the Urbanist cause, and Ceva claimed some time before October 1383 that he knew many secret Urbanists on Cyprus and that he could bring over that island; Ceva was to keep his Urbanist nomination secret. Ceva secured from Rhodes a licence for Vagnone to travel to Sicily taking with him letters from Urban VI to Caracciolo and to others. Fr. Giorgio de Ceva stayed on Cyprus, ascribing his failure to visit Urban to the lack of a ship and to the need to harvest the sugar crop on Cyprus. Vagnone went back to Italy and then returned to Rhodes where his plot was uncovered and immediately collapsed.[46]

Ceva had left Cyprus by 20 July 1384 when he was near Salerno with the Urbanist Master Caracciolo who then entitled him Commander of Cyprus; on 8 September 1384 Pozzo's proctor, Fr. Petrus Tordella, also swore obedience to Caracciolo. By 16 July 1385 Caracciolo had recognized Ceva as Prior of Messina and on 8 May 1386 Caracciolo received monies sent from Palermo.[47] Preparations of some sort for a Genoese and Urbanist control of the Commandery of Cyprus were under way. King Jacques was in Genoa in 1383 and 1384; the Genoese may have been involved in the plot of Vagnone who had indeed threatened that they would capture Rhodes.[48] From 23 September 1385 to 16 December 1386 Urban VI was uninterruptedly in Genoa and resident at the

42. Malta, Cod. 322, f. 255-255v.

43. A. Esch, *Carafa, Bartolomeo*, in *Dizionario Biografico degli Italiani*, XIX, Rome, 1976, p. 495, dates to 1378/83 a text of Urban VI, in Biblioteca Vaticana, Ms. Vat. Lat. 6330, f. 62-63, naming Carafa as Commander of Cyprus; the appointment presumably preceded Ceva's appointment made by Urban VI, apparently in mid-1383, as *administrator* in Cyprus. In fact Urban VI addressed Carafa as Prior of Rome on 27 June 1382: Reg. Vat. 310, f. 256v-257.

44. Malta, Cod. 281, f. 1.

45. Luttrell, 1966, *op.cit.,* pp. 45-46.

46. *Ibid.*, pp. 42-44.

47. Malta, Cod. 281, f. 9v, 49-49v, 64-65, 93.

48. Luttrell, 1966, *op.cit.,* pp. 45-46.

Hospitallers' commandery there,[49] and at least from 10 December 1385 to 29 November 1386 Caracciolo was with him.[50]

Fr. Giorgio de Ceva apparently left Cyprus owing monies as *responsiones* to Rhodes. On 24 February 1385 an assembly of priors and other Hospitallers meeting in Paris advised the Master in Avignon to write amicably to Ceva with the suggestion that, in view of his seniority and experience and of the goods and honours he had received from the Hospital, he should pay the Cypriot *responsiones* to the Convent which was suffering seriously from the papal schism, for which it was in no way responsible.[51] An arrangement was eventually reached and on 20 January 1386, following its resignation by Fr. Domenico de Alamania, Fr. Juan Fernández de Heredia at Avignon granted the Cypriot commandery, together with the *responsiones* of Anoyira and Phinikas, for ten years to Fr. Giorgio de Ceva, whom he recognized as Prior of Messina. On account of wars and devastation in the commandery its *responsiones* had been lowered to 5,000 florins a year but after five years they were to rise to 7,000 florins; the lease by the Master and Convent of certain casals to Fr. Giovanni de Pozzo was to run for the term conceded, and the *presteria* or *prasteia* of *Chierinis* was excluded. On 26 January Pozzo, by then Commander of Milan, was instructed to hand over the commandery, of which he was governor, to Ceva.[52] The Genoese war of 1373/4 and other disasters must have created genuine financial difficulties; this switch of 1386 was presumably the result of some tacit compromise to secure payment to Rhodes of at least some part of the Cypriot *responsiones*. Two months later Fr. Riccardo Caracciolo at Genoa also granted Ceva the *regimen* of the Commandery of Cyprus, with Anoyira and Phinikas.[53]

Ceva did in the following years control the commandery and *responsiones* were sent to Rhodes; Ceva was still recognized as commander by the Convent at Rhodes as late as 1402.[54] Fr. Bertrand de Orsanis, who held Anoyira and Phinikas in 1365[55] and still held it in 1383,[56] died some time before 1 May 1387, on which date the two were granted by the Master in Avignon at *responsiones* of 6,000 white besants of Cyprus, roughly 1,500 florins, to Fr. Palamedo di Gio-

49. L. Tacchella, *Il Pontificato di Urbano VI a Genova (1385-1386) e l'Eccidio dei Cardinali*, Genoa, 1976, pp. 47-48.

50. Delaville, *op.cit.*, pp. 256-257.

51. Marseilles, 56 H 4090 (transcript most kindly supplied by Anne-Marie Legras).

52. Malta, Cod. 323, f. 209-209v, 210. The *prestaria* of *Charentis* had been exempted from the grant of the commandery in 1365: Luttrell, 1987, *op.cit.*, p. 172 n. 100.

53. Malta, Cod. 281, f. 82v-83.

54. Malta, Cod. 332, f. 174v-175.

55. Luttrell, 1987, *op.cit.*, p. 171.

56. Malta, Cod. 322, f. 283.

vanni, Prior of Venice and Admiral of the Hospital.[57] This led in 1389 and 1390 to a quarrel with Ceva over the *responsiones* which was adjudicated by the Master at Avignon with the decision that since Anoyira and Phinikas had also suffered devastations their *responsiones* should also be reduced, in a way not clearly expressed, by an eighth part.[58] Clearly at least some part of the Cypriot *responsiones* was reaching Rhodes.

The papal schism produced ambiguity and confusion in Cyprus where clear allegiances and obediences were rarely evident; the fluctuating affairs of the Hospitaller commandery demonstrated that. The split within the Hospital over its Cypriot commandery did not come until 1383, and by early 1386 it had been settled by compromise, tacit or agreed, rather than by outright confrontation. The chief protagonist, Fr. Giorgio de Ceva, was apparently drawn by his Genoese connections towards the Urbanist tendency, while the Convent at Rhodes remained firmly for Avignon. For the Convent and brethren at Rhodes the Commandery of Cyprus was important for its wealth which was derived especially from its sugar. In the end, Ceva secured the commandery and its incomes but apparently he did pay some *responsiones* to Rhodes.

57. Malta, Cod. 324, f. 135-135v.

58. Malta, Cod. 324, f. 110, 110v-111; Luttrell, 1987, *op.cit.*, p. 173 n. 106, incorrectly states that Ceva was said to have succeeded Orsanis as ruler of Anoyira and Phinikas.

V

The Hospitallers in Cyprus after 1386*

The Latin military–religious orders orginated in Jerusalem with the emergence of the Temple early in the twelfth century. In 1191 the Templars briefly acquired Cyprus by purchase in what was probably the earliest attempt by a military order to set up an independent state, but they lacked the money or manpower to sustain their rule on the island.[1] The Hospitallers held lands in the Diocese of Limassol by 1203 and were granted the *casale* of Kolossi near Limassol by the king in 1210;[2] when Kolossi was fortified with a tower is uncertain.[3] The Hospitallers increased their privileges and holdings on Cyprus, especially around Limassol where the port was important to them as a stage along their lines of communication from the West. After the fall of Acre and the surviving remnants of the mainland Latin kingdom in 1291, the Hospital and the Temple both set up their Convent or headquarters at Limassol on Cyprus where they found themselves partly subordinate to a hostile monarchy which imposed restrictions upon them. The Hospitallers made some moves towards the adoption of a new role in the defence of the Christian Kingdom of Cilician Armenia, while in 1300 the Templars initiated a return to Syria by occupying and defending the small island of Ruad off Tortosa on the mainland due east of Limassol, an initiative which

---

*This paper is a revised version of one published, with numerous printing errors and omissions, in N. Coureas and J. Riley-Smith (eds), *Cyprus and the Crusades* (Nicosia, 1995); and that version should henceforth be ignored.

[1] This article continues three previous publications covering the Hospitallers in Cyprus from 1291 to 1386: A. Luttrell, *The Hospitallers in Cyprus, Rhodes, Greece and the West: 1291–1440* (London, 1978), II; idem, *The Hospitallers of Rhodes and their Mediterranean World* (Aldershot, 1992), IX; idem, 'Sugar and Schism: the Hospitallers in Cyprus from 1378 to 1386', in A. Bryer and G. Georghallides (eds), *'The Sweet Land of Cyprus'* (Nicosia, 1993). See also idem, 'Ta Stratiotika Tagmata', in T. Papadopoulos (ed.), *Istoria tes Kyprou*, IV, part 1 (Nicosia, 1995).

[2] Texts in *Cartulaire général de l'Ordre des Hospitaliers de S. Jean de Jérusalem: 1100–1310*, J. Delaville le Roulx (ed.), 4 vols (Paris, 1894–1906), nos 1176, 1354; cf. G. Hill, *A History of Cyprus*, II (Cambridge, 1947), p. 22. The most detailed treatment is now that in N. Coureas, *The Latin Church in Cyprus: 1195–1312* (Aldershot, 1997), pp. 121–186.

[3] In 1452 Kolossi had a ruined *turris* which it was then decided should be replaced by a *castrum* with a tower at each of its four corners: Valletta, National Library of Malta, Archives of the Order of St John, Cod. 363, f. 142–144. The pre-1452 tower was apparently round: E. Aristidou, *Kolossi Castle through the Centuries* (Nicosia, 1983), pp. 13, 17–19, 32 (plan).

ended disastrously with the loss of Ruad to the Egyptian Mamluks in 1302. In 1307 the Master of the Temple and many of its brethren were arrested in France and in 1312 the whole order was suppressed.[4] The Hospitallers had meanwhile invaded Rhodes in 1306 and by about 1309 they were setting up a virtually independent regime there.

When the Hospitallers transferred their Convent to Rhodes they retained their properties on Cyprus and in 1313 they acquired the bulk of the Templars' possessions there. From 1310 onwards they enjoyed close and friendly relations with the Lusignan dynasty. The Hospital's Cypriot commandery was rich, thanks especially to its sugar plantations around Kolossi. In 1317 and 1330 the annual payments or responsions supposedly due from it to the Convent at Rhodes were set at 10,000 florins, a greater sum than that owed by any single Western priory. In 1329 the knowledgeable Venetian Marino Sanudo considered that Cyprus provided 20,000 florins or one ninth of what he estimated to be the Order's total income of 180,000 florins, and in 1374 the Hospital was said to have over sixty *casali* on Cyprus. The two island governments repeatedly collaborated in leagues and expeditions against Mamluks and Turks, especially in 1365 when a Cypriot crusade sailed from Rhodes to sack Alexandria in Egypt; in 1374 the Master of the Hospital went to Nicosia in an attempt to settle the king's quarrels with the Genoese. Famagusta was important to the Hospital as a financial centre where the commandery's incomes could be pledged in advance to raise money and through which bankers and merchants could transfer the Order's Western incomes to Rhodes.

Rhodes and Cyprus were large islands which possessed important ports on the Latins' mercantile routes to Syria and Egypt. Both had large Greek-speaking populations which were Orthodox in religion but which, unlike Crete for example, had not been subjected to Latin rule in consequence of the Western conquests in *Romania* in and after 1204. Cyprus received certain laws and institutions deriving from the Latin state in Jerusalem, some of

---

[4]A. Luttrell, 'Gli Ospitalieri di San Giovanni di Gerusalemme dal Continente alle Isole', in F. Tommasi (ed.), *Acri 1291: la Fine della Presenza degli Ordini Militari in Terra Santa e i Nuovi Orientamenti nel Secolo XIV* (Perugia, 1996). See also P. Edbury, 'The Templars in Cyprus', A. Gilmour-Bryson, 'Testimony of non-Templar Witnesses in Cyprus', and A. Iliéva, 'The Suppression of the Templars in Cyprus according to the Chronicle of Leontios Makhairas', all three in M. Barber (ed.), *The Military Orders: Fighting for the Faith and Caring for the Sick* (Aldershot, 1994). L. Imperio, *Il Tramonto dei Templari: il Processo di Cipro - Uomini e Vicende dell'Ordine nei suoi ultimi anni di vita* (Latina, 1992), is useful but requires caution. A Templar interrogated in 1309 stated that there were 400 (*quadringinti*) Templars on Cyprus in 1292: text in J. Michelet, *Procès des Templiers*, II (Paris, 1851), p.139. However forty (*quadraginta*) seems probable. Forty was the number of *freres cheualiers* together with ten *freres sergens darmes*, which the Hospital decided to keep on Cyprus in 1292: Marseilles, Archives départementales des Bouches-du-Rhône, 56 H 4055.

which the Hospital apparently transferred to Rhodes. Both islands were governed not as colonies but as their own metropolis. Both were controlled by a predominantly French-speaking ruling class; important groups of Italians, Catalans and other Latins who were merchants, bureaucrats, ecclesiastics, mercenaries, pirates and so on were established on Cyprus and Rhodes, but fundamentally there was a Francophone entente between the two island regimes which showed itself in their repeated co-operation. Communication between them could be rapid but in winter there were difficulties. Thus an envoy of the Duke of Bourbon who arrived on Rhodes on 29 November 1398 had to wait until 29 January 1399 for a ship to Cyprus, his passage costing three ducats; he reached Limassol on 3 February. On 27 October he was at Famagusta where he was unable to take a Venetian galley, and so the king provided a royal galley on which he left Kyrenia on 2 November to reach Rhodes again six days later.[5]

The largely settled relationship between the two islands was partly disrupted by the schism in the papacy created by the election of Clement VII in September 1378. Since 1365 the popes had been exercising their apostolic powers by providing to the rich Cypriot commandery various Italian Hospitallers who were acting as papal servants in the West. On the death in 1378 of the absentee commander, Fr Daniele del Carretto, his lieutenant in Cyprus was Fr Giorgio de Ceva, who was also Prior of Messina, that is of Sicily. The bulk of the Hospitallers at Rhodes were French and they supported the Avignonese pope, Clement VII, against the Roman pope, Urban VI; the Hospital's Master, Fr Juan Fernández de Heredia, actually resided at Avignon from 1382 until his death there in 1396. However, a number of Italian brethren supported Urban VI, and on Cyprus the Ligurian Fr Giorgio de Ceva was involved during 1384 in an abortive Genoese plot to win over the Rhodian Convent to the Urbanist cause. As also happened elsewhere, this led to a confused competition for control of the commandery's incomes which was settled in 1386 through a compromise by which Ceva retained the Commandery of Cyprus but sent its responsions to Rhodes.[6]

*

* *

The arrangement of 1386 worked successfully. At Avignon on 20 January 1386 the Master accepted Fr Giorgio de Ceva, despite his recent defection,

---

[5]Text in L. de Mas Latrie, *Histoire de l'île de Chypre sous le Règne des Princes de la Maison de Lusignan*, 3 vols (Paris, 1852–1861), II, pp. 449-450.

[6]The Hospital in Cyprus from 1291 to 1386 is covered in Luttrell (1978), II, pp. 166–171; idem (1992), IX; and idem (1993); a complete list of the Hospital's Cypriot possessions is still to be established.

recognising him as Prior of Messina and naming him as Commander of Cyprus for ten years. On account of unspecified wars *et alia inordinata*, the Master lowered the responsions to 5000 florins a year for the first five years; for the second five years they were to be 7000 florins. Ceva was to receive the responsions of the lesser Cypriot Commandery of Phinikas and Anoyira but the Hospital's *presteria* or hamlet of *Chierinis*, perhaps somewhere near Kyrenia, was to be held by Fr Giovanni de Pozzo, Commander of Milan. Pozzo, who was governor of the Commandery of Cyprus, was to hand it over to Ceva on 1 September of that year.[7] Presumably Ceva had in reality retained control of the commandery and at Genoa on 20 March 1386 the Urbanist 'anti-Master', Fr Riccardo Caracciolo, also granted Ceva, whom he too recognised as Prior of Messina, the Commandery of Cyprus together with Phinikas and Anoyira at 5000 florins of responsions a year.[8] Here at least the schism within the Hospital was settled by compromise. Another example of such admirable ambiguity was provided by Richard II of England, who supported the Roman pope but was prepared to give priority to the defence of 'a frontier of Christianity' by allowing English Hospitallers and their money to go to Rhodes as long as neither passed through Avignon.[9] In February 1386 Fr John Raddington, Prior of England, was due to leave England as royal ambassador with undisclosed business on both Rhodes and Cyprus.[10] Late in 1392 Raddington was accompanying Richard II's cousin Henry of Derby to Jerusalem,[11] and on the way back Derby sent him from Famagusta on a mission to the king at Nicosia.[12] Until August 1396, when his representative declared for Pope Benedict XIII at Avignon, King Jacques of Cyprus managed to avoid any commitment to either pope[13] and Raddington's two missions conceivably involved English attempts to secure the king's allegiance to the Roman pope.

The lesser Commandery of Phinikas and Anoyira was held separately from the Commandery of Cyprus, though it owed responsions to the latter's

---

[7]Malta, Cod. 323, f. 209–209v; Cod. 324, f. 110v–111. The location of *Chierinis* (Kyrenia?) is uncertain. It was also given as *Charentis:* Luttrell (1992), IX p. 172 n. 100.

[8]Malta, Cod. 281, f. 82v–83.

[9]Luttrell (1978), V, p.199; C. Tipton, 'The English Hospitallers during the Great Schism', *Studies in Medieval and Renaissance History*, IV (1967).

[10]Ibid., p. 109; text in Mas Latrie, II, p. 401.

[11]Text in E. Perroy, *The Diplomatic Correspondence of Richard II* (London, 1933), pp. 114–115.

[12]*Item in expensis domini prioris Sancti Johannis, domini Otes Graunson, et aliorum militum et scutiferorum euntium versus regem Cyprie de Famagost vsque Nikasye, vna cum conductione equorum ...*: in L. Toulmin Smith (ed.), *Expeditions to Prussia and the Holy Land by Henry, Earl of Derby* (London, 1894), p. 226. C. Tyerman, *England and the Crusades: 1095–1588* (Chicago, 1988), p. 296, suggests that this embassy might have been connected with some crusade proposal.

[13]Luttrell (1993), pp. 156–160; J. Richard, 'Le Royaume de Chypre et le Grand Schisme: à propos d'un Document récemment découvert', *Académie des Inscriptions et Belles-Lettres: Comptes Rendus* (1965).

commander. Phinikas and Anoyira had been held since 1365 at latest by Fr Bertrand de Orsanis[14] but he died before 1 May 1387, on which date the Master at Avignon granted the lesser commandery to Fr Palamedo di Giovanni, Prior of Venice and Admiral of the Hospital, presumably because the latter had lost control of his priory and its incomes to the Urbanists. Like his predecessor, he was to pay 1500 florins to the Commander of Cyprus, but since the latter's responsions had been lowered the Master decreed on 20 January 1389 that Fr Palamedo should pay the commander one eighth of what the latter paid, since Phinikas and Anoyira had also been damaged and destroyed.[15] Fr Giorgio de Ceva did apparently pay responsions to Rhodes, though on 24 November 1400 the new Master Fr Philibert de Naillac and the Convent at Rhodes empowered Fr Baudouin de *Nouauiletta*, who was presumably from Northern France, to secure the arrears due for the financial year 1399/1400 from Ceva or from his lieutenant Fr Ruffino de Biandrate; two days later they instructed Fr Ruffino to transfer to Fr Baudouin the quantities due in grain, barley or cash.[16] On 3 May 1401 Fr Baudouin and the lawyer Bernard de Saint Saturnin were appointed as procurators to rule Phinikas and Anoyira.[17]

Fr Palamedo di Giovanni was dead by 17 February 1402 on which day Phinikas and Anoyira were granted *ad vitam* to another important Italian Hospitaller, Fr Domenico de Alamania, technically at 1000 florins a year of responsions and free of any other impositions. Since Alamania had advanced 11,200 florins to the Order for the defence of Smyrna, he was considered to have paid his Cypriot responsions for the next eleven years; for some reason not explained in the grant, he was, however, to pay 500 florins a year for the next six years.[18] On 1 June 1402 Fr Antonio de Riva, Prior of Venice, whom Alamania had named as his lieutenant in Phinikas and Anoyira, was licensed to go to Cyprus and to remain there to rule Phinikas and Anoyira, while Fr Cencio di Giovanni was commissioned to determine another dispute over rights and incomes between the Commander of Cyprus and the Commander of Phinikas and Anoyira. Four days later, on 5 June, the *prestaria* of *Cherinis* was granted to Fr Buffilo Pannizati, the new Admiral of Rhodes who was also Prior of Barletta. Cyprus was still being reserved for leading Italians on Rhodes who must have been deprived by the schism of incomes from their own priories. Ceva died at some point before 15 September 1402, on which date Fr Jean Grivel, Castellan of Rhodes and Seneschal of the Master, was named as lieutenant to rule the Cypriot commandery and to collect Ceva's spolia.[19]

---

[14]Luttrell (1992), IX, pp. 170–172.
[15]Malta, Cod. 324, f. 110v–111, 135–135v.
[16]Malta, Cod. 330, f. 92, 119.
[17]Malta, Cod. 331, f. 159–159v.
[18]Malta, Cod. 331, f. 167v.
[19]Malta, Cod. 332, f. 164, 164v, 166v.

6

The Commander of Cyprus was often an absentee who governed through a lieutenant. The number of Hospitaller brethren on the island must have been limited, partly because service on Cyprus did not necessarily qualify for seniority in the Convent which was vital for matters of promotion. In fact on 30 October 1405, at the instance of Fr Raymond de Lescure, the Prior of Toulouse who was also Commander of Cyprus, and with the agreement of the brethren of the *langue* of Provence, the Master and Convent accepted that service on Cyprus by brethren of that *langue* should qualify for seniority at Rhodes.[20] Hospitallers did go back and forth. On 22 July and again on 26 November 1399 Fr Cencio di Giovanni was licensed to leave Rhodes for Cyprus, and on 11 February 1400 a Fr Hugo was granted a licence to go from Rhodes to reside in the Cypriot commandery and to assure divine service as prior of the Hospital's church at Nicosia.[21] The administration of the estates naturally caused difficulties, though the unspecified destructions and damages mentioned in 1389 may well have been exaggerated in order to justify the reduction of the responsions. There were also problems with the crown. On 29 January 1400 the Master and Convent empowered the Commander of Cyprus, Fr Giorgio de Ceva, and the Prior of Lombardy, Fr Lodovico de Valperga, to appear at the royal court to defend the Hospital's rights and demand the commandery's *libertates, servitutes, bona et emolumenta.*[22] Some property was let out to secular tenants. Thus on 20 August 1400, after consulting with the commander by letter, the Master and Convent reduced from 50 to 25 besants of Nicosia the annual census owed by the noble *miles* Paulus de Acrolissa who held from the Hopital certain lands and houses near Nicosia which had all been destroyed and needed repairs.[23]

Cyprus remained an important and convenient financial centre. For example, on 20 February 1401 Ceva's lieutenant, Fr Ruffino de Biandrate, was instructed, together with Fr Baudouin de *Nouaviletta*, to pay in Famagusta to Henricus Lecanora, inhabitant of Famagusta, 1620 gold ducats in the name of Fr Domenico de Alamania, and on 5 March the same two were to pay Lecanora 700 ducats to be taken from the arrears of the Cypriot commandery for 1399/1400, this time in the name of the Rhodian financier Dragonetto Clavelli. On 19 March orders were given for Ceva or Biandrate to repay 2000 ducats to Jacopo Ricci or Vettore Bragadino, two Venetians who had handed over woollen cloth to that value in Rhodes; the money was to be paid in Nicosia from the Cypriot

---

[20]Malta, Cod. 333, f. 33.

[21]Malta, Cod. 331, f. 119, 138.

[22]Malta, Cod. 330, f. 122v.

[23]Malta, Cod. 330, f. 125–125v: the property was *confrontata cum campo du balle eundo rectum iter ad flumen Nicossie vsque ad hospicium de Quiriaco et versus jardinum dominj Petrj Pisanj et redeundo per iter rectum ad campum supradictum.*

responsions.[24] On 20 January 1402 Biandrate was ordered to pay, from the 1400/01 responsions, 2000 ducats owed to Dragonetto Clavelli for cloth and grain imported into Rhodes, and on 13 March Ceva, Biandrate or whoever might be governing in Cyprus was to pay, out of the incomes for 1401/02, 2200 ducats advanced in Rhodes by Filipo di Pietro of Florence, *civis* and *habitator* of Rhodes, on behalf of Silvestro Morosini, a Venetian of Cyprus who was to be repaid in Cyprus.[25] On 5 June 1402 Ceva or his lieutenant Biandrate were instructed to pay, again from the 1401/02 incomes, 740 gold ducats owed by the Hospital's Treasury at Rhodes to Fr Buffilo Pannizatti, Admiral and Prior of Barletta, to refund expenses he had incurred for the defence of Smyrna. On 15 September, following Ceva's death, the mandates of 13 March and 5 June, evidently not yet fulfilled, were repeated to Biandrate.[26] In such ways the Commandery of Cyprus was used to raise quick money in Rhodes.

*
* *

Cyprus was party to an anti-Turkish league, concluded at Rhodes on 1 December 1388, which provided for ships of Cyprus, of Rhodes and of the Genoese of Chios, Mytilini and Pera to patrol Turkish waters between Constantinople and Gorighos on the mainland due north of Cyprus; the league's vessels were to have the use of the harbour at Kyrenia.[27] Fourteen years later the close alliance between Rhodes and Cyprus came under strain as a result of renewed Genoese aggression on Cyprus. The problems of the schism within the Hospital had largely been overcome. The majority of Hospitallers remained close to the papacy at Avignon where the Aragonese Benedict XIII was elected pope in 1394, and when the Romanist 'anti-Master' Fr Riccardo Caracciolo died in 1395 he was replaced by a lieutenant rather than by a new 'anti-Master'. At Rhodes the Frenchman Fr Philibert de Naillac was elected Master in mid-1396, and in August of that year the Cypriot crown declared its support for Benedict XIII.[28] In 1402, however, the Hospital was involved in a new conflict between the Cypriot crown and the Genoese, who remained powerful in their privileged base at Famagusta. Several decades earlier, in 1374, the Hospitallers had faced embarrassment when they were forced by the Genoese to hand over Jacques de Lusignan, uncle of the young King Pierre II, and to give all Cypriots on Rhodes three days in which to leave the island.[29] In July 1402 the Hospitaller Commander of Genoa, Fr Antonio Grimaldi, left Genoa and took three

[24]Malta, Cod. 330, f. 126v, 135.

[25]Malta, Cod. 331, f. 167, 176.

[26]Malta, Cod. 332, f. 166v, 174v–175.

[27]Hill, II, pp. 439–440.

[28]Richard, p. 500.

[29]Luttrell (1992), IX, p. 175.

Genoese galleys to Famagusta which in August he relieved from its siege by King Janus; subsequently Grimaldi also attacked Venetian shipping, but then died at Famagusta some time before 15 January 1403.[30] Grimaldi had been acting as a Genoese rather than as a Hospitaller, and in inflicting a serious blow on the king he had created an awkward breach of Hospitaller neutrality.

In June 1403 a much larger Genoese fleet reached Rhodes under the command of Jean de Boucicaut who was both Marshal of France and Governor of Genoa. Once at Rhodes Boucicaut prepared to attack Janus. The Master Fr Philibert de Naillac had been with Boucicaut in the great crusading battle against the Turks at Nikopolis and had subsequently helped to raise a ransom for the captured Boucicaut, who had visited Rhodes following his release by the Turks in 1397.[31] Naillac was able to dissuade the Marshal from an assault on Cyprus, and Boucicaut sailed instead to attack the Turks in Southern Anatolia while Naillac went to Cyprus in June to negotiate a settlement with Janus.[32] The Master was accompanied by Fr Walter Grendon, Prior of England, Fr Raymond de Lescure, Prior of Toulouse, and Fr Pierre de Bauffremont, who held the office of Hospitaller with charge of the hospital at Rhodes.[33] Boucicaut's forces attacked Alanya on the southern coast of Anatolia on 29 June and sacked it, after which he made peace with the local Muslim leader, possibly Savgi Beg of Tekke or his son Qaramani. Meanwhile Naillac persuaded Janus to accept Boucicaut's demands. Boucicaut then left Alanya for Cyprus where he met Naillac at Pendayia on the north coast; the two travelled to Nicosia where peace terms were agreed with the king on 7 July. Janus was to pay the Genoese 150,000 ducats and in part security for this sum he pledged his crown jewels and plate, worth 70,000 ducats, which were to be held by the Hospital until the contracting parties had fulfilled their obligations.[34]

---

[30]Hill, II, pp. 450–452. Grimaldi was dead by 15 January 1403: Malta, Cod. 332, f. 146. Amend J. Delaville le Roulx, *La France en Orient au XIVe siècle: Expéditions du Maréchal Boucicaut*, 2 vols (Paris, 1886), I, p. 411, giving this date, from Cod. 332, f. 136, as 26 March 1402.

[31]Delaville (1913), pp. 235–237, 271–272; K. Setton, *The Papacy and the Levant: 1204–1571*, 4 vols (Philadelphia, 1976–84), I, pp. 360–361. Boucicaut had already visited Rhodes on pilgrimage in 1389, while two Hospitaller galleys had served with him at Constantinople in 1399: D. Lalande (ed.), *Le Livre des Fais du bon messire Jehan le Maingre, dit Bouciquaut* (Geneva, 1985), pp. 64, 138, and Setton, I, 371.

[32]Hill, II, pp. 453–454; Setton, I, pp. 385–386.

[33]Grendon, Lescure and Bauffremont were at Nicosia on 7 July 1403: text in Mas Latrie, II, pp. 466–471. Delaville (1886), I, p. 427, adds Fr Domenico de Alamania and Dragonetto Clavelli, but these are merely taken from the text given at Rhodes on 19 September in Malta, Cod. 332, f. 168v.

[34]Details in Hill, II, pp. 454–455, 460; Setton, I, pp. 385–387. On the Emirs of Tekke, B. Flemming, *Landschaftsgeschichte von Pamphilien, Pisidien und Lykien im Spätmittelalter* (Wiesbaden, 1964), p. 114. By the treaty of 7 July 1403 Janus was to pay 150,000 ducats in instalments. 70,000 ducats were pledged on the crown jewels and plate to be held by Naillac, and

Boucicaut next planned an assault on Alexandria but that was foiled by bad weather and he had to return to Rhodes. During August 1403 he pillaged Tripoli, Botrun, Beirut, Sidon and Lattakia. Some Cypriot forces, accompanied by the Master Naillac, Lescure, Bauffremont and two Hospitaller galleys, took part in this campaign.[35] The Hospitallers were involved in the seizure of Venetian property at Beirut and elsewhere, incidents which were to cause prolonged troubles with Venice. Thereafter Naillac went to Kyrenia, where Fr Domenico de Alamania, Commander of Naples and Avignon, was with him, and then left for Rhodes on about 21 August.[36] On Boucicaut's return voyage he stayed at Rhodes and was feasted there for ten or twelve days.[37] The Hospital had balanced its obligations to attack the infidel with its interest in preserving the Lusignan monarchy and the need to satisfy Franco-Genoese demands. From his home in Egypt, Emmanuele Piloti was later to claim that Boucicaut had agreed to hand Alexandria over to the Hospital for 40,000 ducats.[38] That seems most unlikely, though a Hospitaller tenure of Alanya might conceivably have been envisaged as a replacement for Smyrna, which had been lost to Timur in December 1402. The Hospital needed a token bridgehead on the mainland which would

---

80,000 on crown property; Janus would also pay 121,000 old besants of Nicosia, about 30,000 ducats, to the Genoese of Famagusta: text in Mas Latrie, II, pp. 466–471. Naillac's registers provide further information. Presumably following Boucicaut's ransom after his capture at Nikopolis in 1396, he owed Naillac 2000 florins, which on 25 August 1400 Naillac empowered l'Hermite de la Faye to collect: Cod. 330, f. 122. At Rhodes on 17 September Naillac recognised the receipt from Boucicaut of 4400 ducats plus 2000 ducats which Naillac had earlier lent him. On 19 September Naillac recognised that he owed Boucicaut 10,000 ducats as part of 25,000 ducats for which he was Janus' guarantor. A few days later (date partly illegible) Naillac recognized a debt to Boucicault, his *consanguinus*, of 15,000 ducats (presumably the 25,000 less the 10,000) for which the guarantors were Alamania, Grendon, Bauffremont and Dragonetto Clavelli: Cod. 332, f. 168v. Instructions of 22 September arranged for this sum to be paid in unspecified yearly instalments from the incomes of the priories of the three French *langues*: Cod. 332, f. 169. Since he had not been accompanied to Cyprus by proctors of the Convent, Naillac formally declared on 15 October that he and the Convent held pledges from Janus worth 70,000 ducats, the jewels and the plate valued at 45,000 ducats, plus 25,000 ducats described as *de nostris pignoribus per ipsum dominum Regem nobis bene securatis*; from the 25,000 were deducted 4000 ducats already paid to certain Genoese: Cod. 332, f. 169v (text in S. Paoli, *Codice Diplomatico del Sacro Militare Ordine Gerosolimitano, oggi di Malta*, II [Lucca, 1737], pp. 107–108).

[35]*Livre des Fais*, p. 239; Setton, I, pp. 386–388. Bernardo Morosini reported two Hospitaller galleys: text in L. Muratori, *Rerum Italicarum Scriptores*, XXII (Milan, 1733), pp. 800–801.

[36]Text ibid., pp. 800–801; cf. F. Surdich, *Genova e Venezia fra tre e quattrocento* (Genoa, 1970), pp. 90–91.

[37]*Livre des Fais*, p. 253.

[38]P.-H. Dopp (ed.), *Traité d'Emmanuel Piloti sur le Passage en Terre Sainte (1420)* (Louvain–Paris, 1958), pp. 193–194.

demonstrate the Order's permanent dedication to a direct confrontation with the infidel.

The next nine years of Rhodian-Cypriot relations were dominated by the figure of Fr Raymond de Lescure. Quite probably from the region of Albi, he had been Prior of Toulouse since 1396 and between 1400 and 1402 he was active on missions in the Morea.[39] In 1403 the Hospital made an exceptional agreement with the Sultan of Egypt which would have granted it rights to take pilgrims to Jerusalem and other holy places and to have consuls and tax advantages in Mamluk ports. This treaty, which could have given the Hospital control of much of the lucrative pilgrim traffic to Syria, eventually came to nothing, perhaps because of the Hospital's participation in Boucicaut's raids, but in November the Hospital was sending the Prior of Toulouse to Egypt to secure ratification of the treaty which had recently been agreed in Rhodes by the sultan's envoys. This mission resulted in Lescure being held hostage in Egypt. On 9 August 1404 the Master and Convent wrote to the Venetian, Genoese, Catalan and French merchants and consuls resident at Alexandria asking them to advance 6000 ducats to ransom Lescure and his retinue who were detained as prisoners there; Lescure was free by December 1404.[40]

Meanwhile the vacancy in the Cypriot commandery caused by Ceva's death in or before 1402 was evidently causing perplexities or disputes in the Convent on Rhodes. Two Hospitaller brethren, Fr Odetus de Badeto and Fr Hugues Ricart, were licensed to leave Rhodes for Cyprus on 19 November 1403, and on 16 February 1404 Fr Ruffino de Biandrate, *gubernator* of the *baiulia* of Cyprus, was instructed to repay 300 ducats to the Cypriot agent of Nicolino de Leone who had lent the money at Rhodes.[41] On the following 8 March the Master and Convent empowered Fr Pierre Gache, the lieutenant of the Grand Preceptor at Rhodes, and Fr Pierre Galoys to rule the Cypriot commandery, to collect all monies owed to Ceva together with Ceva's *spolia* and other dues, and to demand accounts from Biandrate. On 17 March the same two brethren were instructed, as visitors and procurators in Cyprus, to pay on behalf of the Rhodian Treasury 700 ducats of the commandery's incomes to Domenico di Giovanni of Florence.[42] At about this time the

---

[39]Delaville (1913), pp. 278–281.

[40]Luttrell (1992), X, pp. 194–198. The *Livre des Fais*, pp. 358–360, later stated that Janus paid 25,000 ducats to ransom Lescure who had been detained in Alexandria and then taken to Cairo, but the passage, which wrongly places his mission in about 1407, seems confused and unreliable; Delaville (1886), I, p. 506 n. 3, and Hill, II, p. 468, deduce that Lescure had been sent to negotiate a treaty on Janus' behalf.

[41]Malta, Cod. 332, f. 57, 182.

[42]Malta, Cod. 332, f. 171v–172, 182. The same two were instructed on 5 April 1404 to pay, from the Hospital's Cypriot incomes, 1100 Venetian ducats to Gaspare and Mellado Pallavisino of Genoa: Cod. 333, f. 130.

Master's lieutenant and the council at Rhodes issued instructions for the two commissioners. They were neither to accept nor to deal with Lescure as Commander of Cyprus unless he first observed a certain unspecified promise he had made to the council. The two visitors were to receive the commander's incomes from 1 January to September 1404 in barley, oats, cotton, wine and other items which included the *catapenagium,* that is the personal tax paid by the serfs in cash as opposed to what they owed in kind. They should elect others to govern the commandery on behalf of the Treasury at Rhodes. The two were to furnish the commandery with meat, barley, and other things necessary for the coming year. They were also to collect the dues in kind owed by the *rustici* and *servi* of the Hospital's *casali*. If possible they should sell this produce to merchants or others and send the money to the Treasury either by letters of change or in cash sent at the Treasury's risk; otherwise they should load the produce on a ship they should hire. The two visitors were, furthermore, empowered to inspect all accounts and to issue receipts.[43] On 18 June 1404 Fr Odetus de Badeto and Fr Hugues Ricart, who had been licensed to go to Cyprus in the previous November, were instructed not to interfere in the affairs of the commandery or its members and to pay over any monies they had received to the two visitors.[44] On 6 August 1404 Fr Elie de Fossat *alias* Picon, the Grand Preceptor of Rhodes, was created lieutenant and procurator in the *baiulia* of Cyprus with powers to reform it, to depose rebels, check accounts, receive debts, hold assemblies, control castles and deal with the king and with the Hospital's subjects.[45]

Precisely what had gone wrong was not clarified. Fr Raymond de Lescure was back on Rhodes by late October 1404 and on 17 December he and Fr Elie de Fossat were summoned without delay to the Master's presence.[46] On the same day Biandrate was addressed as the commandery's *gubernator* and was ordered to leave it vacant and to present full accounts for it; yet nine days later on 26 December he was appointed lieutenant and procurator of the Master and Convent in Cyprus.[47] Lescure clearly wanted the Cypriot commandery and its incomes. Ten months later on 22 October 1405, following a request from Pope Benedict XIII, he was eventually granted the commandery, technically vacant through Ceva's death, for ten years at 6000 florins a year; the Master's bull of appointment mentioned Lescure's repeated services against the Turks.[48] On 23 October Lescure was licensed to leave for Cyprus, and a few days later on 30 October Fr Daudeneto Herailh, Fr Jean *Alespee,*

---

[43]Malta, Cod. 332, f. 156v.
[44]Malta, Cod. 333, f. 118v.
[45]Malta, Cod. 333, f. 120.
[46]Malta, Cod. 333, f. 33, 121.
[47]Malta, Cod. 333, f. 121.
[48]Malta, Cod. 333, f. 123.

12

Fr Jean Claret and Fr Bernard Roux were all four, at Lescure's request, granted licences to travel to Cyprus; at the same time the brethren of the *langue* of Provence were permitted to count time spent on Cyprus towards their seniority in the Rhodian Convent.[49] On 6 November 1405 Biandrate was summoned to Rhodes, but contacts with Cyprus continued regularly; for example, on 13 August 1406 Fr Antonio *Zeni* received a licence to sail from Rhodes to act as prior or senior priest in the church of Saint John at Famagusta, that is to maintain the spiritual side of the Hospital's presence on Cyprus.[50] In 1411 the prior of the Order's church in Nicosia was Fr Agoy de Lozaco.[51] In 1418 a traveller from Famagusta to Nicosia stayed with the Hospitallers at a place called *Mores*, presumably Mora, and in Nicosia he lodged in the *grant hostel* of the Hospital's commandery where he found in the chapel an arm of Saint George and part of his lance, a head of Saint Anne, a body of Saint Euphemia and other holy relics.[52]

King Janus maintained contacts with the French crown and shortly before 8 October 1405 Fr Pierre de Bauffremont, who had become Commander of Beaune and Lorraine, was at Basel accompanying a mission from the King of Cyprus to the King of France.[53] Lescure was a more important envoy who was sent West two years later to seek a bride for King Janus; he was also to redeem the royal jewels, presumably still at Rhodes, according to the terms of the treaty of 1403.[54] Lescure was in Genoa in August 1407, at which time the Venetians were prepared to accept him as an arbitrator in their disputes with the Genoese.[55] Boucicaut discussed his schemes for a new attack on Alexandria with Lescure, who was there in Genoa as an envoy from Janus and whom Boucicaut's contemporary biographer described as 'a man of great honour, wise, prudent, and expert in all things'. As a result Boucicaut's squire Jean de Ony and Fr Jean de *Vogon* or *Vienne*, Commander of Belleville, were sent from Genoa to the Master at Rhodes and to the king in Cyprus to discuss the proposed expedition and also the question of the Genoese debt and the royal jewels. At Rhodes Fr Jean de *Vogon* was to ask the Master for a ship if no other was available to take him to Cyprus, and on reaching Nicosia he was to go to the *hostel de Sainct-Jean* and send a message to the king through Lescure's lieutenant there. Many details

---

[49]Malta, Cod. 333, f. 33, 123v.

[50]Malta, Cod. 333, f. 124, 127v.

[51]Text in L. de Mas Latrie, 'Nouvelles Preuves de l'Histoire de Chypre', *Bibliothèque de l'École de Chartes*, XXXV (1874), pp. 124–128.

[52]P. Noble (ed.), *Le Voyatge d'Oultremer en Jherusalem de Nompar, Seigneur de Caumont* (Oxford, 1975), p. 49. The *domus More* was granted to the Hospital in 1210: text in *Cartulaire*, no. 1354.

[53]R. Wackernagel (ed.), *Urkundenbuch der Stadt Basel*, V (Basel, 1900), pp. 355–356.

[54]Hill, II, p. 466.

[55]Delaville (1886), I, p. 499.

concerning the proposed fleet, which it was planned should assemble at the island of Kastellorizzo between Rhodes and Cyprus, were worked out, and Lescure declared that if the king could not pay half the estimated cost of 132,000 ducats, then he himself would raise the first 18,000 or 20,000 florins in the West, since he had royal authority to do so. The Hospitallers on Rhodes possibly agreed to such schemes, but Janus, after some indecision, rejected them.[56] Fr Jean de *Vogon* of the Priory of Auvergne was licensed to leave Rhodes for the West on 7 November 1407.[57]

On 25 April 1408 Lescure left Portovenere, on the coast east of Genoa, accompanying Boucicaut, who was sailing to Rome, as captain of one of his galleys; but Boucicaut was blown onto the coast at Motrone in Northern Tuscany and then returned to Provence.[58] At some point between 5 July and 26 August 1408 Lescure was in Venice with a large retinue, requesting permission to arm a galley and to sail to Rhodes in company with the Venetian merchant galleys; he was thought in Venice to have an annual income of 40,000 ducats and was treated with great honour there.[59] Lescure seems next to have returned to Cyprus to report on the marriage negotiations; at any rate he and two Hospitaller brethren accompanying him left Rhodes for the West with yet another licence dated at Rhodes on 20 November 1408.[60] On 10 January 1409 the Venetian authorities agreed to a request from Lescure, who had presumably reached Venice and who was acting for King Janus, for the transit from Venice to Cyprus of Charlotte de Bourbon;[61] she married the king by proxy at Melun in France on 2 August 1409.[62] Meanwhile a general council, which opened at Pisa on 25 March 1409 and which was attended by the Master of the Hospital Fr Philibert de Naillac, elected a new pope, Alexander V, on 26 June; this achievement accelerated the movement towards unity within the Hospital, a development which was consolidated at a chapter-general of the Order which met at Aix-en-Provence in April and May 1410. There Lescure was elected as one of three magistral lieutenants who presided over the chapter, and on 21 May he was appointed both to negotiate with certain schismatic Hospitallers and also

---

[56]*Livre des Fais*, pp. 344–363, with much detail. The *Livre* spoke of *Vienne* or *Viegne*, but the registers had *Vogon* or *Vigon*: Malta, Cod. 334, f. 56; Cod. 339 f. 233. Belleville is in the district of Villefranche (Rhône).

[57]Malta, Cod. 334, f. 56.

[58]*Livre des Fais*, pp. 374–375. Lescure and others founded a hospital or hospice at Toulouse in 1408: text in M. du Bourg, *Histoire du Grand-Prieuré de Toulouse* (Toulouse, 1883), pièces justicatives, pp. xvii–xviii (wrongly dated 1413 and 1508).

[59]L. Dorez (ed.), *Chronique d'Antonio Morosini: Extraits relatifs à l'Histoire de la France*, I (Paris, 1898), p. 240.

[60]Malta, Cod. 334, f. 45v; Lescure's return to Cyprus in 1408 has been overlooked.

[61]Text in Mas Latrie, II, pp. 494–495.

[62]Hill, II, p. 466.

to reform the Hospital's Treasury.[63] Lescure was apparently on Rhodes on 15 March 1411.[64] On 6 June 1411, again at Lescure's request, the Venetians advanced the departure date of two galleys destined for Beirut so that they could take Charlotte de Bourbon to Cyprus.[65] Lescure was said to have accompanied her to Cyprus where she was married to Janus on 25 August 1411; he may in fact have travelled with her from Rhodes rather than from France or Venice.[66]

Lescure, like Ceva, paid the Cypriot responsions but not always on time or in full. He too was able to advance funds to the Master and Convent. At the time of his return to France the Hospital's Treasurer in the West was instructed on 22 November 1408 to repay Lescure 1000 francs; in the register this was then altered to 1500 francs, changed back to 1000, and finally crossed out. By 1 February 1409 Lescure had recently advanced 4000 ducats to the Master's lieutenant on Rhodes, who lent the money to the Order; 2400 ducats of this was to be recouped by Lescure out of the future responsions he would owe for Cyprus.[67] On 26 September 1409 the same lieutenant, Fr Jean de Claret, was instructed urgently to send, on the first Venetian galleys leaving Cyprus, both the responsions for the year 1408/09 and 750 ducats as a composition for earlier arrears still owing, but a year later on 22 October 1410 the lieutenant of the Master at Rhodes was complaining to Lescure that the Venetian galleys had brought little from Lescure's proctors on Cyprus who refused to make any payment without Lescure's mandate; Lescure was called upon to send the necessary instructions at once. Finally on 20 November 1410 the Master's lieutenant quit Lescure for a total of 9000 ducats received, that was for 7500 ducats, at 32 *asperi* of Rhodes per ducat, making 12,000 florins of Rhodes which he owed for the Cypriot responsions at 6000 florins a year for the two years 1408/09 and 1409/10, plus 1500 ducats of arrears partly owed for Cyprus and partly for his Priory of Toulouse; of the 9000 ducats owing, he had paid 4000 ducats on or before 1 February 1409 and the remaining 5000 ducats by November 1410.[68] Some time before Lescure's death in about September 1411 he gave Fr Pierre Molezini of the Priory of Toulouse the administration of the Hospital's *domus* in Nicosia.[69]

---

[63]Delaville (1913), pp. 304–316.

[64]Two documents of Lescure copied, apparently with the erroneous date of 15 March 1412, in Malta, Cod. 339, f. 122–123; they show that he had the register of the Priory of Toulouse with him on Rhodes.

[65]Mas Latrie, II, p. 495 n. 1.

[66]Francesco Amadi, in R. de Mas Latrie (ed.), *Chroniques de Chypre d'Amadi et de Strambaldi*, 2 vols (Paris, 1891–93), I, p. 498, stated that Charlotte came to Cyprus accompanied by Lescure, Prior of Toulouse, and was married on 25 August 1411; Diomede Strambaldi, ibid., II, p. 265, added that Lescure, the *comandator de Cipro*, brought her *de Italia*.

[67]Malta, Cod. 334, f. 173, 174v–175v.

[68]Malta, Cod. 339, f. 144v–145, 196v, 219v.

[69]Malta, Cod. 339, f. 173–173v. During the earlier part of 1411 Lescure was governor and

The Commander of Cyprus had to deal with the local inhabitants and with the king. Thus on 30 July 1406 Fr. Antonio de Riva, Prior of Venice, Fr Jean de Claret, lieutenant of the Commandery of Cyprus, and a certain Johannes de Plesente were empowered to settle in the royal court a dispute with the noble Philippus *Dyscolaunery* over lands in the Commandery of Phinikas and Anoyira.[70] On 21 February 1410 King Janus requested that the sister of Theodore Sozomeno, Bailiff of Commerce at Nicosia, be permitted to go with her children to live in Cyprus, a request granted at Rhodes on 26 October.[71] Some time before 25 September 1411 Fr Raymond de Lescure was killed fighting the Turks at Makri and on 1 October the king exempted the Hospital from its annual obligation to pay the royal *dime* or tenth, listing barley, linen, cotton, beans, peas, carrots, sesame, almonds, olives and other items, including 10 quintars, 18 ratals and 9 onques of sugar, 6 quintars, 96 ratals of *calamela* or sugar molasses, and 2526 besants in cash. On 3 October, following the death of Fr Jean de *Vigon*, who had been Commander of Belleville as well as of Phinikas and Anoyira and who presumably had also been killed at Makri, the king made similar annulments for the Commandery of Phinikas and for that of Templos; Phinikas and Anoyira had owed lesser quantities of similar items, including 2 quintars, 25 ratals and 6 onques of sugar and 1 quintar, 28 ratals and 6 onques of molasses. Phinikas and Anoyira had owed 251 besants and so had Templos; those amounts were one fifth of what was owed by the main or grand commandery. On 15 December the Lieutenant Master at Rhodes wrote thanking the king and announcing that, in response to a royal request, the Convent had written urging the Master, then in the West, to grant Phinikas and Anoyira to someone unnamed.[72]

Fr Raymond de Lescure, together with other Hospitallers and a certain Viscount *Dacy*, was killed by the Turks in an attack on Makri on the Turkish mainland shortly before 25 September 1411; they were probably engaged in an otherwise unknown Cypriot expedition.[73] Lescure had played a leading role in Janus' policies which may have furthered the Hospital's interests, and at the time of his death the king owed him 12,000 Venetian

---

administrator of the Hospital's Treasury (Cod. 337, f. 134) but his movements are unknown.

[70]Malta, Cod. 333, f. 127v.

[71]Malta, Cod. 339, f. 168v–169 (text *infra*, p. 20).

[72]Malta, Cod. 339, f. 232v, 233, 234v–235 (two latter texts in Mas Latrie, II, pp. 499–502).

[73]A letter of Janus of 1 October 1411 mentioned that Lescure's death was known by 25 September: Malta, Cod. 339, f. 232v (text in Mas Latrie, II, pp. 498–499). A Hospitaller text of 21 April 1412 stated that he was cruelly killed in battle fought against the Turks *vnacum suis militibus socijs ac fratribus nostre religionis*: Cod. 339, f. 239v. Another Hospitaller text, of 11 November 1413, said that he had died at Makri (Fetiye) with other Hospitallers and seculars: Cod. 339, f. 247. The unidentified Viscount *dacy* or *d'acy* is mentioned in Lyons, Archives départementales du Rhône, 48 H pièce 1.

ducats.[74] After some dispute over the succession to the commandery, it transpired that the king had paid 6000 ducats to Alexander V's successor, the new Pope John XXIII whom the Hospital had recognised, in order to purchase the expectation of the commandery for his seven-year-old natural son Louis de Lusignan. The Hospitallers on Rhodes, deprived of their richest benefice, actually threatened to leave Rhodes and in 1414 they recalled all their brethren from Cyprus in a bitter dispute with the crown which dragged on until 1421.[75]

At stake in many of these issues was the wealth derived from the Hospital's sugar plantations. The Order had held Kolossi, the main centre of production, since 1210, and may well have been growing sugar there in the thirteenth century. The levels of responsions expected from the commandery, which stood at 10,000 florins a year in 1317, and the total estimated income of 20,000 florins in 1329[76] suggest a considerable output of sugar. In 1343 the commander delivered 571 ratals or about 1300 kilos of sugar worth 800 besants, maybe 190 florins, to a Catalan merchant at Famagusta, and thereafter sugar was mentioned from time to time;[77] in 1384 the commander excused himself for not visiting Pope Urban VI with the claim that he had to stay in Cyprus to harvest his sugar crop.[78] The protracted law suit of 1401 between the Cornaro family of Episkopi and the Hospital at Kolossi over the use of river water, a matter which the crown had already adjudicated in the Hospital's favour some twenty-seven years earlier, also implied a considerable production.[79] Since in 1411 the various commanderies owed a royal *desme* or tithe of some 210 quintars or 4600 kilos of sugar and mollasses, their total production must have been very much greater than that. Much later, in 1464, the estimated total was about 800 quintars a year.[80]

*
* *

There was at least one Western source which reflected something of Rhodian-Cypriot relations in this period. That was the quasi-historical fairy

[74]Malta, Cod. 346, f. 165v.

[75]Details in Delaville (1913), pp. 319–321, 324–325; Hill, II, pp. 461–464.

[76]*Supra*, p. 2.

[77]Luttrell (1992), IX, pp. 165, 172, 184.

[78]Luttrell (1978), XXIII, p. 43.

[79]Text of 19 August 1401 summarised in Mas Latrie, II, pp. 455–456; text of 31 August 1406 in H. Noiret, *Documents inédits pour servir à l'Histoire de la Domination venétienne en Crète de 1380 à 1485* (Paris, 1892), pp. 167–174.

[80]Mas Latrie, III, pp. 86–90; cf. A. Luttrell, 'The Sugar Industry and its Importance for the Economy of Cyprus during the Frankish Period', in *The Development of the Cypriot Economy from the Prehistoric Period to the Present Day* (Nicosia, 1996).

story about *Mélusine*, the mermaid Lusignan princess, written during 1392 and 1393 by Jean d'Arras.[81] His sources for Rhodian events are not known. He could not have found his information in the known writings of Jean de Mandeville, Jean Froissart, Guillaume Machaut or Philippe de Mézières.[82] Froissart's knowledge of Eastern affairs was extraordinarily confused,[83] but Guillaume Machaut was better informed, and was perhaps even the author of a lost earlier version of *Mélusine* written before 1358, probably between 1342 and 1356.[84] Jean d'Arras had extensive access to courts, libraries and chronicles, and he could have spoken with Philippe de Mézières, the former Chancellor of Cyprus and companion of Pierre I de Lusignan, or with Leo VI, the exiled Lusignan king of Cilician Armenia who was in Paris from 1384 to 1393. Furthermore, in 1382 a Jean d'Arras was occupying a house at Arras for which he paid dues to the Hospitallers;[85] and, if that tenant was indeed the author of *Mélusine*, he could have received some information about the East from some Hospitaller who had been there. Any genuine Rhodian events reflected in *Mélusine* must, of course, have occurred between the Hospitaller conquest of the island in 1309 circa and the fall in 1375 of the Armenian kingdom which figured prominently in the story.

In outline, the Rhodian aspects of *Mélusine* are that her sons Urian and Guion, who are to become Kings of Cyprus and Armenia, sail from La Rochelle to defend Cyprus and find two Hospitaller vessels fighting many Mamluks who are attacking Famagusta. The Mamluks use a captured Rhodian *vaissel* as a fireship but are defeated. Urian and Guion go to Rhodes and give the Hospitallers the ships known as *fustes* which they have captured; they are received with a great feast after which the Master sends a force of Hospitaller brethren with about six galleys, troops and crossbowmen, to the aid of Cyprus. They sail to the isle of *Coles* or *Collos*, possibly near Gorighos in Cilicia, the Master travelling on Urian's galley. The Hospitallers participate in a great victory and the Master leads the entry into Famagusta; the Master then sails to Damascus, Beirut, Tripoli and Damietta. Following a new victory, the Hospital is given two captured *nefs* and also 100 Muslim prisoners to exchange for Hospitaller brethren and others

---

[81] Text in L. Stouff, *Mélusine: Roman du XIVe siècle par Jean d'Arras* (Dijon, 1932), and study in idem, *Essai sur Mélusine Roman du XIVe siècle par Jean d'Arras* (Dijon–Paris, 1930); bibliography in J. le Goff and E. le Roy Ladurie, 'Mélusine maternelle et défricheuse', *Annales: Économies, Sociétés, Civilisations*, XXVI (1971).

[82] For the sources and contacts, Stouff (1930), pp. 43–71.

[83] A. Luttrell, 'Latin Responses to Ottoman Expansion before 1389', in E. Zachariadou (ed.), *The Ottoman Emirate: 1300–1389*, (Rethymnon, 1993), pp. 132–133.

[84] R. Nolan, 'The Roman de Mélusine: Evidence for an Early Missing Version', *Fabula*, XV, (1974).

[85] J. Baudot, *Les Princesses Yolande et les Ducs de Bar de la Famille des Valois*, part 1: *Mélusine* (Paris, 1900), p. 257.

taken at sea by the Turks of Karaman. Next the Hospitallers are sent to *Cruq*, also possibly Gorighos, and the Master goes with 100 brethren first to Cyprus and then to Armenia. The sultan forms a great alliance stretching from North Africa to Kurdistan and swears to destroy first Rhodes and then Armenia and Cyprus, but the Hospital is warned by an Arabic-speaking spy who learns the news and takes it to Beirut and thence to Rhodes on a ship bound for *Turquie*. The Master writes to warn the Kings of Cyprus and Armenia, and the latter reaches Rhodes with his army. 4000 men, including Hospitaller knights and *freres sergens d'armes*, various adventurers and 600 or 700 crossbowmen, reach Jaffa. The Master commands a division in various battles; the Latins cry 'Lusegnen et Saint Jehan de Rodes' and 'Rodes et Lusegnen'. There are naval victories, but with losses; the Muslims pay tribute; the Master visits Jerusalem and Armenia; and then there are four days of feasting at Rhodes.[86]

Most of this account was fantasy, though certain details rang true. The Hospitallers had provided some help to the Lusignans of Armenia between 1291 and about 1324 and again in 1346 or 1347,[87] and in 1374 the Master did go to Cyprus where he died, but that was to negotiate with the Genoese and not to oppose the infidel.[88] There was Hospitaller participation, first in the Cypriot crusade which in 1365 assembled at Rhodes and then sailed with four Hospitaller galleys and 100 Hospitaller brethren to sack Alexandria in Egypt; and, secondly, in the Cypriot campaigns along the Southern Anatolian and Syrian coasts during 1367 in which the Hospitaller Turcopolier was killed at Tripoli.[89] It was also true that, as in 1403 when the Master received news of the movements of Timur in Anatolia, the Hospital had spies on the Muslim mainland.[90] However, none of this was of the scale or intensity suggested by Jean d'Arras, in whose work the Master continually played a leading role in councils of war and military actions. Jean d'Arras was writing a dynastic fairy story in which he combined some notions of Hospitaller activities in an exaggerated mixture of fantasy and veracity, twisting elements of Cypriot history and conflating its personalities.[91] His

---

[86]Stouff (1932), pp. 82, 88–94, 98, 101, 108, 111, 123–144, 213–221, 227–230, 235–238. Baudot, p. 258, suggests that the island of *Coles* or *Collos* represented Kolossi on Cyprus.

[87]A. Luttrell, *Latin Greece, the Hospitallers and the Crusades: 1291–1440* (London, 1982), V, pp. 121–130; the Hospitallers seem to have sent some help to Armenia in 1346 or 1347, but there is no evidence for the notion in Stouff (1930), p. 109, that they 'purged' Armenia of the infidel.

[88]Luttrell (1992), IX, p. 174.

[89]Delaville (1913), pp. 152–160; Luttrell (1992), II, p. 95. Stouff (1930), p. 102, wrongly states that it was the Master who took the Hospitallers to Gorighos in 1367.

[90]Luttrell (1992), II, p.100.

[91]Apart from Stouff (1930), pp. 106–110, only Baudot, pp. 189–247 *et passim*, really discusses the Hospitallers' appearances in *Mélusine*. Baudot, p. 258, regards the place given in the story to the Hospitallers as 'excessive'.

Mélusine presented a certain Western image of Eastern affairs; perhaps Jean de Boucicaut had read it before 1403. The historical reality which the inventions of Jean d'Arras did reflect was that of a community of interests between the Hospitallers and the Lusignans. This collaboration continued to be fundamental to the Hospitallers since Cyprus formed a bulwark between Rhodes and the Mamluks, while it was also important to the Hospital on account the sugar plantations centred on Kolossi. During the years after 1386 the Hospital's difficulties in Cyprus lay in the problems provoked by the papal schism, by the Genoese and by the increasing instability of Lusignan government.

DOCUMENT

Malta, Cod. 339, f. 168v-169 (Nicosia, 21 February 1410: Rhodes, 26 October 1410)

Frater Domenicus de Alamania sacre domus hospitalis sancti Johannis Jherusalem preceptor sancti Stephanj prope Monopolum et locumtenens Reuerendissimi in Christo patris et dominj dominj fratris Philibertj de Nelihaco dei gracia dicte sacre domus magistrj dignissimj, et pauperum Christi custodis Ceterique bailliuj priores et procheres conuentus Rodj in consilio congregati vniuersis et singulis ad quos presentes peruenerint, Salutem et sinceram in domino caritatem. notum facemus quatenus Nicolaus Rotondo burgensis et habitator Rodj in conspectu nostrj locumtenentis et consillij literas Serenissimj et Illustrissimj dominj dominj Jennij dei gracia Regis Cipri et Jherusalem presentauerat sigillatas ipsius Serenissimj dominj regis sigillo cuius tenor talis est // Treschers et bien ames nostre ame et feal Thodre Sozomeno baillj de nostre comerchi de Nicosia nous a donne entendre que Fenne Sozomeno suer de cellui Thodre et espouze de Nicola Rotondo a present demorente en Rodes du consentiment de celluj Rotondo est envolente de venir habiter a nostre Royaume de Chippre et demorer entre ses parens de pardessa, Et comme auons entendu celle Fenne ne puet partir de Rodes sans auoir Vostre bonne licence pource vous prions affectueusement que pour amor et contemplacion de nous jcelle Fenne auecques ses enfans soufres et laissies venir pardessa sans lui donne aucun empachement Et vous nous feres singulier plaisir prester de auons conplaire en semblables et plus grans choses dieu soit garde de vous. donne a Nicosia le xxᵉj jour de feurier .m. iiijᶜ. ix // Indorso vero ipsius litere erant descripta uerba subsequentes // A nos th[re]scher et bien ames les baillis et conseil du conuent de Rodes // Janus par la dieu gracia Roy de Jherusalem de Chipre et dArmenia.

Quibus litteris visis et intelectis ob contemplationem ipsius Serenissimj dominj Regis Cipri tibj Nicolao predicto cum tua vxore tuisque filijs et bonis eundj recedendj de insulla Rodj et redeundj et cohabitandj si tibj placuerit in insulla Cipri auctoritate presentium damus et concedimus licenciam et parabollam omni contradictione cesante. In cuius rey testimonium sigillum nostrj dicti locumtenentis quo vtimur presentibus in ciera viridj est appesum. datum in prefato conuentu Rodj die vigesima sexta octobris millesimo Anno Incarnacionis dominj quatercentessimo decimo

VI

The Building of the Castle of the Hospitallers at Bodrum

(i) Hospitaller Policy in Anatolia: 1291-1421

The Hospital of St. John of Jerusalem was founded in Syria at the time of the First Crusade and gradually became military in character, acquiring extensive properties, privileges and exemptions in the Christian West which helped to make it a major power in Latin Syria. After the fall of Acre in 1291 the Hospitallers withdrew to Cyprus, but this proved an unsatisfactory base from which to continue that armed religious warfare which gave the military orders their principal *raison d'être*. In the decades following 1291 the Hospitallers sent several expeditions to Cilician Armenia, where they continued to make occasional interventions until the Armenian kingdom fell to the Mamluks in 1375. In 1306 the Order initiated the conquest of the offshore island of Rhodes and thereafter the island was governed in effective independence by the Hospitallers, whose power was in theory limited only by their subjection to the pope. In reality the Hospital depended on its resources and manpower from the West, and it had to justify the continued retention of its Western lands and incomes by an appearance of military activity; this made the Order particularly susceptible to papal pressures for it actively to combat the Turks.[1]

Technically Rhodes had formed part of Byzantium but during the decade before 1306 it had been ravaged, and perhaps even partly occupied, by the Turks of the Emirate of Menteshe on the coasts opposite Rhodes. In the years following the conquest the Hospitallers defeated the Turks at sea and there is considerable evidence that they also occupied certain unidentified places on the mainland during the period until about 1344. A contemporary chronicle stated that the Hospitallers "reduced to their obedience several places in Turkey which gave them tribute."[2] A brief official compilation of obituaries reported that they captured from the Turks and held "many castles in Turkey."[3] An appeal issued in Rhodes on 14 May 1313 called for settlers to inhabit places taken from Greeks and from Turks "both in the islands and on the mainland."[4] Ludolf de Sudheim, who was in the East between 1336 and 1341, also mentioned that the Hospital held "a small

and very powerful castle in Turkey."[5] There is no evidence as to whereabouts along a very considerable stretch of coast this castle may have been.[6] The Hospitallers initially captured the island of Kos, but they lost control of it some time before 1319 and did not recover it until about 1336[7] so that it is unlikely that the Hospital held the nearby site of Halikarnassos during that period, though the possibility cannot entirely be excluded.[8]

The Hospital had already played a considerable role in bottling up the naval aggression of the Anatolian emirates when in 1344 a Latin crusade captured the castle by the sea in Smyrna harbour from the Emir of Aydin. Thenceforth the Order was increasingly involved in the problems and expenses of the garrison and fortification of Smyrna castle, and in 1374 the pope made the castle's defence the sole responsibility of the Hospital which was to receive a papal subsidy for it. These difficulties were aggravated after 1378 by the schism in the papacy, and after 1389 by the conquests of the Ottomans on the mainland opposite Rhodes which allowed them to attack the Latins at sea in the Aegean. By 1391 the Ottoman ruler Bayazid had subdued the Emirates of Aydin and Menteshe, and much of the rest of Anatolia had been conquered by 1400. The Hospitallers had to restrict the perimeter of the castle at Smyrna; they rejected an Ottoman ultimatum towards the beginning of 1393 and successfully resisted attacks on the fortress by Bayazid, who also cut off the annual grain shipments from the mainland to Rhodes and to the other Latin islands. In July 1402, however, Bayazid was defeated and captured near Ankara by the Mongol khan Timur, who then marched on Smyrna and in December blocked the harbour, mined the walls and destroyed the Latin castle; survivors of the Hospitaller garrison escaped by sea.[9] A Western source stated that the Hospitallers themselves estimated that it would cost more than 100,000 gold florins to rebuild the castle.[10] The brethren were left with no outpost on the Turkish mainland which would help to justify their Western privileges and wealth, and they stood to lose the incomes from the sales of the papal indulgences granted in 1390 for the defence of Smyrna; these had brought in several thousand florins a year,[11] a significant sum when the average annual income from the West apparently stood at around 38,500 florins.[12] The establishment of a castle at Bodrum may have been in part an attempt to repair this financial loss.

The chronology of the construction of Bodrum castle is uncertain. Its foundation followed Timur's capture of Smyrna in December 1402, and it could not, therefore, have been begun before 1403; work probably commenced in 1406 or 1407 and on 17 March 1408 the Master visited the castle and dated a document there *in nostro castro sancti petri in turquia.*[13] The major source for the building of St. Peter's is the Greek writer Doukas whose grandfather settled in Ephesus after 1346; Doukas first appears in Phocaea and he composed his confusing but valuable history between 1453 and about 1462.[14] Doukas explained how, after the battle at Ankara in 1402, Ephesus and Smyrna were disputed between Umur son of the Emir of Aydin and an upstart named Junayd. Strife among these Turks and the struggle among Bayazid's sons continued for a decade. In a later passage, Doukas described how, at a moment which he wrongly implied had been in about 1415, Bayazid's son Mehmet went to Smyrna to oust Junayd. At Smyrna various Latin and Turkish leaders, including the Emir of Menteshe and the Master of the Hospital who had with him three galleys, "all came to make Mehmet obeisance and to offer him assistance in destroying the tyrant Junayd." The Master, who apparently assisted Mehmet in his capture of Smyrna from Junayd, had previously, against Junayd's wishes according to Doukas, been rebuilding the castle by the sea which had been destroyed by Timur and he had half completed an enormous tower at the harbour mouth. Mehmet had this razed, upon which the Master at once protested vehemently that the castle had originally been built at the Hospital's expense and that unless Mehmet allowed its reconstruction "there would be resentment between Mehmet's dominion and the most blessed pope; a great force would be despatched from the nations of the West which would destroy his realm." Mehmet replied that the destruction of the castle was considered to have been Timur's one good deed, for the castle had allowed the slaves of Ionia to escape to the Hospitallers who were the Turks' implacable enemies on land and sea, and therefore he could not allow its rebuilding:

"None the less, let us do as you wish but without annoying

the Turks. I offer you as much land as you require on the borders of Caria and Lycia. Go and build whatever kind of fortress you desire." After giving careful consideration to these words, the Grand Master replied to Mehmet, "Ruler, give me instead a portion of the lands under your dominion and do not send me to foreign provinces." Mehmet replied, "But I am giving you what is mine since I have awarded the province to Menteshe. Have no further concern." Requesting first a written decree, which he received, the Grand Master then departed.

Subsequently the Hospitallers constructed their castle at Bodrum, which is situated well to the south of Smyrna, Ephesus and Miletus, despite opposition from Ilyas, the Emir of Menteshe within whose lands the castle was built.[15]

Notwithstanding the chronological and other confusions so typical of Doukas, and indeed of many medieval and modern accounts of Anatolia in this chaotic period, much of this story rings true. The incidents cannot, however, date to 1415 as Doukas' account would imply; they must be placed between 1403 and 1407, since the castle certainly existed by early 1408. Once Timur had withdrawn to Samarkand, leaving the Ottomans in disorder, the Hospitallers would naturally have sought to safeguard their image in the West by reoccupying and refortifying Smyrna; the Turks would have been likely to oppose them; and Mehmet might well have proposed a compromise which involved moving the Hospitallers to territory not under Ottoman control. In order to establish a chronology for these events, it is necessary to consider them from both the Hospitaller and the Turkish viewpoints.

After the loss of Smyrna, the Hospitallers were engaged elsewhere. They were a party to the treaty which Bayazid's son Sulaiman, who had fled to the Balkans, made with the Christian powers in January or February 1403. In April it was reported that the Hospital had renewed its ancient truce with Miletus; that there were 400 soldiers at Rhodes en route for Cyprus; and that the Hospital was sending some ships and a small force to Clarenza in the Latin Principality of the Morea. From July to August 1403 the Master and Hospitaller galleys were campaigning on the Syrian and Cilician coasts. The Hospital was also defending Corinth and the Despotate of the Morea, which it did not evacuate until 1404.[16] It is unlikely that it was also active at Smyrna in that year and the Castilian Ruy González de Clavijo, who sailed northwards from Rhodes and stopped at Kos in September 1403, made no mention either of Bodrum castle or of Smyrna.[17] By 1405 the Hospitallers were free of their involvements in Greece and could look elsewhere for a field of action. That summer they proposed to build a castle at their own expense on the island of Tenedos in the Dardanelles, but the Venetians, who controlled the island, rejected the suggestion on 21 September;[18] this decision presumably reached Rhodes late in October. It was probably after that date, and definitely before 1408, that the Hospitallers attempted to restore their position at Smyrna and subsequently founded a fortress at Bodrum.

From the Turkish point of view, the destructions effected by Timur's forces in 1402 had disrupted Ottoman rule in Anatolia. Miletus and the Emirate of Menteshe passed to Ilyas, a nephew of its former emir, and the Emirate of Aydin to Isa and Umur, sons of its former emir. Isa and Umur, however, lost Smyrna and Ephesus to Junayd, and Isa was killed. Doukas described in detail how Umur appealed for help "to his uncle, Menteshe Ilyas Beg, the ruler of Caria," who marched to recapture Ephesus. Junayd sought aid from Bayazid's son Sulaiman, who was ruling Ottoman Europe; with Sulaiman's help he recaptured Ephesus, married Umur's daughter and, on Umur's death, became sole ruler of Aydin. The chronology and many of the details of these events, which depend upon Doukas' account, remain obscure, but Junayd's recapture of Ephesus probably occurred at the beginning of winter late in 1405. It was followed by struggles between Sulaiman and his brother Mehmet, who had come to Smyrna and subdued Junayd. Apparently early in 1406, Sulaiman left for Asia Minor and, according to Doukas, took Smyrna and attacked Ephesus; Junayd then went over to Sulaiman and they both departed for Europe. Then, probably in 1407, Sulaiman launched a new campaign in Asia.[19] By 2 September 1407 news had reached Venice that Sulaiman's fleet of twenty vessels had left Gallipoli both to attack Ephesus and Miletus and to build a walled fortress at Smyrna.[20]

If the incident in which Mehmet led a coalition against Junayd and razed the Hospitaller tower at Smyrna did occur roughly as described by Doukas, it must be dated not to 1415 but probably to a time in or before 1407, the most probable year of Sulaiman's defeat of Mehmet and the latest year in which the castle could have been begun. Assuming that Doukas really was describing an attack on Smyrna by the Ottoman Mehmet, and not that of Sulaiman in 1407, and that Doukas' chronology for events in Aydin from 1403 to 1406 was approximately correct, then it may well have been 1406 when Mehmet dismantled the Hospital's new tower at Smyrna. In any case, the Master was justified in protesting that

Caria, the region to the south of Aydin, was not within Mehmet's dominions, and Mehmet's claim to have awarded Menteshe to Ilyas was probably an empty one. Ilyas seems to have rejected Mehmet's award, for Doukas described how he "arrived with a large force" to prevent the Hospitallers from building the new castle at Bodrum.[21] There is evidence that the building of the castle involved fighting with the Turks,[22] but Doukas was definitely wrong to place the incident around 1415, though that was the moment at which the Ottoman Mehmet reduced Ilyas of Menteshe to tributary status.[23] Bodrum castle was probably begun in 1406 or 1407, but the exact date remains uncertain.

The new castle at Bodrum was clearly intended to replace the fortress at Smyrna and was given the same dedication to St. Peter. There is no evidence that the strategic position of Bodrum was, as is so often asserted, a particularly significant one.[24] The straits between Kos and Bodrum could perfectly well be controlled from Kos, and there is no reason to suppose that the construction of a castle on the out-of-the-way site at Bodrum assured the security of the whole Rhodian peninsula. Nor was there any question, as at Smyrna, of denying the Turks the use of a valuable port, for the site was almost completely unknown and was located on a barren waterless peninsula covered with scrub and stunted pines which had no notable settlement. This was probably its chief attraction; if the Hospital needed an outpost on the mainland, Bodrum offered not only a position which could be fortified strongly but also one that was so far from any mainland centre as not to provoke any massive reaction from the Turks. Furthermore it was very close to the strong castle on Kos from which it could be supplied and supported. The possession of a bridgehead on the mainland was probably a matter of propaganda and prestige for the Hospital. The castle also constituted a financial advantage, and in 1409 the Order secured a papal faculty to sell plenary indulgences to pay for its defence. Among those who lent money for the construction of the castle were Fr. Domenico de Alamania, Commander of San Stefano Monopoli, who advanced a loan *pro necessariis castri*, and Fr. Lodovico Vaignon, Admiral of the Order; mandates were issued early in 1409 for them both to be repaid.[25] The maintenance of a foothold on the mainland also had certain practical advantages. It allowed Christians and slaves to escape from Turkish rule,[26] a point emphasized by many travellers in their accounts of the dogs who acted as guides for escaping Christians.[27] It may also have provided an opportunity for a minor trade in items, such as grain or horses, needed by the Hospital.[28]

Unfortunately the most explicit and most closely contemporary evidence concerning the origins of the castle is found in Western documents which granted the Hospital a variety of benefits on account of its actions and expenses at St. Peter's and which are somewhat suspect, since they are evidently based on information provided by the Hospitallers who would naturally have tended to inflate their own achievements and losses in order to secure advantageous financial concessions. Thus on 30 July 1409 Pope Alexander V, newly elected in the council at Pisa, granted the Master Fr. Philibert de Naillac and the Hospital faculties to sell indulgences for five years. The Hospitallers had declared that they were so reduced as a result of the schism in the Church, by wars and plagues in the West and by the struggle in the East that they were unable to continue either the war against the Turks or their charitable activities. Special reference was made to the "capture" and construction of St. Peter's Castle "two years ago", that is in 1407, to the loss of manpower involved and to the 70,000 florins expended:

... quam propter captionem, constructionem, et edifica-tionem castri sancti Petri, quod dicti hospitalis fratres vi armorum, non sine magna strage et effusione sanguinis hominum in terra dicta Turcarum, a duobus annis citra, contra ipsos Turchos ceperunt, ad quod de hostium man-ibus fugientes Christi pauperes refugium saluberrimum habere noscuntur, indeque hostes ipsi permaxime impug-nantur, ad etiam reprimuntur, ipsumque suis repararunt, construxerunt, et edificarunt sumptibus et expensis, et ad ejus fortificationem constructionem, ac defensam, preter et ultra personas neci ibi expositas, consumpserunt usque ad summam septuaginta millium florenorum, ...[29]

This indulgence was confirmed at some date before 30 August 1412 by Alexander V's successor Pope John XXIII *pro augmentacione et reparatione et tuitione nostrj castrj sanctj petrj*.[30]

The founding of St. Peter's was also mentioned in a number of documents issued by the King of France to exempt the Hospital from various taxes. The earl-iest of these, dated 3 December 1408, declared:

lesdiz mastre et freres du conuent de Rodes depuis pou de temps enca ont prins et gaigne sur les mescreans en tur-quie certainne place a terre ferme ou ilz font fere et ediffier ung chastel appelle saint pierre pour illecques recueillir et receuoir les christiens prisonniers desdizs turqs quant ilz se pouuent eschaper de leurs mains, Et que pour ledit chastel faire construire et bastir il leur a conuenu et con-uient chacun jour fere grandes mises et despens ...

A number of French Hospitallers had sailed from Aigues Mortes in October to defend the castle.[31] A later royal exemption of 23 June 1414 referred to the effects of war and schism, claiming that while the Hospital had lost more than half its incomes it had great expenses:

attendu les dictes grans frais et charges quilz ont continu a supporter pour la garde et deffense de nostre foy christ-ienne et mesmement pour la garde et deffense du chastel saint pierre quilz ont puis peu de temps enca conqueste sur les mescreans de nostre foy, En quoy ilz ont expose frays et despendu plus de cent mil frans, ...[32]

Yet another exemption, of 26 July 1416, made simil-ar claims and spoke of the reduction in income due to non-payments in lands obedient to Pope Benedict XIII; again there was a brief reference to St. Peter's as *acquis sur les mescreans a grans frais mises et despens*.[33] It was believed, at least in the West, that the site at Bodrum had been taken from the Turks by force and with considerable losses and that the castle had been constructed and defended at a cost of 70,000 florins or, later, of more than 100,000 francs. However, according to the Greek chronicler Doukas and the pilgrim Felix Faber, the fighting occurred after the building of the fortress had begun.[34] Whether these royal and papal texts really constitute reliable evid-ence for the existence of any Turkish fortifications at Bodrum before 1407 is very doubtful. If Turkish resistance occurred only after the Hospital's castle was partly built, then presumably there were no Turkish defences of any substance on the site before 1407, though there may well have been a small com-munity of Greeks and Turks living amid the ruins of the ancient city and they may have offered some initial opposition to the Hospitallers. Even if there was resistance in 1407 there may have been no fort-ifications, and if there were towers or walls they were not necessarily on the castle site on the peninsula but would more probably have been on the mainland where, later in the fifteenth century, the Turks were certainly were established in some strength.[35]

The Castle of St. Peter was scarcely a major thorn in Turkish flesh. Indeed on 14 December 1409 its Captain was instructed to remain strictly on the defensive inside the fortress and to put a stop to the dangerous and provocative practice of skirmishing with the Turks – *ad belum seu ad scarmucam cum turcis.* There were problems with the mercenaries or *stipendarii* in the garrison in 1409 and even, in 1412, a quarrel between the Captain and certain Hospital-lers. The troops must have had lodgings within the walls of the castle, and in 1416 the Treasury of the

Hospital was licensed to sell a house there. In 1409 the yearly expenses at Bodrum were 6000 ducats for the *stipendarii* and 1000 ducats for the Hospitallers stationed there.[36] During these years Ilyas, Emir of Menteshe, was making piratical sorties from Miletus.[37] On 24 July 1410 the Venetians were prepared to send a fleet either to compel the Turks of Ephesus and Miletus to make peace or to destroy them, suggesting that the Rhodian galley should also participate.[38] The Hospitallers seem, in fact, to have intervened a little further to the south. In about 1411 the Prior of Toulouse, Fr. Raymond de Lescure, was killed along with several other Hospitallers and with others who included the Viscount *dacy* while fighting the Turks at Makri, the modern Fetiye, which was part of the Emirate of Menteshe.[39] At the end of 1411 the Hospital was at peace with the Turks *de jurisdictione altologj ubi pacem habemus*, that is with Ephesus, but other Turks were reported on 8 January 1412 to be near the Castle of St. Peter and ready to attack it; these were thought to be of the "Emirate of *Palatia*", that is of Miletus, and presumably they were men of Ilyas of Menteshe who ruled Miletus.[40] On 15 January essential supplies and the Hospital's "guard galley" were being sent to the castle, the galley being given the task of defending Syme and the other islands which had been ravaged by certain "Turks" whose origin was not indicated.[41] The Hospital practised its own brand of piracy and St. Peter's Castle was used as a base. Early in 1412 the *galiotta* armed by the men of the castle at Bodrum seized a "Turkish" *galiotta* at Lesbos since the peace with the Turks held good only on land but not at sea outside the Dardanelles, and this led the Hospital into quarrels with the Latins of Lesbos.[42] The *galiotta* armed at the castle by its garrison, the *consocii et marinarii*, also attacked a *grippus* from Chios, and as a result the Hospitallers at Rhodes had to return the goods seized and to explain that they had constructed the Castle of St. Peter in order to attack the infidel and not "for assaulting other Christians."[43]

The balance of power in Anatolia was shifting. Bayazid's son Sulaiman was killed in 1411 and his brother Musa then attacked Thessalonika and Constantinople; in July 1412 Musa defeated another brother Mehmet, whose power was very firmly based in Asia; and Musa himself was subsequently killed by Mehmet's soldiers on 5 July 1413.[44] On 1 February 1413 the Hospital was seeking help from Cyprus after receiving a report that Musa had prepared thirty galleys which, it was pretended, were meant to attack Constantinople or Thessalonika but which the Hospitallers feared would attack them.[45]

On 13 February the Hospital was proposing urgently to arm two galleys and to reconstitute the league with Chios, Lesbos and others, while help was sought from the rulers of Cyprus, Crete and Naxos.[46] Musa's fleet must in fact have been directed against his brother Mehmet who, after defeating Musa, spread his power over Anatolia.[47] In about April 1415 Mehmet repeated a request that two Hospitaller galleys should assist the Ottomans against *Jannici de Altoloco*, presumably Junayd of Ephesus, and against Mehmet's other Turkish enemies, who presumably included Ilyas. The Hospital's "guard galley" was at Chios and the Hospitallers at Rhodes reacted evasively; Chios was at peace with the Turks on land and sea while the Hospital was at peace with them on land, and the Captain of the Hospitaller galleys was therefore instructed to reply to Mehmet that he was guarding the sea against a possible escape of Mehmet's enemies.[48] By 26 April 1415 the Hospitallers had decided that Mehmet had subjugated all *Turquia* and *Grecia* except the Emirate of "Miletus", that is of Ilyas, and that the Hospital was at peace with Mehmet and all the other eastern infidels; they concluded from this that the time was ripe for an attack on the Mamluks of Egypt and Syria.[49] By March 1416 Ilyas had been reduced to tributary status by Mehmet,[50] but there were still rumours of danger and a document of Charles VI issued at Paris on 26 July 1416 spoke of a great fleet with which Mehmet was ravaging the Aegean and which was expected to attack Rhodes or the Castle of St. Peter.[51] This fleet was defeated off Gallipoli by the Venetians in June. The Hospital none the less retained, and doubtless continued to strengthen, St. Peter's Castle until the first period of its history came to a close in 1421, when Fr. Philibert de Naillac, who had been Master of Rhodes since 1396, and Ilyas, who had been Emir of Menteshe since about 1403, both died, as also did the Sultan Mehmet.

(ii) Possible pre-1407 Structures[52]

The peninsula of Zephyria on which the castle was built formed a natural defensive site and the written sources suggest that it was fortified as an akropolis on the initiative of Maussollos. It was sufficiently strong for the Persians to defend for some time when Alexander had captured the rest of the town in 334 BC, and by that time a channel had been cut across the natural rock of the narrow isthmus which may have stood rather higher above sea-level than it does now.[53] A small trial excavation in the centre of the site revealed a stretch of ancient wall in isodomic work described as "perhaps of the fourth century BC, easily recognizable as a large terrace wall;" this is visible beneath the modern Underwater Archaeology Museum.[54] A similar stretch of wall stands nearby, while in the adjoining area some slabs of Green Lava stone have been noticed clamped together and still *in situ*. In the same area, also *in situ*, is a small patch of tessellated flooring datable to the fourth century AD or later.[56] Along the south and east sides of the peninsula are the footings for a double line of Hellenistic walling which were cut into the rock and are still clearly visible a few metres above sea-level.[57] Some of the vast cisterns may also be ancient in origin. At no point, however, is there any clear sign that parts of the medieval fortifications incorporated ancient work which was still *in situ*, though this may well have happened. Most probably the Hospitallers found piles of ancient stone; they may have built on classical foundations; and conceivably they dismantled any surviving stretches of the Hellenistic outer walling in order to build their own initial works at the summit of the site.

Byzantine and subsequent Turkish tenure of the town presumably involved some occupation of the peninsula. Byzantine life in the town probably consisted of the continued use of any surviving classical buildings and the construction of at least one church or monastery. There is no clear evidence that the Hospitallers' earliest towers and walls were either Byzantine or Turkish in origin, though again this is not impossible, nothing definite being known about any Turkish presence in Bodrum before 1407; there is only a faint possibility that there was pre-1407 Hospitaller work there.[58] The idea of a pre-1407 Turkish castle was advanced by Pullan, who thought that those stretches of the main castle walls which are built of enormous Hellenistic blocks were pre-Hospitaller work in which the Turks had re-used ancient materials probably taken from the town walls. Pullan referred to the main south wall, the lower parts of the east and west walls, and to a portion of the north-east angle where the lowest six metres of walling is in Green Lava stone. For Pullan "this proves that the Knights were not the first to destroy the Mausoleum for the sake of building materials."[59] This is mere speculation. These walls could in theory have been Hellenistic work still *in situ* but the joins and rearrangements in the stonework, especially at the foot of the west wall, suggest that

the stones were re-used classical pieces; this re-use could, however, have been the work of the Hospitallers rather than of the Turks, and indeed it probably occurred at a comparatively late stage in the post-1421 construction sequence.[60] Pullan's theory about the Green Lava stone assumes that all such stone must have come from the Maussolleion, which is by no means the case;[61] that there was a Turkish castle, which seems unlikely; and that the outermost north-east works were part of the original Hospitaller castle, which they clearly were not, the earliest work in that area being at Tower E which is almost certainly datable to 1407/21.[62] And since the main east wall is built around Tower E, that wall is presumably post-1407 and not Hellenistic.

Maiuri used a quite different reasoning for his argument, which was that the Hospitallers re-used or simply adopted pieces of existing work which Maiuri sometimes called Byzantine, sometimes Turkish. Maiuri was a distinguished classical archaeologist who saw the castle in a state of damage and disrepair in 1919 when such work may have been more easily distinguishable, but his assumption was based only on the evidence of the stonework and on the re-used Arabic inscriptions which he mistakenly thought were Seljuk; and as an Italian he may subconsciously have rejected certain clumsy pieces of building as being unworthy of Latin authorship.[63] The early Arabic inscriptions are not *in situ*; they were built into the castle in and after 1497, and presumably came from a building in the town. Maiuri's thesis must therefore rest on an analysis of the building itself. He postulated pre-1407 work in:

(i)   the wall running south from the French Tower;
(ii) the inner east side of the double west curtain, especially in the north-west and south-west corners of the outer keep;
(iii) Tower D and Gate 3;
(iv) Tower G;
(v)   Tower H;
(vi) the work below the guardhouse approached through Gate 4.

Maiuri regarded (i) and (iv) as Byzantine, and (iii), (v) and (vi) as Seljuk, concluding that the Hospitallers re-used a Byzantine castle and, in part, "a fortress of the Seljuk period of the eleventh-twelfth century."[64] It remains to examine his six sections and with them (vii) the French Tower itself, remembering that there is no other firm evidence for any Byzantine or Seljuk fortress.

(i)   The wall running southwards from the French

Tower is very crudely constructed, much of it having been rebuilt. None of its stones is particularly large; it contains a considerable quantity of tile and pottery, and in the stretch adjacent to the French Tower there is even some Green Lava stone which is presumably datable post-1494.[65] The wall is not bonded into the French Tower, and it contains two shields datable 1433/5 [cvii, cviii]. A pre-1407 origin seems unlikely though possible.

(ii) The east side of the west curtain, which was later thickened to the west, has only one shield on it; it is in the lower passageway at its extreme north and is datable 1421/54 [xcix a]. The east face of this wall is obscured with post-1522 rebuilding and plaster, and its southern section is now built over; the north-ernmost stretch is crudely built, or rebuilt, with tile. A pre-1407 origin remains unproven.

(iii) Tower D, which is the round Maritime Tower, the wall to its east and Gate 3 are all of one build and are datable pre-1421. The tower and adjoining wall are constructed of clumsy but not irregular courses of thick, large stones, with no use of tile and pottery. At Rhodes there were three round towers, the Tower of St. Paul, the Tower of St. Peter and the Tower of the Mills, all three probably datable to the mid-fifteenth century, though none of them is really similar to the solid Tower D; two of them had interior vaulted chambers and two stood in front of their curtain wall while the other was sited on a mole.[66] There is no com-pelling reason to date Tower D, the adjoining wall or Gate 3 before 1407.

(iv) Tower G, datable pre-1412, is a round tower built with irregular courses and a great deal of tile and pottery, especially on the interior; it has been considerably rebuilt and obscured with plaster, and its two chambers now have domed roofing. It could date before 1407, but there is no indication that it did.

(v) Tower H, which seems to be datable 1421/40, is square and very crudely built or rebuilt with unequal and clumsy stones, irregular courses, and much use of tile (Plate V). It is not unlike Turkish work, for example that at Pechin some 40 kilometres north-east of Bodrum (Plate VI), and it could well be pre-1407, but its origin remains unproven.

(vi) The guardhouse approached through Gate 4 has walls which look much like those of Tower H and of the French Tower, but they are of clumsy work with much tile and so heavily repaired, partly with Green Lava stone pre-sumably datable post-1494, that they cannot confidently be attributed to any period.

(vii) The French Tower, datable 1407/15, is very untidily built with irregular courses of not very large stones and with much use of tile, while the walls have a rough rubble core with a heavy use of mortar (Plate IV). It could be pre-1407, but there is no evidence that it was.[67]

It would be a reasonable supposition that the Hospitallers in and after 1407 found and utilized earlier structures or ruins, conceivably Towers G and H and the French Tower; there is also a slight possibility that there was a Hospitaller occupation and some construction work in the early fourteenth century. However, there is no proof for such hypoth-eses, and Doukas' story that the Hospitallers took building materials to Bodrum and constructed the castle from its foundations tells against such theories, especially as his remark is partly corrobor-ated by the account of 1483 given by Felix Faber.[68] Square towers, round towers and possibly gun plat-forms are datable at Rhodes not only to a time which at Bodrum was the first building period but also to the decades before and after 1407.[69] At Bodrum there seems to be no building in a demonstrably Seljuk style,[70] though Tower H in particular constit-utes a possible exception. Clumsy "Byzantine" building with the re-use of classical stonework and much tile and pottery is rare within the town of Rhodes, but common enough in the castles spread around Rhodes, Kos and the other islands where the Hospitallers may on occasion have used pre-existing structures but where they also built with classical stones found on the spot and used indigenous work-manship functioning in a "Byzantine" manner.[71] It is doubtful whether any walls at Bodrum can at pre-sent confidently be dated pre-1407 or pre-1421 sim-ply through an investigation of their stonework.[72] Quite possibly the earliest surviving work in the castle does in fact date to the period between 1407 and 1421 when work was done hurriedly and clums-ily using rough materials which lay conveniently to hand but which could not easily be utilized to create regular courses.

(iii) The Earliest Fortifications to 1421

The archives contain no useful material concerning

the initial construction of the castle at Bodrum, but there are written accounts by the Greek chronicler Doukas, writing after 1453 but knowledgeable about the area, and by the German pilgrim Felix Faber, who visited Rhodes in 1483. Neither author was contemporary with the building of the castle. Doukas seems to have had the date of construction wrong, but his account is detailed and in some ways convincing:

In that same year the Grand Master fitted out a fleet of three biremes and several galleys. He loaded them with all kinds of building materials, such as unslaked lime, squared stones, timber, planks and anything else needed for the construction of a fortress, and went to the borders of the province of Caria. Here on a promontory he erected a fortress in honour of Peter, the Prince of the Apostles, naming it Petrónion. When he had laid down strong foundations and begun to erect the walls, the ruler of Menteshe Ilyas Beg arrived with a large force determined to obstruct the work under way, but he accomplished nothing. After the Grand Master had completed the fortress to his satisfaction, to which he had added very high towers, he returned to Rhodes but only after installing Hospitallers within as sentinels. He charged the custodians of the fortress to be sober and vigilant according to law and custom, and to take care of escaped captives by offering them help and safety inside the fortress and, furthermore, by emancipating them in writing in the name of St. Peter. The fortress survives to this day.[73]

The quantity of stone, lime and other material taken to Bodrum suggests that, if Doukas is reliable, no defensible buildings were already standing there. To have carried ordinary ashlars to a classical site presumably littered with ruins might seem strange. Possibly the Hospitallers were badly informed or uncertain about the exact spot where they would be building, or maybe they needed to build defences very rapidly in order to establish an initial bridgehead and to defend the narrow isthmus against the Turks who presumably controlled the rest of the ancient town site. Alternatively, the Hospitallers re-used classical ashlars for ordinary wall-building but needed specially pre-prepared pieces cut by skilled master masons at Rhodes for the delicate ribbing of their intersecting ribbed groined vaults. They did build such vaults at Bodrum in the hall or loggia between the French and Italian Towers but at a later date, and it is unlikely that they erected such delicate work while hurrying to create a fortified bridgehead in enemy territory; possibly Doukas' chronology was once again confused. Whether the Emir of Menteshe attacked the Hospitallers or simply withdrew is not reported by Doukas. One "very high" tower, the French Tower, is indubitably datable to

this initial period though Tower E may also have been built at that time. In fact, apart from its implied date which is clearly erroneous, Doukas' story is entirely acceptable.[74]

Felix Faber's information was probably gathered while he was at Rhodes on his second pilgrimage of 1483. He was much concerned with the dogs which rescued fugitives and with the tale that the founder of the castle was supposedly a fellow-German, Fr. Johannes Schlegelholtz. According to Felix Faber, this Hospitaller took a group of brethren or *milites* and workmen or *servi* to Bodrum, a place where numerous Turks had for some years periodically been gathering for a fair and which was thought in Felix Faber's time to be Tarsus. The Hospitallers chose a *pecia campi* as a suitable place and, despite dire threats from the Turks, they began digging ditches and constructing a wall or palisade, after which they erected a wooden fortress. Then they laid the foundations for very strong walls and slowly built a wall, presumably of stone. The Turks, perhaps because they were waiting for the Emir Ilyas to arrive with sufficient force, did not attack the castle until it was finished, but then found it impregnable; they were never able to take it by force, by night attack or by treachery. Incidentally, Felix Faber not only referred to Bodrum as Tarsus but on a different page he wrote of Halikarnassos and the Maussolleion in a way which made his ignorance of its site quite plain: *In hac Caria est civitas Halicarnassus* ...[75] The accounts of Doukas and Felix Faber seem to be independent of one another; they provide evidence for a ditch, for walls built on strong foundations, for an initial construction of wood and for high towers. They suggest that no existing buildings were available, though doubtless there were ruins and loose stones which were re-used. It seems that considerable quantities of wood were also used, since on 24 September 1418 the Venetian Senate permitted the Bishop of Winchester, uncle to the King of England, to export from Crete 200 beams, 300 smaller beams and 500 planks of cypress to be used in Bodrum Castle.[76] Pending excavation, the only other evidence is that of the surviving stonework itself and of the shields fixed upon it. The reference by Felix Faber to Fr. Johannes Schlegelholtz presumably derived from the presence in the castle of the arms of Fr. Hesso Schlegelholtz;[77] a similar mistake was made in 1524 by Jacques Fontaine, who had been a judge at Rhodes and who attributed the beginnings of the castle to a Fr. *Henricus* Schlegelholtz.[78] Felix Faber's account tends to confirm the evidence of Doukas and of the papal and other documents that

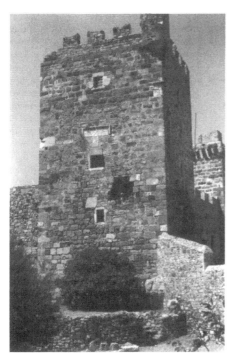

Pl. IV: St. Peter's Castle: the French Tower from the East showing Stonework and Shields

earlier gate had Naillac's arms upon it. Possibly shields were coloured as at Rhodes where some shields are made of different coloured stones. However this colouring is found at Bodrum on only two shields of Fr. Jacques de Milly, Master from 1454 to 1461,[80] and it is, therefore, impossible to differentiate between the similar arms of two successive Masters, Fr. Antoni Fluviá, from 1421 to 1436, and Fr. Jean de Lastic, 1436 to 1454, though at Rhodes Lastic occasionally used a coloured intarsia work to indicate the difference; certain structures, therefore, are only datable between 1421 and 1454. For the later fifteenth century the problem is more simple as many shields had inscriptions with names and precise dates, and furthermore it was the practice to erect the arms of the Captain of the Castle who was often appointed for two years, so that an accurate dating is possible. At Rhodes there are problems as to whether shields have been detached from the walls or buildings, or even been incorrectly replaced.[81] Unfortunately some shields at Bodrum are standing on the ground no longer *in situ*, and in theory there is also the possibility that the post-1407 builders simply affixed their arms to earlier work which they may have modified or repaired. Deductions from the shields must therefore be made with some caution.

Any assessment of the earliest work in the castle must consider six buildings and, in some cases, their adjoining walls:

the construction of the castle involved military action against the Turks.

To some extent the dating of these early buildings depends upon the shields found on or near them. The buildings involved are the French Tower, Towers D, E, G and H, Gate 3 and the presumed early chapel. At this early period many of the shields indicated that the individual involved, not always the Master, was ruling or commanding at Rhodes at the time of the work.[79] Sometimes an individual's arms may show that their owner paid part of the cost of the building, in which case the actual work had not necessarily been completed, or even begun, at the time of his death. In the case of Tower E, Fr. Philibert de Naillac's arms, though not on the original building, are now built into the wall nearby and it seems likely that they were on the earlier construction which that wall replaced. On Gate 3 Naillac's arms are not in their original place but on the rebuilt gate nearby together with the unidentified arms of whoever rebuilt it; again it may well be that the

(i) *The French Tower.*[82] This square tower stands at the highest point on the castle peninsula. Its main shield [cvi] carries the arms of Fr. Philibert de Naillac, Master from 1396 to 1421, and of Fr. Hesso Schlegelholtz, who was Preceptor of nearby Kos from 1386 to 1412 and Lieutenant at Rhodes from May 1411 until his death in May 1412, and who may well have had a leading role in the foundatio.. of the castle. The arms of the Rhodian financier Dragonetto Clavelli, who was the Receiver or financial agent of the Master from 1382 until his death in 1414/5 and who may have paid for part of the tower, are on a separate stone below the others (Plate IV). These shields suggest a date before 1412 for the tower's foundation, Clavelli's shield possibly being a later insertion. Two other shields datable 1421/51 [cv, cvi b] presumably record additions; indeed the tower was considerably rebuilt, especially in its upper section. The tower is in some ways comparable to the Naillac Tower at Rhodes, though the latter was placed at the end of a mole.[83] The French Tower is entered from the west at first floor level, while an inside staircase which leads up to another floor and then to the roof is entered from the south. This tower is mostly built rather untidily with irregular courses of not very large stones probably found on or near the site, with much use of tile and some classical fragments; the walls have a rough rubble core and much mortar was used. The basement room is now entered from a rectangular chamber at the lowest level through a west doorway with illegible Gothic inscriptions; a slab above this doorway is 170 cms. in length, 70 high and 28 wide, and the west wall of the room is 210 cms. thick. The room has a vault running east-west made of carefully-shaped soft, grey stones of irregular sizes, some 20, 30 or even 40 cms. long. It may have been this type of squared limestone needed for vaulting, rather than the clumsier stones available on the spot and used in building the walls, which the Hospitallers, if Doukas was correct, brought with them from Rhodes.[84] The wall to the south of the tower is not bonded into it, and the adjacent rectangular chamber, the vaulted hallway and the belvedere which join it to the Italian Tower to its west are apparently later in date. The French Tower seems originally to have stood by itself. The two arms of France in its main shield [cvi] may indicate French finance for its construction or its use by the French brethren in residence, or both.[85]

(ii) *The Naillac Building.* This rectangular building to the north-west of the Italian Tower still carries the arms [cii] of the Master Naillac and of Fr. Hesso Schlegelholtz who died in 1412. Its south end has been badly damaged and clumsily restored; the north end, restored with Green Lava stone presumably after 1494, had a door inserted into it which was subsequently blocked up; the lower part of the west wall was buttressed with a battered wall built onto footings of Green Lava, probably in the time of Fr. Antoni de San Martí Captain between 1510 and 1512, whose arms [ci, ci a] are above the doorway and on the north wall; the interior is now largely obscured with whitewash. The upper portion of the west façade seems to be the original work still visible in carefully-shaped, squared, small grey stones laid in courses varying between 23 and 40 cms. At

Rhodes the courses datable between 1421 and 1436 are of 40 cms. and employ fragments of tile in their mortar, while those datable between 1436 and 1454 are only 25 cms. in height.[86] The upper western face is topped with square merlons which may not be in their original condition;[87] the two southernmost merlons with arrow-slits are clearly restored, while that next to them carries the arms of Naillac and Schlegelholtz. This shield is not placed centrally in the building or even centrally on the merlon, to which it may have been moved when the arms of San Martí and of Fr. Aimeric d'Amboise, Master from 1503 to 1512, were placed on the building. The inside is roofed by a rounded barrel-vault with a faintly pointed arch all built in small grey stone blocks; two moulded strips run across the curve of the barrel from east to west and rest on ancient, early Christian or Byzantine capitals which have been re-used by incorporating them into the side wall. In the north end of the east wall is a small niche, and in the centre of the wall is a much larger niche with strangely contrived "sagging" vaulting. The small niche to the north is framed by two columns 170 cms. high which have engaged capitals composed of re-used classical or early Christian pieces, the southern capital having a Hospitaller-type "Maltese" cross on it. The interior cannot be dated, but the building was possibly the castle's earliest chapel or maybe some kind of chapter-house with altars in the niches.[88] It contains quantities of the small, squared limestone blocks of the type which may have been brought in from Rhodes in 1407 or soon after.

(iii) *Tower E.* This was a tall tower with a gunport just below its top, most of it encased within the massive outer east curtain, from which a rounded section now protrudes slightly on the exterior (Fig. 4).[89] The lower part of the tower, which is possibly somewhat different in build from the largely invisible upper part, is built of clumsy stones in fairly regular courses, the courses and mortaring being rather like that of Tower D. At the present ground level of the interior of the castle at the top of the tower at [a], but not now *in situ*, is a shield of Naillac, Master from 1396 to 1421 [cviii d]. The external diameter of the top of the tower, only part of which is visible, is approximately 6.70 metres. Beneath the jamb of the door built

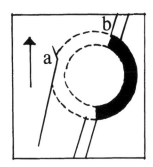

Fig. 4: Sketch Plan of Tower E at its Summit

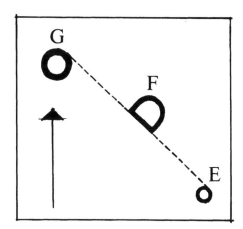

Fig. 5: Sketch Plan of Part of the Hypothetical Original North Castle Wall with Towers E, F and G

above the tower the partially uncovered top of a piece of shield [cviii e] was recently visible in the ground at [b]. It seems possible that the lower part of this tower dates to the original Naillac period.

Before the construction of Tower F some time after 1421 there was presumably a wall which ran in a straight line directly from the northern side of Tower G to that of Tower E (Fig. 5), for such a line would run absolutely flush along the south face of Tower F, which is datable to 1437/54 by a shield [xcii]; if this hypothesis is correct, Tower F was built out from such an early wall along this line. On either side of Tower F, which was presumably built onto the original wall, are two gun-ports which would have enfiladed this original wall. Subsequently new walls were built from Towers E and G to meet Tower F at points close to its gun-ports. These two stretches of wall, which carry shields [xci, xciii] datable 1454/61 and 1460 which make them later than Tower F, do not constitute a continuous straight line; they seem to have had gun embrasures and they are not bonded into Tower F. The original wall could possibly be found by excavating inside the existing walls.

(iv) *Tower G*. This round tower, datable to 1407/12

by the shields on it, including one of Fr. Hesso Schlegelholtz [xcv, xcvi], shows no sign in itself of having formed part of a system of walls though it may in fact have done so. Its rebuilding is documented by a shield [xcv] dated 1462, while the Green Lava stone at the top is presumably post-1494. The tower is clumsily built with much use of tile, especially on the inside; it does not have regular courses of large stone as does Tower D. The ground floor room has a separate entrance at the south and has two windows or embrasures pointing north and north-east; it has a domed roof, which has been repaired with square limestone blocks. The upper room is approached by climbing an outside ramp, and some protruding stones near the entrance suggest that there was some sort of barrier across the ramp. This upper room has walls some 2.15 metres thick and is also domed, though much of the ceiling is obscured by modern plaster; an internal staircase leads to the roof. Three large square windows, one of which has been filled in, do not seem to have been defensive and may be additions. This tower was apparently there in Naillac's time, and it could have been there before 1407; it is difficult to interpret a building apparently so extensively altered.

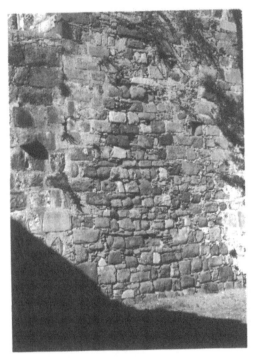

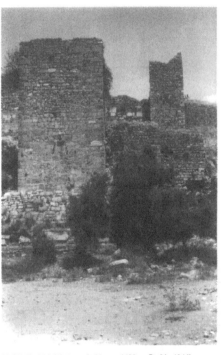

Pl. V: St. Peter's Castle: the South Face of Tower H

Pl. VI: Turkish Work, probably pre-1400, at Pechin 40 kilometres inland from Bodrum

(v) *Tower H*. This rectangular tower is evidently older than the stretches of wall to the east and the west of it, which are not bonded into this tower and do not meet it neatly. The wall to the west has gun embrasures which may suggest a post-1421 date; that to the east carries a shield [xcv a] datable 1461/7. On the inner, south face of this east stretch, which is narrower than the tower, are one shield datable ca. 1440 [xcvii] and another, closer to the tower, dated 1440 [xcviii]; a shield [xcix] on the tower itself is datable 1421/54 and presumably pre-1440. The top part of the tower is rebuilt; the tower can be entered only from the top. The rest of it is constructed crudely with no regular courses, clumsy stones many of them unsquared, and much use of tile (Plate V). It apparently dates to 1421/40, but could have been even earlier and have formed part of an original defence curtain.

(vi) *Tower D and Gate 3*. This tower, the Maritime Tower, is a round tower bonded into the wall running eastwards to Gate 3; the whole stretch from tower to gate is of one build, though the join is somewhat clumsy where the wall meets the tower on its north side (Fig. 6). Since the gate is datable to the Mastership of Naillac from 1396 to 1421 by a shield [xviii], the tower probably dates before 1421. The stretch of wall east of the gate was rebuilt, but the foundations on its south face seem to be part of the original work, which suggests that the original wall extended east of the gate, as would have been natural. The tower is solid and has no entrance, its platform, which must have controlled the port, presumably being reached along the walk along the top of the wall. Tower and wall were built of large, thick clumsily-squared stones laid in roughly regular courses with thick irregular mortaring, but with no tile or pottery; two bollards, possibly for mooring ships, protrude from the west and north of the foot of the tower. The tower was repaired in 1469, as indicated by a shield [xix] at [a], and much of the upper work on the tower and the wall is late in date, though parts of the inner work of the steps up to it may be original. The Hospitallers built round towers at Rhodes late in the fifteenth century and, after 1440, on Kos,[90] so there is no reason to date this tower before 1407.

The gate was rebuilt at an unknown date, and while the wall to its east may be datable 1476/95 by shield [xvii] at [b], the whole stretch of wall which contained Gate 3 had a parapet and other details added in Green Lava stone, presumably post-1494. At the east end of the walk along the wall from the tower there were probably steps, and maybe a draw-bridge, leading up to the level of the inner courtyard; little more can be said about this area. The north face of the wall seems originally to have re-entered at [c], where there is a clear break in the masonry. The line of the original wall is apparently visible inside the present gate where there are also sockets for a heavy bar and a shaft or chute at [d] for dropping liquids or stones on attackers. When the new gate was built forward in front of the original one a new shaft was made at [e] and a portcullis inserted, while the arms of Naillac

Master from 1396 to 1421, which must have been above the original gateway, were presumably brought forward and placed on the new section on the outside at [f] together with the unidentified arms [xviii] belonging to the period of the new work.

If those structures which can be dated with reasonable security before 1421 are placed on a plan, the result is a defensive line across the peninsula running from Tower E on the east to Tower G, and – in a way which cannot at present be established – from Tower G to Gate 3 which was connected by a wall to Tower D on the sea. On the summit was the French Tower with the Naillac Building, perhaps a chapel or chapter-house, below it to the west. There must also have been houses behind the wall, such as the *domus* mentioned in 1416.[91] Doukas spoke of walls and high towers, while Felix Faber mentioned ditches and very strong walls. There is therefore no evidence that there was originally an inner keep or redoubt, or that there was more than a north wall with a fosse in front of it; there is no evidence for the utilization of earlier structures; and, in particular, there is no recognizable Maussolleion stone in any of this early work. At Rhodes the two rectangular towers datable between 1377 and 1396 and another type datable between 1396 and 1421 are all built into the ramparts, but in the south-western corner of Rhodes town a series of relatively tall towers datable from

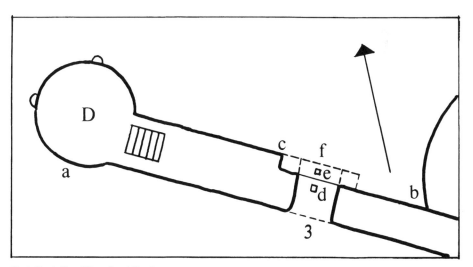

Fig. 6: Sketch Plan of Tower D and Gate 3

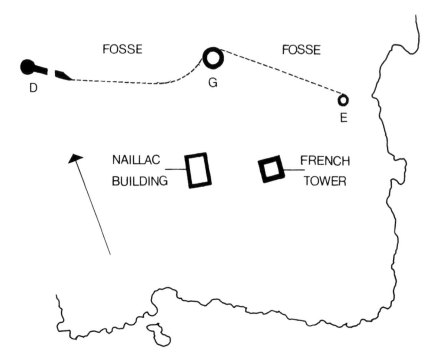

Fig. 7: Hypothetical Sketch Plan of the Earliest Work at St. Peter's Castle: 1407-1421

1421 to 1436 were detached from the curtain and stood in front of it, originally communicating with the town walls merely by bridges.[92] At Bodrum the Hospital had a small plateau to defend. Though any original wooden defences have gone and subsequent fortifications have obscured the lie of the land, it seems likely that in the central section of the peninsula the earliest Hospitaller work exploited the minor scarp at the northern edge of this plateau, using it as a natural wall and building towers on the solid rock above it.

More considerable building came later. The shields suggest that the eastern curtain running south from Tower E dates to ca. 1454/60, the southern curtain to 1461/7, the tower once at the southwest corner to roughly the same period, and the west wall to 1472 though the passage at the northern end of the west wall is datable before 1454.[93] These dates

would imply further work on the north curtain between 1421 and mid-century, but no enclosure of the whole peninsula before about 1460. Tower H was presumably built as a gun platform and enfilading bastion; the "English" and Italian Towers were constructed, the former some time before 1437 and the latter in 1436; and periodic, probably almost continuous, repairs and additions were made. These changes were made in reaction to increased Turkish pressures, to the development of Ottoman seapower and to the need to resist ever larger cannon. After the unsuccessful Turkish siege of Rhodes in 1480, Bodrum was relatively safe for a while because the Hospitallers had control of the Sultan's brother Jem who was kept in France until he was handed over to the pope in 1489. Soon after, in 1494, the Hospital began to fortify St. Peter's Castle even more strongly.[94] Since the fortifications were built on ris-

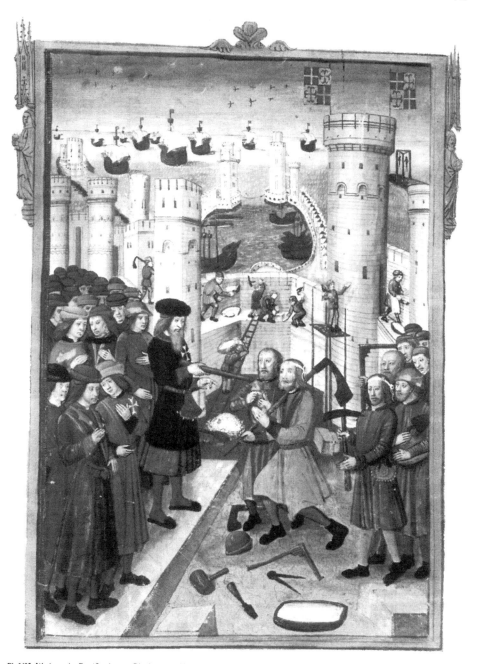

Pl. VII: Work on the Fortifications at Rhodes ca. 1480 from a French Illuminated Manuscript (Paris, Bibliothèque Nationale, Ms. Latin, 6067, f. 9v)

ing rock, the walls could not be lowered to reduce their vulnerability to cannon, but they were vastly strengthened with heavy gunports and interior passages which obscured much earlier work. The southwest corner was rebuilt with a covered battery around 1494/6; the west end of the north curtain was newly built as an outer curtain in 1498/9; the powerful Opertis Revellino created a small inner harbour to the west in about 1505/6; the Gattineau Bastion and the casemate to the north were constructed in 1512/3; and really heavy gunpowder defences came with a great deal more building between 1512 and 1522, producing massive artillery works which contrast completely with the clumsy medieval walls of the first decades of the fifteenth century.[95] During the siege of Rhodes in 1522 the castle was defended strongly under the Captaincy of Fr. Bernardino de Airasca[96] and considerable reinforcements of men and munitions were sent from Bodrum to Rhodes.[97] When the Master surrendered and left Rhodes on 1 January 1523 he sent instructions to the Captain and garrison at Bodrum to abandon the castle, and they arrived in Crete around the middle of January 1523.[98]

Notes

1. Luttrell (1978), I *passim*, and (1982), I *passim*. E. Zachariadou, *Trade and Crusade: Venetian Crete and the Emirates of Menteshe and Aydin (1300-1415)* (Venice, 1983), did not appear in time to be used in this chapter.
2. *Les Gestes des Chiprois*, 865.
3. These obituaries survive in many variant texts; for a text of 1357, see L. de Mas Latrie, "Notice sur les Archives de Malte à Cité-la-Valette," *Archives des Missions scientifiques et littéraires*, 1 ser., vi (1857), 29.
4. Text in Luttrell (1978), III 771-773.
5. Ludolphus de Suchem, *De itinere Terrae Sanctae liber*, ed. F. Deycks (Stuttgart, 1851), 27.
6. Çifitkalesi, some 12 kilometres south-west of Bodrum, has medieval remains: *supra*, 140 n. 68. Hamilton, ii. 38, spoke of a "small castle built by the Turks or by the Knights of Rhodes" at Çifitkalesi. Foss [forthcoming] reports a possible castle at Kadikalesi just south of Myndos and cites a seventeenth-century reference to Çifitkalesi itself being captured from the Venetians by the Hospitallers who lost it to the Emirs of Menteshe.
7. Cf. Luttrell (1978), I 293 and n. 27.
8. The archaeological evidence is altogether inconclusive: *infra*, 147-149.
9. Details in Luttrell [forthcoming]. On the Hospitaller fortifications, see W. Müller-Wiener, "Die Stadtbefestigungen von Ismir, Siğacik und Çandarli: Bemerkungen zur mittelalterlichen Topographie des nördlichen Jonien," *Istanbuler Mitteilungen*, xii (1962).
10. ... *cum centum milibus florenorum auri in statum pristinum reduci non*

posset: Theodoricus de Nyem, *De Schismate libri tres*, ed. G. Erler (Leipzig, 1890), 173.
11. This sum is difficult to calculate, and must be set against the apparent failure of the Avignonese pope to pay his share of the costs: text of 1398 in J. Miret y Sans, *Les cases de Templers y Hospitalers en Catalunya* (Barcelona, 1910), 456-458. Accounts of 26 April 1392 showed that nine priories had produced 25,353 florins of income from the indulgences out of a total income received in the West of 73,085 florins, that is roughly a third of the total: Valletta, National Library of Malta, Archives of the Order of St. John, cod. 326, f. 68v-70. This, however, was for the first years of the indulgence, and returns soon fell. Four priories and a certain *bon homme* produced 2383 florins in 1394/5, while in 1396/7 various priories provided 565 florins, and in 1398 the Priory of Auvergne produced 52 florins, 1 gros: cod. 329, f. 67; cod. 330, f. 17-17v. The indulgence was first granted not in 1391 but on 19 April 1390: cod. 11 nos. 10, 17.
12. Very crudely, the average income of the Receiver in the West from 1378 to 1394 was about 38,500 florins, calculating from figures in J. Nisbet, "Treasury Records of the Knights of St. John in Rhodes," *Melita Historica*, ii no. 2 (1957), 102-104.
13. Malta, cod. 334, f. 150. A number of other documents confirm the date: *infra*, 145-147. On Christoforo Buondelmonti's evidence, *infra*, 189-190.
14. D. Polemis, *The Doukai* (London, 1968), 196, 198-199.
15. According at least to Ducas, *Istoria Turco-Bizantină: 1341-1462*, ed. V. Grecu (Bucarest, 1958); xviii 3-11, xxi 2, 4-5, xxii 1; see also Doukas, *Decline and Fall of Byzantium to the Ottoman Turks*, trans. H. Magoulias (Detroit, 1975).
16. Luttrell (1978), I 307-308; *idem* [forthcoming].
17. Ruy González de Clavijo, in *Embajada a Tamerlán*, ed. F. López Estrada (Madrid, 1943), 22-23.
18. Text in K. Sathas, *Documents inédits relatifs à l'Histoire de la Grèce au moyen âge*, ii (Paris, 1881), 11-12.
19. Details from Doukas in Foss (1979), 164-168, and Luttrell [forthcoming]; the whole question and its chronology remain extraordinarily confused.
20. ... *pro acquirendo loca de altoloco et palathia, et etiam debent ire ad smirnas, ubi Zalapinus dominus turchorum vult facere fabricarj quoddam fortilicium de muro:* Venice, Archivio di Stato, Misti del Senato, 47, f. 138v.
21. Doukas, xxii 1.
22. Eg. texts *supra*, 146, 150; *infra*, 185-186.
23. P. Wittek, *Das Fürstentum Mentesche: Studie zur Geschichte Westkleinasiens im 13.-15. Jh.* (Istanbul, 1934), 97-98, where, however, he wrongly accepts Doukas' implied date of 1415 for the year of the castle's construction.
24. By Delaville, 287, and Maiuri, 291, to give just two among numerous examples.
25. Malta, cod. 334, f. 173v, 174v (22 Jan., 1 Feb. 1409). E. Bernareggi, "Gigliati del Gran Maestro dei Cavalieri di Rodi Philibert de Naillac," *Rivista Italiana di Numismatica*, lxvi (1964), 134-136, suggests that the expenses of Bodrum castle may explain the hurried and heavy emission of coins made possibly at that time.
26. Escaped slaves were a continual preoccupation, for example to Bayazid ca. 1393 (Delaville, 233) and to Sulaiman in 1403; text in G. Dennis, "The Byzantine-Turkish Treaty of 1403," *Orientalia Christiana Periodica*, xxxiii (1967), 77-80. Slaves also worried Ilyas of Miletus in 1403: text in G. Thomas, *Diplomatarium Veneto-Levantinum*, ii (Venice, 1899), 293-296; see also *supra*, 144, and *infra*, 165-166, 180 n. 53.
27. Eg. *infra*, 185-186, 186.

28. On Latin trade in this area, see Zachariadou (1976) and *idem,* "Prix et Marchés des Céréales en Romanie: 1343-1405," *Nuova Rivista Storica,* lxi (1977).

29. Text in D. Wilkins, *Concilia Magnae Britanniae et Hiberniae,* iii (London, 1737), 131-132; another copy in Lyons, Archives Départementales du Rhône, 48 H 31 pièce 1. Delaville, 318 n.1, cited a copy of one such indulgence issued at Rhodes on 23 April 1410, preserved in Arnheim, Archives of Province of Guelders: S. Jan. no. 147. A similar indulgence with beautifully illuminated initials was issued at Clerkenwell in London for Sir William Fitzhugh and his wife Margary in 1414 in the name of Pope Alexander V: London, British Library, Cotton Charters, IV. 31, published in A. Oliver, "Notes on the Heraldry at the Castle of Bodrum," *Ars Quatuor Coronatorum: Transactions of the Quatuor Coronati Lodge no. 2076, London,* xxi (1908), 86-87. On 24 October and 3 November 1409 Sir Henry Fitzhugh was exempted from customs dues in England on a considerable quantity of arms to be sent to Bodrum: A. Reeves, *Lancastrian Englishmen* (Washington, 1981), 81. The Fitzhugh arms were among the many English arms on the "English" Tower: C. Markham, "The Display of English Heraldry at the Castle of Budrum (or Halicarnassus) in Asia Minor," *Proceedings of the Society of Antiquaries of London,* 2 ser., xiv (1891-1893), 285-287. E. Jacob, *The Fifteenth Century: 1399-1485* (2nd ed: Oxford, 1961), 326, incorrectly said that Henry Fitzhugh "built a castle in Rhodes." In 1415 the Hospital borrowed 2000 ducats sent to Rhodes by the English king, barons, knights and merchants for the papal indulgences for building Bodrum castle: Malta, cod. 339, f. 301v. An undated text shows these indulgences being collected in the West at that time: cod. 339, f. 293v-294.

30. Mentioned in Malta, cod. 339, f. 156v-157.

31. Toulouse, Archives Départementales de la Haute-Garonne, H 139 pièce 8.

32. Lyons, 48 H pièce 1.

33. Lyons, 48 H pièce 2.

34. Texts *supra,* 150; *infra,* 185-186.

35. *Infra,* 164-166.

36. Malta, cod. 339, f. 240-241 (2/12 Nov. 1409), f. 245v (14 Dec. 1409), 269v (15 Jan. 1412), 299 (24 Apr. 1416). Antonius Ruffinus held an *apotheca* in the castle in 1410: cod. 339, f. 168v-170.

37. Turkish raids were launched from Miletus: Luttrell (1978), I 312.

38. Text in Sathas, ii. 246-247.

39. Lyons, 48 H pièce 1 (23 June 1414); the expedition had occurred *depuis deux ou trois ans.* Lescure died before 25 Sept. 1411: Delaville, 278/9 n. 7.

40. ... *ex auditu percepimus qualiter non nullj turchj fuerunt circa castrum sanctj petrj vbj putatur quod sit exercitus admiratj palatie pro expugnando dictum castrum:* Malta, cod. 339, f. 268.

41. ... *expedire fecimus galeam nostram gardie et cum aliqua dampna passi fuimus a turchis cum earum lignis depredatj fuerunt aliquos homines de symia et de alijs insulis nostris quare velit[...] expedire galeam, cum intendimus ipsam mittere in gardia pro custodia et saluatione aliarum nostrarum insularum:* Malta, cod. 339, f. 269v (with evidently incorrect grammar).

42. ... *cum notorium sit quod galee nostre armate quando reperiuntur in marj extra strictum Roman[ie] cum aliquibus lignis turchorum armatis iuste poste [sic] capere et lucrarj,* ... The Latins of Lesbos imprisoned and tortured the Hospitaller crew in retaliation: Malta, cod. 339, f. 270v-271 (ca. Feb. 1412).

43. Malta, cod. 339, f. 267v-268 (8 Jan.), 271, 271v (ca. Feb. 1412).

44. In addition to the standard works of Iorga, Wittek and others, more modern references are given in J. Barker, *Manuel II Palaeologus 1391-1425: A Study in Late Byzantine Statesmanship* (New Brunswick, 1969), 284-288.

45. ... *qualiter in partibus galipolj jlle perfidus mossy Sap', quj nimium christianos habet exosos galeas et ligna usque ad numerum xxx, ex quibus extant galee ix nititur armare, se suum ducere iter usque constan-[tinopolim] uel saloniqui fingendum:* Malta, cod. 339, f. 283v.

46. Malta, cod. 339, f. 283v-284.

47. On 19 July 1414 the Venetian Senate considered that the rulers of Ephesus and Miletus might make peace with Mehmet, as he had demanded; Venice wanted peace with these rulers, the end of piracy and the return of captives, and was prepared to use force if need be: texts calendared in N. Iorga, *Notes et Extraits pour servir à l'Histoire des Croisades au XVi siècle,* i (Paris, 1899), 220-221.

48. Malta, cod. 399, f. 297; the document does not mention Ilyas, as Delaville, 328, implies. For subsequent details on the anti-Turkish league, see references in Schreiner, ii. 402, 405. The coin showing Junayd in control of Ephesus but in subservience to Mehmet cannot be dated with precision despite attempts to do so, as is made clear in G. Miles, "Note on Islamic Coins", in appendix to G. Hanfmann, "The Fifth Campaign at Sardis: 1962," *Bulletin of the American Schools of Oriental Research,* clxx (1963), 33-35 and Fig. 23.

49. ... *qualiter Soldanus quericj totam turquiam et greciam, nisi dumtaxat territorium admiratj palatie subiugauit, cum quo omnibus que alijs infidelibus orientalibus presentialiter pacem ferimus:* Malta, cod. 339, f. 297-297v. Coins of 1419 show Ephesus under Mehmet's control: C. Ölçer, *Yildirim Bayezid'in Oğullarina ait Akçe ve Mangirlar* (Istanbul, 1968), 72-75.

50. Ilyas had made a treaty with Venice on 17 October 1414: text in Thomas, ii. 305-306. He had become subservient to Mehmet by some point in the year 13 March 1415 to 1 March 1416: coin of 1415/6 published in Wittek, 161 [for "817" read "818"]. Mehmet was at Bursa occupied with an attack by the Emir of Karaman during summer 1415: Barker, 341 n. 81.

51. Lyons, 48 H 37 pièce 2.

52. In what follows, "dated" means that the work carries a written date; "datable" means that the date can be deduced.

53. References in Bean – Cook, 86-87, 89, 93; *supra,* 128.

54. Fig. 11: cf. Maiuri, 328, and *idem,* "Il Castello dei Cavalieri di Rodi a Budrúm," *Clara Rhodos,* i (1928), 181.

55. Information from Professor Kristian Jeppesen.

56. *Supra,* 130.

57. Newton, ii. 275.

58. *Supra,* 143.

59. Newton, ii. 645, 647, 653. E. Akurgal, *Ancient Civilizations and Ruins of Turkey* (Istanbul, 1973), 250, considers the foundations of the west side of the main west curtain to be pre-1400 "Turkish" work.

60. *Supra,* 156.

61. *Infra,* 203.

62. *Supra,* 152-153.

63. Maiuri, 295, 304-305, 314, 320, 323.

64. Maiuri, 328.

65. On the dating of work containing Green Lava stone, see *infra,* 203-204.

66. Gabriel, i. 59-61, 70-72, 75; Figs. 33, 40-41; Plates XVI, XVII (1), XXV (1,3); ii. 232. No work in the castle at Kos is datable before ca. 1400: Maiuri, 276-286.

67. Towers D, G, H and the French Tower are described and dated *supra,* 151-155.

68. Text *infra,* 185-186.

159

VI

69. There seems to be no way of identifying or dating the earliest gun platforms at Rhodes; even if identifiable, they could be later than the towers which support them. Gabriel discusses round towers, some of them standing free in front of the curtain, datable to the mid-fifteenth century (i. 43-44 and Fig. 17, 44-45 and Fig. 18, 55-57 and Figs. 30-31, 70-72 and Fig. 40, 75-76 and Fig. 41); two rectangular towers datable 1377/96 (i. 74 and Plate XV [2]) and one of 1396/1421 (i. 72-73); and a rectangular tower, datable 1396/1421, with a platform (i. 67, 127 and Fig. 38). There were rectangular and rounded towers in the Hospitaller work at Smyrna castle, probably datable 1390/6: Müller-Wiener (1962), Fig. 3. A gun platform at Corinth, datable ca. 1400, might be Hospitaller work: K. Andrews, *Castles of the Morea* (Princeton, 1953), 141. The Hospital was acquiring *bombarde* by 1381: Malta, cod. 321, f. 204v. Cannon were widely in use by Europeans and Ottomans by ca. 1400: D. Petrovic, "Fire-arms in the Balkans on the Eve of and after the Ottoman Conquests...," in *War, Technology and Society in the Middle East*, ed. V. Parry – M. Yapp (London, 1975). A small fifteenth-century bombard (78.3 cm. long, 21 cm. maximum width, 7 cm. bore) survives within Bodrum castle.

70. Assuming such a style can be recognized: cf. Müller-Wiener (1961) and (1962).

71. G. Gerola, "I Monumenti medioevali delle Tredici Sporadi," *Annuario della R. Scuola archeologica di Atene*, i-ii (1914-1916); on local workmen, *infra*, 169 n. 84.

72. No attempt is made here to establish any rigid typology or chronology of the medieval stonework at Bodrum along the somewhat debatable lines suggested in Müller-Wiener (1961) and (1962). Such work would require extensive study on the spot; it is difficult to make stylistic judgements when ancient materials have been re-used; and the dating of the various pieces of work being compared with one another is often uncertain. The different types of work from Smyrna illustrated in Müller-Wiener (1962), Tafeln 15-16, are not particularly like any of the putative early work at Bodrum, which is mostly much less regular and uses less tile, though really clumsy works of any sort tend to look similar. The stonework in the "English" Tower is well illustrated in E. King – H. Luke, *The Knights of St. John in the British Realm* (revised ed: London, 1967), 56. For datable Seljuk work see, for example, S. Lloyd – D.S. Rice, *Alanya ('Alā'iyya)* (London, 1958).

73. Doukas, xxii 1 (trans. Magoulias, 122), using the words *lithoi akrogōniaioi*. This is a Biblical phrase with a symbolic meaning, as in Ephesians 2.20 and the Septuagint Isaiah 28.16, which may have meant corner stones, capping stones or foundation stones: cf. E. Good, "Cornerstone", *The Interpreter's Dictionary of the Bible*, i (New York, 1962), 700. Doukas wrote some fifty years after the event and it might be best to translate "carefully-squared stones" (the Italian translation gave *piere quatrangulare*) such as would have been ready for immediate use; carefully-squared stones are noted in early buildings in the castle: *infra*, n. 84. According to H. Liddell – R. Scott, *A Greek-English Lexicon*, i (revised ed: Oxford, 1968), 56, *akrogoniaios* could mean "at the extreme angle," which might conceivably imply a stone intended for vaulting or ribbing.

74. Bosio, ii. 158, wrote that the Master of Rhodes himself sailed to Halikarnassos and took the castle from the Turks by force, implying that a castle already existed there; neither point can be proved. On the emancipation of slaves in general, see Luttrell (1982), VI *passim*.

75. *Fratris Felicis Fabri Evagatorium in Terrae Sanctae, Arabiae et Egypti peregrinationem*, ed. C. Hassler, iii (Stuttgart, 1849), 261-

262 (reproduced *infra*, 185-186), 265. According to Cristoforo Buondelmonti, writing in about 1420, the work force included "innumerable Turks": text *infra*, 189.

76. Text in G. Fedalto, *La Chiesa Latina in Oriente*, iii: *Documenti Veneziani* (Verona, 1978), 186-187.

77. *Infra*, 198.

78. ... *struere coepit Henricus Sclegelholt eques Germanus:* J. Fontanus, *De Bello Rhodio libri tres* (Rome, 1524), H. i.

79. On the arms and shields at Rhodes, see G. Gerola, "Gli Stemmi superstiti nei Monumenti delle Sporadi appartenute ai Cavalieri di Rodi," *Rivista del Collegio Araldico*, xi-xii (1913-1914), and Gabriel, i. 91-104, 119 and n. 4, 144-145 *et passim*; ii. 232; on those in Cyprus, see W. Rüdt de Collenberg, "L'Heraldique de Chypre," *Cahiers d'Heraldique*, iii (1977), Fig. 27 nos. 4, 29, 44; on those at Smyrna, see *infra*, 169 n. 85.

80. Gerola, 71, 77.

81. On Rhodes, see Gerola (1913-1914), xi. 731 n. 4, 738, and Gabriel, i. 107; on Gate 3 at Bodrum, see *supra*, 154-155.

82. Tower J described and illustrated in Maiuri, 295-297 and Figs. 11-12; the interior stonework is shown in Newton, Plate XXVI, and Karo, Fig. 7.

83. Gabriel, i. 72-73; Fig. 40; Plate XXIV.

84. This limestone is soft and greyish, and was cut into carefully-squared rectangular blocks; it was used for external walls, as in the Naillac building and the façade of the church at Bodrum, as well as for vaulting. The loggia between the French and Italian Towers has rounded ribbed vaultings which spring from plain engaged capitals resting on engaged columns, and are constructed of smallish squared rectangular limestone blocks, the masonry of the rib vaults being separate from that of the walls; Miss Sally Dyer of St. John's Gate, Clerkenwell, London, most kindly supplied photographs. This work is roughly similar to the undated vaultings once in the loggia of St. John at Rhodes, except that the latter were markedly ogival and the capitals were decorated: Gabriel, ii. 71-72, and B. Rottiers, *Description des Monumens de Rhodes* (Brussels, 1838), atlas, Plates XXXVIII-XXXIX. Much fourteenth-century work at Rhodes used large, clumsily-squared blocks, many of them doubtless ancient, with occasional use of tile. Towers and walls, however, often used this standard squared and smoothed limestone, which could have been found in the vicinity of Bodrum. At Bodrum some of this work seems to be datable to 1407/12. Gabriel, i, Figs. 42, 44, 46, 49, shows ribbed vaulting in the Tower of St. Nicholas at Rhodes founded in 1464. For earlier types of Hospitaller groin vaulting and rib vaulting springing from corbelled supports see, in addition to Gabriel on Rhodes, P. Lojacano, "La Chiesa Conventuale di S. Giovanni dei Cavalieri di Rodi: Studio storico-architettonico," and *idem*, "Il Palazzo del Gran Maestro in Rodi: Studio storico-architettonico," both in *Clara Rhodos*, viii (1964); H. Balducci, *Il Santuario di Nostra Signora di Tutte le Grazie sul Fileremo presso di Rodi* (Rhodes, 1931); *idem*, *La Chiesa di S. Maria del Borgo in Rodi fondata dal Gran Maestro Hélion de Villeneuve* (Pavia, 1933); F. Fasolo, "La Chiesa di S. Maria del Castello di Rodi," *L'Architettura a Malta dalla Preistoria all'Ottocento = Atti del XV Congresso di Storia dell'Architettura* (Rome, 1970); A. Orlandos, *Archives des Monuments Byzantins de Grèce* [in Greek], vi part 1-2 (Athens, 1948). Compare photographs of work at Krak, Margat and Acre in Syria: eg. in P. Deschamps, *Terre Sainte Romane*, plates 24-25, 27, 34-35, 44-45; S. Langè, *Architettura delle Crociate in Palestina* (Como, 1965), Plates 25-26, 77; Z. Goldmann, "The Hospice of the Knights of St. John in Akko," *Archaeology*, xix (1966), *passim*; J. Riley-Smith, *The Knights of St. John in Jerusalem and*

Cyprus: c. 1050-1310 (London, 1967), 304; M. Benvenisti, *The Crusaders in the Holy Land* (New York, 1972), 110, 113; R. Smail, *The Crusaders in Syria and the Holy Land* (London, 1973), Plate 34; J. Folda, "Crusader Frescoes at Crac des Chevaliers and Marqab Castle", *Dumbarton Oaks Papers*, xxxvi (1982). To what extent the Hospitallers continued to use the same style of vaulting across several centuries is yet to be established. From 1291 to well after 1310 is a longish period and nothing relevant can be said about Hospitaller building in Cyprus during that time; Gabriel, i. 134, states that the ramparts at Rhodes show none of the essential characteristics of Hospitaller fortifications in Syria. Elements of continuity might imply a tradition maintained by master masons. The *portie maistre* or *protomaestro* of the castle was present, incidentally, with the commissioners who gave instructions for new works at Bodrum in 1495: text *infra*, 187-188. In 1414 two Greek *muratores* of Kos who had worked on the "newly constructed" castle at Bodrum were freed from servitude, though when required they were to serve as builders for two *asperi* and the accustomed victuals per day: Malta, cod. 339, f. 290v. In 1428 the Order freed from the *servitudo marina* the sons of the Rhodian Georgius Singan *alias* Turcho, a *murator et protomagister* who had worked on the fortifications at Rhodes and at Bodrum: cod. 348, f. 160v-161. On the *protomaistro murador* Manoli Counti, presumably a Greek, in 1457, see Gabriel, i. 98, 113; ii. 232. H. Balducci, *Orme del Rinascimento Italiano in Rodi al tempo dei Cavalieri* (Pavia, 1931), 31, assumes Manoli Counti was an Italian. In 1472 various *magistri latomi* declared it inopportune to build a castle on Rhodes in winter because the rain would prevent the mortar from setting: text in Gabriel, i. 145. Investigation is needed of stylistic details, the chemical composition of mortars, the possible tapering of vaulting stones, and so on.

85. A slab at Smyrna castle combined the arms of Fernández de Heredia 1377-1396; the Order of the Hospital; the Papacy; Domenico de Alamania (died 1411); the Baux(?) family; and apparently Innocent VI 1352-1362: F. Hasluck, "Heraldry of the Rhodian Knights formerly in Smyrna Castle," *Annual of the British School at Athens*, xvii (1910-1911), 148-150 and Fig. 2; photograph in Müller-Wiener (1962), Tafel 18 (i). Marie de Baux accompanied her husband Humbert de Viennois who led a crusade to Smyrna in 1346. Probably fourteenth-century are the arms at Rhodes: fleurs-de-lis (England?); the Papacy; England: Gabriel, ii. 174; Fig. 120; Plate XXXVII (4). Also at Smyrna, a papal castle, was a slab with the arms of the Papacy; Innocent VI surmounted by the papal tiara; and Alamania: Hasluck, Fig. 3; photograph in Müller-Wiener (1962), Tafel 18 (ii). Hasluck, 145, incorrectly states that Alamania was Admiral and at Smyrna in 1392: Luttrell (1978), XXIII 47. L. Maggiorotti, *Architetti e Architetture militari*, i (Rome, 1933), 94, mistakenly claims that the arms at Smyrna were taken there from Bodrum. A group of five arms at Rhodes showed: Order; Corneillan 1353-1355; Bérenguer 1365-1374; Pins 1355-1365; and apparently Innocent VI 1352-1362: Gabriel, ii. 175. Papal arms were apparently not otherwise used by the Hospitallers at Rhodes or elsewhere before 1417, possibly because direct papal financial support was not otherwise involved: Gerola (1913-1914), xi. 728. Hasluck and others give Innocent VI's arms at Smyrna as those of Fr. Pierre de Culant, Lieutenant of the Master at Rhodes 1382-1396, but they differ from Culant's arms at Rhodes. Furthermore fortifications were presumably built at Smyrna by the papal captain in Innocent's time: cf. Luttrell (1978), I 297; (1982), XVI 144. It is probably unimportant that both

Smyrna arms lack the chief with three escallops and one lacks the bendlet or bar, while one papal tiara lacks one crown, since Innocent's arms did not always show these elsewhere: D. Galbreath, *Papal Heraldry* (2nd ed: London, 1972), 10, 22, 78. A group of five arms at Rhodes showed: England; Villeneuve 1319-1346 and Order; Order; Gozon 1346-1353; England: Gabriel, ii. 175; Fig. 120; Plate XXXVII (3). A slab at Rhodes bearing five shields included those of Fernández de Heredia and Culant (with lion reversed, that is turned to sinister, apparently without stars or mullets, but with a fillet and cut-off bendlet): Gabriel, i. 67, 101; Fig. 37. A group of seven arms at Rhodes showed: Clavelli; Alamania; Fernández de Heredia (?badly drawn); Order; L'Isle Adam elected 1521 with Order; Culant (with lion reversed and without chief or mullets); Docwra(?): Rottiers, atlas, Plates IX, XI, XXXVI, shows the same lion. Rottiers, atlas, Plate LXXIII (13), shows Culant's arms at Rhodes complete in all details (but with lion reversed) next to the arms of the Order. Balducci, *Fileremo* (1931), 27-29 and Fig. 27, suggests that the arms of Fulques de Villaret 1305-1317 appeared in a fresco together with those of his four successors, but in that case they were painted long after his Mastership.

86. Gabriel, i. 112.

87. These merlons have probably been altered, since square-topped merlons are rare; Gabriel, i. 265 and Fig. 32, provides just one example for Rhodes town.

88. Maiuri, 301, regards it as probably a gatehouse or guardhouse to an inner redoubt, but its interior seems to have been too grandiose for such a use. The stone blocks of the ceiling were seen in 1976 before they were whitewashed; it is now difficult to study the room. On re-used Byzantine and Byzantinesque stone carvings at Rhodes, see Balducci, *Fileremo* (1931), 17-25; Figs. 9-25.

89. More of Tower E is visible than Maiuri's plan (*infra* Fig. 11) suggests.

90. Gabriel, i. 70, 75-77 and Figs. 40-41; Maiuri, 276-286.

91. Malta, cod. 339, f. 299.

92. Gabriel, i. 67, 74, 127-130 *et passim*, and Fig. 4.

93. On Towers F and H, *supra*, 149, 152-154.

94. Plate VII shows work on the fortifications at Rhodes in an illumination in Guillaume Caorsin's history of the 1480 siege of Rhodes: Paris, Bibliothèque Nationale, Ms. latin 6067, f. 9 verso. This manuscript was illuminated by an artist working in Paris soon after 1480: information kindly provided by M. François Avril, Keeper of the Department of Manuscripts. This artist was, however, clearly well informed about conditions at Rhodes.

95. Post-1421 developments can be followed in reasonable detail in Maiuri's text and plan (*infra* Fig. 11); see also *infra*, 199-204.

96. Fontanus, L i verso.

97. Jacques de Bourbon, *La grande et merueilleuse et tres cruelle expugnation de la noble cité de Rhodes* ... (Paris, 1525), 30-30v, 33v, 34v; *I Diarii di Marino Sanuto*, xxxiv (Venice, 1892), 82-87.

98. Bosio, iii. 1-2. According to the Turkish sources, Bodrum was occupied on 5 January: E. Rossi, *Assedio e Conquista di Rodi nel 1522 secondo le Relazioni edite ed inedite dei Turchi* (Rome, 1927), 43 n. 1. *I Diarii di Marino Sanuto*, xxxiv. 67, gave 4 (or 8?) January.

VII

RHODES : BASE MILITAIRE, COLONIE, MÉTROPOLE DE 1306 À 1440

> Qu'une puissance économique comme Gênes entende avant tout assurer au mieux ses intérêts, quoi de plus naturel, et la religion peut donc en être un utile vecteur. Mais le mélange des genres est encore plus subtil lorsqu'il s'agit d'un ordre religieux comme celui de Rhodes, dont l'implantation territoriale a la lutte contre l'Islam pour seule raison d'être, mais dont les réalités temporelles dominent à l'évidence, au point de coûter fort cher au réseau hospitalier du monde occidental.

La conquête de Rhodes, entreprise par les Hospitaliers en 1306, fut une manifestation tardive du processus de colonisation occidentale en Méditerranée orientale, processus commencé avec les premières croisades. Avec une population, des institutions et une Église grecques, Rhodes constituait une partie de l'Empire byzan-

VII

tin, occupée de force par un groupe de Latins qui la gouvernèrent avec des pouvoirs presque illimités, et qui y exerçaient les prérogatives princières : rendre la justice, frapper monnaie, lever des taxes et concéder des biens. L'ordre de l'Hôpital colonisa une grande partie de l'île en y attirant une nouvelle population, en y installant des marchands latins, une bureaucratie latine, une Église latine et d'autres institutions occidentales. Rhodes devint une base militaire et navale puissante et se développa en tant que comptoir commercial et entrepôt à l'avantage principal des Latins, mais ne devint pas une colonie occidentale typique ; de fait, le souci de l'exploitation, qui caractérise d'habitude les régimes coloniaux, fut fortement limité. Les Hospitaliers étaient en gros un instrument de la société occidentale ; en fin de compte ils dépendaient de l'approbation pontificale, comme le leur rappela certainement la dissolution des Templiers en 1312, mais ils ne constituaient pas une partie d'un empire ou d'un système colonial ou commercial normal.

Le gouvernement et le quartier général de l'ordre de l'Hôpital était établi à Rhodes ; mais il n'y avait pas de métropole occidentale pour profiter directement de la position économique ou stratégique de l'île, ni de dynastie occidentale ayant occupé l'île pour en exploiter les revenus et les ressources. L'Hôpital était une institution charitable multinationale, sans but lucratif, un ordre de l'Église romaine, dont les membres avaient prononcé des vœux religieux de célibat, donc sans enfants ou héritiers pouvant revendiquer un intérêt quelconque dans le régime. L'occupation initiale de Rhodes était le résultat d'un compromis avec les habitants, selon lequel les terres étaient réservées aux Grecs dont l'Église conservait une part de ses biens et son indépendance. L'Hôpital adopta une attitude paternaliste à l'égard de la population grecque ce qui fit, qu'à de rares exceptions près, les révoltes furent virtuellement inconnues. L'Hôpital se donna une peine considérable pour protéger ses sujets et défendre la population grecque non seulement contre les razzias turques, mais aussi contre la rapacité des gouverneurs, hospitaliers ou latins, et des capitaines. La vie sur une île méditerranéenne pouvait être dure aussi bien pour les Latins que pour les Grecs ; cependant, comme le rapporte vers 1352 Nicéphore Grégoras, les Rhodiens reconnaissaient que, s'ils avaient perdu quelques libertés, ils étaient bien nourris et bien défendus.

Le rôle particulier de l'Hôpital était de constituer une opposition militaire et navale contre les Infidèles, mais, comme dans le cas des ordres « nationaux » en Aragon, Castille, Portugal et également en Prusse, la reconquête s'accompagnait de repeuplement. Pour Rhodes, cela signifiait attirer des colons latins, faire venir des Grecs et autres esclaves, développer l'agriculture, concéder des terres incultes en emphytéose et construire des châteaux pour défendre la paysannerie. Un *emporium* sûr fut créé dans la ville avec un arsenal et des facilités commerciales favorisées par d'importantes routes maritimes est-ouest et nord-sud. D'autres richesses vinrent de visiteurs occidentaux et surtout de pèlerins allant à Jérusalem, pour lesquels les Hospitaliers créèrent un hospice et d'autres services ; en 1403 même, l'Ordre négociait avec les Mamlûks pour contrôler la circulation des pèlerins en Syrie.

D'une certaine façon, toutes les sociétés sont organisées pour la guerre, mais l'insuffisance des ressources à Rhodes même rendit nécessaire de créer une réserve de richesse et d'effectifs qui pourrait être taxée et mobilisée pour la défense des îles, très exposées aux attaques turques. La population, avec l'aide des prisonniers pris chez les Infidèles, dut travailler aux fortifications qui entouraient la ville portuaire. La paysannerie devait s'acquitter d'un service de garde et de corvées sur les routes, les ponts et les châteaux ruraux qui préservaient la population ou surveillaient la navigation ennemie. Les hommes de Lindos étaient contraints de fournir du bois de charpente pour les constructions navales à Rhodes. Importations et exportations étaient taxées à travers le *commerchium* et par la vente aux enchères des fermes ou des gabelles sur le vin et sur d'autres denrées, afin de financer la galère de garde et de payer la solde des mercenaires. Des impôts particuliers furent consentis par les *cives* latins et grecs à la veille de l'attaque mamlûke de 1440. La galère de garde avait un équipage fourni par des Grecs de Rhodes, dont certains devaient une *servitudo marina* qui évitait à l'Hôpital les dépenses d'entretien d'un équipage permanent de rameurs. Dans les périodes de crise, comme en 1440, des navires génois, catalans ou autres, qu'ils soient ou non pirates, pouvaient être réquisitionnés ou affrétés, tandis qu'à partir de 1413 au plus tard, un armement autorisé pour la course ou *corso* rapportait du butin. La masse de la population, urbaine et rurale, devait une forme de service militaire, mais les tentatives pour établir au début du XIVᵉ siècle, un système de fiefs tenus par les Latins, en échange d'obligations militaires ou, dans le cas de l'île de Nisyros, en échange d'un service de galère, n'eurent qu'un succès très limité[1].

Il y avait un autre front sur lequel il était vital de mener la guerre contre les Infidèles, guerre qui constituait la raison d'être de l'Hôpital et la justification essentielle de sa richesse, de sorte qu'il se finançait en partie lui-même. Les Hospitaliers rendaient à l'Occident latin un service général en défendant Rhodes et ses mers et en combattant pour contenir d'abord les Turcs des émirats côtiers d'Anatolie, ensuite, vers 1389, les Ottomans dans les Balkans. L'Ordre participait aussi à des ligues navales et à des expéditions maritimes de croisade ; après 1344 l'Ordre eut le premier rôle dans la défense de Smyrne[2]. Une démonstration convaincante d'activité contre les Infidèles était nécessaire pour persuader l'opinion publique latine que l'Hôpital méritait bien ses possessions et ses revenus en Occident, ses privilèges et ses exemptions. En particulier l'Hôpital recherchait les indulgences pontificales à vendre au public ; l'indulgence promulguée par Clément VII en 1390 pour Smyrne procura plus de 25 000 florins en 1392[3]. Après la perte de Smyrne au profit de Timour en 1402, l'Hôpital chercha sans succès à s'y rétablir, puis jugea essentiel de prendre pied en territoire turc dans une position de défense, ce qu'il fit en construisant le château de Bodrum en 1407/8. Les frères écrivirent avec éloquence sur le sang et l'argent dépensés à Bodrum, mais en réalité le nouveau château, placé en un lieu où il y avait peu de chances que les Turcs ne pouvaient l'attaquer sérieusement, rapporta à l'ordre des donations, des exemptions et une publicité fructueuse à l'Occident ; il représenta presque certainement un investissement lucratif même à court terme[4].

L'Hôpital ne profita pas de son île comme d'une base coloniale, à la manière dont, par exemple, Vénitiens et Génois exploitaient la Crète et Chio. Rhodes n'était pas une colonie au sens où son gouverneur pouvait en tirer un profit exportable vers un arrière-pays occidental. Au contraire, le maintien de l'Ordre à Rhodes dépendait largement de l'arrivée continuelle de capitaux dans l'île, sous la forme de sommes provenant des impôts et des contributions perçus sur les possessions de l'Hôpital en Occident, prieurés et commanderies qui constituaient en réalité ses « colonies » occidentales ; dans la terminologie officielle de l'Hôpital, *outre-mer* signifiait Europe occidentale. Les revenus occidentaux comprenaient les paiements du *passage* effectué par les frères venant à Rhodes, les dépouilles des frères décédés et diverses autres ressources, mais la masse des revenus provenait des *responsiones* de chaque commanderie, des séries de paiements impliquant un système de collecteurs et de comptes, mais aussi de nombreuses

VII

évasions fiscales et de fréquents arrérages. Les comptes occidentaux des années 1373-74 et 1374-75 mentionnent des revenus respectivement de 42 230 et de 46 820 florins. Ces sommes n'étaient pas toutes envoyées à Rhodes en espèces ; certaines arrivaient sous forme d'argent, de vaisselle d'or, de vêtements ou, venant de Chypre, de sucre[5].

L'Ordre avait besoin de maintenir sa position sur une île qui, tout en étant facilement défendable contre un adversaire doté d'une force navale limitée, disposait d'une population et d'une économie trop restreintes pour produire une richesse suffisante pour payer des armes, des chevaux, des approvisionnements ou de coûteux mercenaires. Malgré un investissement continu dans des fortifications de pierre ne requérant que de petites garnisons, l'Ordre devait maintenir un certain nombre de frères dans le couvent de Rhodes et l'entretien de plusieurs centaines d'Hospitaliers en Orient coûtait fort cher. En certaines occasions, comme en 1352, les frères furent dissuadés de venir servir à Rhodes, à moins d'arriver avec armes et chevaux ; en 1362 au moins cinquante-neuf Hospitaliers et donats, la plupart d'origine française, reçurent l'ordre de quitter Rhodes et Cos pour l'Occident[6]. L'« État-Ordre » rhodien différait beaucoup de l'*ordensstaat* des chevaliers Teutoniques en Prusse, lequel reposait sur une population de plusieurs centaines de milliers de personnes et n'avait pas besoin ou ne recevait pas de revenus de ses commanderies germaniques. L'ordre Teutonique avait besoin d'hommes pour administrer et défendre ses territoires, mais se dispersait dans sa mission contre les Infidèles, luttait contre de trop nombreux ennemis, accroissait trop ses dépenses en louant les services de trop nombreux mercenaires, et s'aliénait les sujets qu'il exploitait. Il ne se remit jamais réellement du désastre militaire subi au Tannenberg en 1410[7].

L'État-Ordre rhodien n'avait besoin que d'un effectif limité d'Hospitaliers pour se maintenir à Rhodes. Théoriquement les frères, qui faisaient vœu de pauvreté et d'obéissance et étaient affectés à la lutte contre les Infidèles, devaient servir sans récompense. En réalité, un système de promotions, compris par tous les frères, garantissait qu'un service de quelques années à Rhodes, des périodes de service sur mer ou dans des châteaux ou îles extérieures, procuraient, à Rhodes, une ancienneté à l'intérieur de chaque *langue* – ou groupe national – des Hospitaliers et l'espoir d'une commanderie en Occident, pour l'avenir. Un tel bénéfice n'était pas nécessairement une sinécure, mais constituait certainement un stimulant. Au cours du XIVe siècle, les détails de ce système furent consignés et fréquemment amendés dans les statuts de l'Ordre. Par exemple, par un décret de 1379 le Maître n'avait pas à octroyer aux offices vacants tant qu'il n'était pas à Rhodes, puisque cela aurait porté préjudice aux droits du Couvent et aurait signifié qu'aucun Hospitalier n'aurait voulu aller à Rhodes tant que ceux qui étaient déjà là auraient voulu partir[8]. La critique de cet arrangement était un peu irréaliste. Vers 1390, Philippe de Mézières, qui a certainement très bien connu Rhodes, se plaignait que les temps avaient changé, car autrefois il y avait eu un petit groupe de soldats hospitaliers capables de porter la terreur au cœur des Turcs : maintenant les frères venaient d'Occident et restaient quatre ou cinq ans afin d'obtenir un bon prieuré ou une bonne commanderie en Occident, et quand c'était chose faite, ils n'avaient plus du tout l'intention de revenir à Rhodes : « c'est une moquerie ou grant derision »[9]. Il y avait des abus, mais c'était le système et, somme toute, cela fonctionnait.

Le système de promotion des Hospitaliers était très complexe. Beaucoup de frères, particulièrement les prêtres, qui étaient généralement plus nombreux que les frères militaires, ne servaient jamais à Rhodes. Il y eut un groupe de frères qui firent la plus grande partie voire toute leur carrière en Orient, tenant garnison dans des châteaux, administrant les îles et aspirant éventuellement à un poste d'officier supérieur du couvent ou même de Maître, à Rhodes. Les offices les plus élevés, y compris les commanderies de Cos et Chypre, étaient souvent occupés par des Français, et en particulier par les nombreux frères de Provence et Languedoc, mais il y avait une législation répétée destinée, avec un certain succès, à empêcher les monopoles et à partager les postes parmi les *langues*[10]. Il y avait aussi un bon nombre d'hommes qui faisaient le va-et-vient entre Rhodes et l'Occident[11]. Quelques frères prirent soin de rester au pays. Ainsi en 1411, six Hospitaliers se rencontrèrent à Trévise et nommèrent quatre frères parmi lesquels le prieur devait choisir celui qui servirait à Rhodes. L'un des quatre, frère Angelo Rossi, était présent et insista pour être dispensé pour plusieurs raisons. Premièrement, il avait déjà servi le prieur en dehors du prieuré, à Rome, pendant dix ans. Deuxièmement, il était engagé dans un procès touchant sa commanderie qui durait depuis trois ans et qui serait perdu, au grand détriment de l'Hôpital, s'il était absent. Troisièmement, il n'avait qu'un frère, un pauvre homme avec une famille nombreuse, qui souffrirait de son absence[12].

Quelques nominations seulement eurent lieu à Rhodes et elles furent organisées de différentes façons. Le Maître « se réserva » un certain nombre de prieurés et commanderies comme « chambres » ou *camere* à la tête desquelles il pouvait personnellement nommer les chapelains, des membres de sa maison et d'autres[13]. Occasionnellement un prieur occidental qui se trouvait en Orient pouvait faire une nomination. Ainsi, en mars 1412, le prieur de Toulouse, agissant avec l'accord du grand commandeur et d'autres officiers de la *langues* de Provence, octroya au commandeur de Bordeaux une commanderie vacante à cause de la mauvaise gestion du commandeur précédent ; le prieur utilisa son sceau personnel et celui de son prieuré, et copia l'acte dans le registre du prieuré qu'il avait apporté avec lui à Rhodes, tandis que le nouveau commandeur enregistrait l'acte du prieur dans le registre du maître, ce qui le faisait confirmer par le Lieutenant Maître et le Couvent[14]. D'autres vacances furent comblées par le Maître et le Couvent suivant les règles d'ancienneté et les décisions prises à l'intérieur de la *langue* concernée. Quand la nouvelle de la mort de frère Pere de Pomers, prieur de Catalogne, parvint à Rhodes vers 1410, le Lieutenant Maître et le Couvent choisirent pour le remplacer le frère Gracian de Messans qui tenait l'office conventuel de drapier à Rhodes et qui était le doyen ou *antiquior* de sa *langue* présente à Rhodes ; ceci fut fait à la requête de « tous les frères de l'*albergia* et *lingua* de Catalogne résidant dans le couvent de Rhodes ». Fr. Antoni Fluvià, futur Maître de Rhodes, fut nommé Drapier et l'on procéda à des nominations pour les commanderies et les *camere* que le dernier prieur avait tenues à l'exception d'une *camera* qui appartenait au Maître[15]. En 1415, il y eut un débat sur une commanderie qu'une réunion de la *langue* de France avait accordée, suivant le statut et la coutume, au candidat qui avait plus d'ancienneté, qui était sergent ; au lieu de cela, le Lieutenant Maître décida en Conseil de l'attribuer à un chevalier qui avait prétendu avoir un droit de priorité en qualité de *miles*, après quoi le sergent en appela au Maître qui était en voyage[16].

Les choix étaient discutés et arrêtés en assemblées plénières de *langues* individuelles. En mai 1399 au moins soixante trois frères de la *langue* de Provence se réunirent dans une de leurs *auberges*[17]. En Février 1403, les vingt et un frères de la *langue* de France se réunirent et se mirent d'accord pour la doyenneté sur le nom de l'un d'entre eux[18]. Une réunion de la *langue* d'Auvergne en 1409 rassembla au moins trente-trois Hospitaliers[19]. La *langue* espagnole comptait seulement dix frères à Rhodes en octobre 1403[20]. Ces quatre *langues* semblent donc avoir rassemblé au moins cent vingt-sept frères, alors que les *langues* d'Angleterre et d'Allemagne envoyèrent peu de frères à Rhodes. Ces chiffres excluaient probablement quelques officiers conventuels, membres de la maison magistrale, certains chapelains et frères dans les châteaux lointains et les îles, à Chypre ou sur mer. Le nombre total des Hospitaliers d'Orient peut avoir atteint les deux cents ou un peu plus[21].

Le système de promotion provoquait des tensions et des querelles, surtout quand les papes mettaient en avant leurs pouvoirs de disposer des postes en faveur d'hommes qui avaient peu ou pas mis les pieds à Rhodes. C'était un sérieux sujet de débat entre les frères conventuels. Ainsi en 1411, ils protestèrent auprès du pape Jean XXIII et de divers cardinaux de ce qu'ils avaient réservé la commanderie d'Avignon pour le frère Pierre de Galbert qui était commandeur en Arles et *pillerius* ou officier doyen de son *auberge* à Rhodes, avait combattu l'Infidèle pendant pas moins de quarante-sept ans, était vieux, borgne et avait de nombreuses autres blessures, et que le pape l'avait donnée à un homme qui était en fait un domestique du pape. Le Couvent en appela à la justice pour qu'elle donne quelque espoir de promotion et des encouragements aux frères de Rhodes qui avaient laissé leurs familles pour une vie de pauvreté et de danger dans un Orient où ils combattaient quotidiennement l'Infidèle et étaient découragés par les ingérences pontificales. Le Couvent exposa péniblement son mécontentement : le pape Benoît XIII avait octroyé des commanderies en Espagne et Catalogne avec, pour résultat, le refus des Hospitaliers espagnols de servir à Rhodes ; les bénéfices occidentaux avaient été originellement donnés par les fidèles pour soutenir la lutte contre l'Infidèle et pour récompenser le service actif, mais les provisions pontificales étaient en train de bouleverser ce système et de détruire l'Ordre ; aucun Hospitalier ne voudrait plus rester à Rhodes qui serait perdue au préjudice de la Chrétienté[22]. Une dernière affaire, interminable et coûteuse, commença en 1413 quand on découvrit, à Rhodes, que Jean XXIII avait vendu au roi Janus pour son fils naturel âgé de cinq ans l'expectative de la riche commanderie de Chypre. En novembre 1413, le Couvent se plaignit de ce que les Hospitaliers de différentes nations protestaient violemment – *alta uoce clamantes* – et demandaient l'autorisation de quitter Rhodes. Ceux, en Occident, qui ne méritaient pas de promotion étaient en train de priver de leurs récompenses les frères conventuels continuellement exposés aux dangers et à la pauvreté ; le Couvent demanda une fois encore que les provisions pontificales ne conduisent pas l'Hôpital à la ruine et la disparition[23].

Les Hospitaliers gouvernèrent, mais n'exploitèrent pas vraiment la population grecque à laquelle ils apportèrent prospérité et sécurité. Ils agissaient, de manière très générale, pour le compte des Latins d'Occident et de l'Église romaine, en défendant Rhodes contre l'expansion turque. Ils apportaient des avantages généraux aux marchands latins sans favoriser aucun groupe particulier de bénéficiaires occidentaux. La défense de Rhodes maintint l'Hôpital en activité et lui permit de continuer à exister en tant qu'Ordre, tandis que la poursuite de la guerrre sainte, de manière seulement défensive, rapporta aux Hospitaliers des avantages économiques en Occident. L'Hôpital maintint une confrontation permanente avec les Infidèles et mit en place un gouvernement assez tolérant et paternaliste à Rhodes dont les dispositions durèrent pendant des siècles[24].

Stratégies et moyens de domination

Notes

1. De nombreux aspects de cette communication ont été développés dans A. Luttrell, « The Military and Naval Organization of the Hospitallers at Rhodes : 1310-1440 », *Das Kriegswesen der Ritterorden im Mittelalter = Ordines Militares – Colloquia Torunensia Historica,* VI, Torun, 1991. D'autres développements sont donnés dans idem, *The Hospitallers in Cyprus, Rhodes, Greece and the West : 1291-1440,* Londres, 1982. Pour le contexte, J. Delaville le Roulx, *Les Hospitaliers à Rhodes jusqu'à la mort de Philibert de Naillac : 1310-1421,* Paris, 1913. Pour l'archéologie, l'art et l'architecture de Rhodes, E. Kollias, *The City of Rhodes and the Palace of the Great Master,* Athènes, 1988, est essentiel, bien que la question des affaires des Hospitaliers ne soit pas directement fondée sur les sources. J. Ch. Poutiers, *Rhodes et ses chevaliers, 1306-1523,* Bruxelles, 1989, contient des intuitions utiles mais est essentiellement un travail de seconde main, à utiliser avec précaution ; cette étude est cependant importante pour son traitement original de la topographie et la typologie des établissements et fortifications éloignés. Ces travaux rassemblent la bibliographie essentielle.

2. Le succès de l'Hôpital dans son action pour freiner l'expansion turque est présenté dans A. Luttrell, « The Hospitallers of Rhodes confront to Turks : 1306-1421 » *in Christians, Jews and other Worlds : Patterns of Conflicts and Accommodation,* éd. P. Gallagher, New York, 1988.

3. *Ibidem,* p. 96 et 103.

VII

4. A. Luttrell, « The Later History of the Maussolleion and its Utilization in the Hospitaller Castle at Bodrum », *Jutland Archaeological Society Publications*, XV, 2, Aarhus, 1986, p. 143-147.

5. Texte dans A. Luttrell, « The Hospitallers' Western Accounts : 1373/4 and 1374/5 », *Camden Miscellany*, XXX, Londres, 1990.

6. Luttrell, 1978, I, p. 296, XXIII, p. 36-37.

7. Pour une interprétation récente, M. Burleigh, *Prussian Society and the German Order : an Aristocratic Corporation in Crisis, c. 1410-1466*, Cambridge, 1984.

8. Strasbourg, Archives départementales du Bas-Rhin, H 2186, fol. 102.

9. *Cf.* A. Luttrell, « Papauté et Hôpital : l'enquête de 1373 », dans A.-M. Legras, *L'enquête pontificale de 1373 sur l'Ordre des Hospitaliers de Saint-Jean de Jérusalem*, I, Paris, 1987, p. 42.

10. Voir Delaville, p. 130, 208-209.

11. Voir les nombreuses courtes biographies données dans le texte et les notes de Delaville.

12. Texte dans A. Luttrell, « Templari e Ospitalieri in Italia », dans *Templari e Ospitalieri in Italia : la Chiesa di San Bevignate a Perugia*, éd. M. Roncetti *et al.*, Pérouse, 1987, p. 26.

13. Voir le texte dans C. Tipton, « The 1330 Chapter General of the Knights Hospitallers at Montpellier », *Traditio*, XXIV, (1968), p. 306-308.

14. Valletta, Bibliothèque Nationale de Malte, Archives de l'Ordre de Saint-Jean, Cod. 339, fol. 122-123.

15. Malte, Cod. 339, fol. 201v°-202, 203, 203v°-204 (sans date).

16. Malte, Cod. 338, fol. 240-240v°.

17. Malte, Cod. 330, fol. 37-38.

18. Malte, Cod. 332, fol. 6v° (aimablement communiqué par Anne-Marie Legras).

19. Malte, Cod. 339, fol. 199v°-201.

20. Malte, Cod. 333, fol. 56.

21. D'autres statistiques sont données par Luttrell dans Legras, p. 39-41.

22. Malte, Cod. 339, fol. 59 v°-60/61, 223-225, 226 v°-227 v° ; *cf.* Delaville, p. 323-324. Le texte du fol. 223 est dans S. Paoli, *Codice Diplomatico del Sacro Militare Ordine Gerosolimitano, oggi di Malta*, II, Lucca, 1737, p. 115-116, daté de manière erronée de 1410, et avec des erreurs.

23. Malte, Cod. 339, fol. 247-247v° ; *cf.* Delaville, p. 319-321.

24. Bien que l'Hôpital quittât Rhodes en 1523, il régna de manière très similaire sur Malte jusqu'en 1798 : A. Luttrell, « Eighteenth-Century Malta : Prosperity and Problems », *Hyphen*, [Malte], III, n° 2, 1982.

VIII

The Earliest Documents on the Hospitaller *Corso* at Rhodes: 1413 and 1416

The Mediterranean world knew many forms of informal naval violence ranging from straightforward piracy to a variety of legalized or quasi-legal activities involving reprisals, privateering and corsairing.[1] The type of *corso* which developed on Rhodes during the fifteenth century was officially licensed by an established authority, the Master of the Hospital, and was limited, in theory at least though often not in practice, to attacks on infidel enemies of the religious order state settled on Rhodes. Such activities fitted into an existing pattern. In the thirteenth century there were already forms of *guerra di corso* in which individuals operated under public control with a licence to attack enemies of the state. Such arrangements may have grown out of permits allowing injured parties to seek indemnities from those who had damaged them, or simply from agreements by which authorities lent vessels to individuals and sometimes financed them. The corsairs had to present *fidejussores* who would guarantee their proper conduct and to promise not to attack subjects or friends of their own state; they were to hand over a portion, often a fifth, of their booty. To profit from this system there emerged professional groups who took high risks and stood to make very considerable gains. The armament of corsair expeditions involved formal notarized contracts and the raising of capital through shares. After expenses had been deducted, profits were divided between the investors, those who played an active role at sea normally receiving a higher return than those who merely provided finance; officers and crews also received shares. Public legislation supposedly controlled such activities, but it could be extremely difficult

1. No attempt is made here to survey the extensive literature on medieval Mediterranean piracy.

178

to prevent corsairs from attacking friendly shipping or seizing the merchandise of third parties.[2]

Before the definitive loss of Latin Syria with the fall of Acre in 1291 the Hospitallers possessed or hired shipping, but that was predominantly for transport and supply.[3] After 1291 the Order moved its headquarters to Limassol on Cyprus, where its island position compelled it to develop a small navy of its own.[4] Following their establishment on Rhodes after 1309 the Hospitallers naturally found themselves operating within a maritime milieu in an area in which Latin shipping was involved in innumerable minor actions and assaults, and these frequently led to reprisals, to protests from third parties, and to prolonged court cases and quarrels over jurisdictions. In such situations, the dividing lines between piracy, indiscriminate raiding, corsair ventures carried out under licence, and justifiable attacks on infidel shipping were seldom clear. Around Rhodes the Hospital was initially involved both in sea battles with the Turks, who conducted their own piratical razzias in the Aegean, and in attacks on Christian ships which were breaking the papal prohibitions against transporting slaves and war materials to the infidel.[5]

The old principle that the military orders could retain lands won from the infidel was recognized in 1307 in a papal confirmation of the Hospital's rights to Rhodes which it had conquered from enemies of Christendom, that is from 'schismatic Greeks' and from 'infidels' who must have been Turks.[6] A statute passed in 1293, the year after

2. See, for example, L. Balletto, *Genova nel Duecento: Uomini nel Porto e Uomini sul Mare* (Genoa, 1983); H. Bresc, 'La course méditerranée au miroir sicilien (XIIIe - XVe siècles),' in *L'exploitation de la mer: la mer, moyen d'échange et de communication* (Juan-les-Pins, 1986).
3. A. Luttrell, 'Gli Ospitalieri di S. Giovanni di Gerusalemme dal continente alle isole' (forthcoming).
4. A. Luttrell, *The Hospitallers in Cyprus, Rhodes, Greece and the West: 1291-1440* (London, 1978), No. II, pp. 162-3.
5. A. Luttrell, *The Hospitallers of Rhodes and their Mediterranean World* (Aldershot, 1992), Nos. II and XIX.
6. J. Delaville le Roulx (ed.), *Cartulaire générale de l'Ordre des Hospitaliers de S. Jean de Jérusalem: 1100-1310*, 4 vols. (Paris, 1894-1906), No. 4751. A papal privilege to the Temple of 1139 permitted it to retain properties won from the 'enemies of the cross' — *Ea etiam, que de eorum spoliis ceperitis, fidentur in usos uestros conuertatis*: text in R. Hiestand, *Papsturkunden für Templer und Johanniter: Neue Folge* (Göttingen, 1984), pp. 96-103. Cf. J. Brundage, 'Humbert of Romans and the Legitimacy of Crusader Conquests', in *The Horns of Hatṭīn*, ed. B. Kedar (Jerusalem – London, 1992).

the Hospitallers moved to Cyprus, showed that the Order
was organizing a naval force and that Hospitaller brethren
were commanding vessels. It also indicated that on occasions
when there were no *freres darmes*, that is no military Hospitaller
brethren, on board, then the *frere de marine* appointed by the
comandor, perhaps by the Grand Commander of the Hospital,[7] should
command the galleys and other vessels, and that any booty taken should
pass to the Hospital's treasury. The implication was that if military
brethren of the Order were in command, then they would receive some
part of the prizes taken. The statute read:

> Item establi est que quant il couendra faire armement de Galee
> ou dautre vasaus, le comandeor les doie faire aparailler et garner
> de ce que besoing sera et de mariners. Et se il couient ametre
> gens darmes que le mareschal les doye retenir, e soient payes au
> tresor et soient a son comandement. Et si freres uont sur les
> galees que le mareschal puisse metre .vn frere chevalier sur
> tout larmement. Et si freres darmes non y uont sur les galees, que
> le frere de marine que le comandor jmetra soit bailli sur tout
> larmement et que le gaaign que les galees ou uaisseaus feront
> que il ueigne tout au tresor.[8]

This statute was soon suppressed,[9] and was evidently replaced by that
of 1300 which defined the powers of the Admiral. The office of
Admiral had been created in or shortly before 1299,[10] and the new
regulations of 1300 explicitly established that he should receive 100
besants a year from prizes taken by the Hospital's galleys and *lins*.[11]
These regulations of 1293 and 1300 applied to vessels armed by the
Hospital in its role as an institution. Hospitaller brethren were members
of a religious order and subject to their Master and, ultimately, to the
Pope, but there was apparently no obstacle in canon law to individual
members of a military order being licensed for the equivalent of
a corsair expedition. Furthermore, at a time when the papacy was

---

7. However, there were officers who were the Commander of the Ship or the
   Commander of the Brethren: J. Riley-Smith, *The Knights of St John in
   Jerusalem and Cyprus: c.1050-1310* (London, 1967), pp. 329-30.
8. A hitherto unpublished statute of 1293 in Marseilles, Archives départementales
   des Bouches-du-Rhône, 56 H 4055.
9. It is not found in later compilations: *Cartulaire*, No. 4234.
10. Ibid., Nos. 4464, 4469.
11. Statute of 1300 in ibid., No. 4515, para. 13.

encouraging the military orders to seize any Latin shipping infringing the papal prohibitions against trade with the Mamluks and other infidels,[12] it was licit for their members to attack Christian vessels which were breaking those prohibitions. In 1306, for example, Imbert Blanc, the Templar *preceptor* of Auvergne, and Pierre de Lengres, *civis* of Marseilles, who were joint *admirati* of certain galleys destined in *subsidio Terre Sancte*, together with those in their service, were granted by Pope Clement V the right to retain any goods they might take either from *infideles* or from *impii christiani* who were taking prohibited materials to infidel parts.[13] A papal letter of 1311 asserted the canonical legality of the detention of Genoese shipping breaking the embargo on infidel trade, and in this case such disciplinary action had been carried out by galleys of the Hospital and of others deputed by the papacy for that purpose *ad reprimendum et impediendum transgressores*.[14]

The riches to be gained from a major prize could be enormous. An extreme case occurred at Rhodes in 1379 when three Venetian galleys arrived in search of bread and found in the harbour a Genoese *chocha*, the *Bichignona*, with 300 fighting men aboard; it was said to be the largest in the world and worth 500,000 ducats. The Genoese unloaded 18,000 ducats worth of goods and fled; the Venetians commandeered a reluctant Catalan *cocha* in the port with its 200 fighting men and chased the *Bichignona*, capturing it together with 222 prisoners of whom 160 were merchants. The Venetians then sold part of the prize at Rhodes for 80,000 ducats, said to be half of the sale's real worth, and demanded 18,000 ducats from the Master for the goods previously unloaded there.[15] These were not acts of piracy, since Venice and Genoa were at war, but on other occasions the religious aspect of naval operations continued to be emphasized. For example, instructions

12. Luttrell, *The Hospitallers in Cyprus*, No. V, pp. 196-7; id., *The Hospitallers of Rhodes*, No. II, pp. 83-5, 110 n. 3; cf. E. Ashtor, *Levant Trade in the Later Middle Ages* (Princeton, 1983), pp. 17-44; J. Richard, 'Le Royaume de Chypre et l'Embargo sur le Commerce avec l'Egypte (fin XIIIe - début XIVe siècle)', *Académie des Inscriptions et Belles-Lettres: Comptes Rendus* (1984), and S. Schein, *Fideles Crucis: The Papacy, the West, and the Recovery of the Holy Land, 1274-1314* (Oxford, 1991), pp. 193-4, 231-3.

13. *Registrum Clementis Papae V*, 8 vols. (Rome, 1885-92), Vol. I, Nos. 1034-35.

14. Ibid., Vol. VI, No. 7118.

15. Daniele di Chinazzo, *Cronica de la Guerra da Veniciani a Zenovesi*, ed. V. Lazzarini (Venice, 1958), pp. 218-20; cf. B. Kedar, *Merchants in Crisis: Genoese and Venetian Men of Affairs and the Fourteenth-Century Depression* (New Haven – London, 1976), pp. 77-8, 198-9.

to Venetian captains in 1402 ordered them — acting if possible in collaboration with the forces of Chios, of the Archipelago and of Rhodes — to attack the Turks and their subjects in defence of Christian interests:

> debeat ire et discurere et cursizare partes et loca maritima Turchorum et subiectorum Turchis, inferendo eis et galeis et locis atque navigiis et rebus suis quam plura damna poterit pro terrore et exterminio suo et conforto et asecuratione locorum et navigiorum christianorum.[16]

However the Venetians, like everyone else, suffered from Christians as well as from Turks. Thus, between 1417 and 1429 they were protesting against attacks by Catalan pirates who were based on Rhodes and who on occasion actually assaulted Venetian shipping in the port there.[17]

There was always scope for individual Hospitaller brethren to profit from piratical activities. For example, in 1392 Fr. Adhémar Broutin alias Talebart of the Priory of Auvergne was actively engaged in piracy in the Western Mediterranean, but his unofficial activities were disavowed by the Order.[18] On other occasions the Hospital's own vessels were responsible for piratical attacks, as in 1390 when Genoese envoys obtained the restitution of a galliot from Chios taken by the galleys of the Order which had been conducting the Emperor Manuel II back to Constantinople to restore him to his throne.[19] In or just before 1403 *le galie de Rodi*, presumably the galleys of the Order, had captured a *grande chocha de saraceni* at Damietta in Egypt and many of those on board had been imprisoned in Rhodes; as part of a peace settlement advantageous to the merchants of Rhodes, the Master had subsequently returned the *chocha,* its goods and the prisoners, but

16. Text in H. Noiret, *Documents inédits pour servir à l'histoire de la domination vénitienne en Crète de 1380 à 1485* (Paris, 1892), pp. 129-31.
17. A. Tenenti, 'Venezia e la Pirateria nel Levante: 1300 c.-1460 c.', in A. Pertusi (ed.), *Venezia e il Levante fino al secolo XV*, Vol. I, Pt. 2 (Florence, 1973), pp. 743, 762-3.
18. J. Delaville le Roulx, *Mélanges sur l'Ordre de S. Jean de Jérusalem* (Paris, 1910), No. XVII; Hospitaller corsairs in Sicilian waters between 1433 and 1444 are noted in H. Bresc, *Un Monde méditerranéen: Economie et société en Sicile, 1300-1450*, Vol. I (Rome, 1986), pp. 341, 344, n. 162.
19. M. Balard, *La Romanie génoise (XIIe - début du XVe siècle)*, Vol. I (Rome–Genoa, 1978), p. 95.

he then imposed a four per cent tax on the merchandise of all those inhabitants of Rhodes who sailed to Mamluk parts. This tax was to last until it had raised the 12,000 or 16,000 ducats needed to compensate for the loss of the profits from the ship and its goods. The inhabitants stood to gain from the establishment of Rhodian consulates and from favourable tax arrangements in Mamluk ports, and they were apparently being expected to make good the profits which the Order was to lose through the peace settlement.[20] To the north in the Aegean the Hospital's ships were also seen as a threat, and in 1415 the Greek monks of the monastery of Saint George on the island of Skyros felt it necessary to issue their ships with safe conducts addressed to the captains of Hospitaller ships which the monks described as carrying the flag bearing the cross and as fighting the infidel.[21]

Such piratical practices initiated by individual Hospitallers apparently developed during the period of great financial strain at Rhodes caused by the schism in the papacy after 1378; this divided the Western priories and greatly reduced the amount of money reaching Rhodes. In 1397, for example, the Catalan brethren complained that the costs of the Order's activities in the East, which included the defence of Smyrna, were being borne by only nine out of twenty-one priories.[22] In 1410 there was a serious plague on Rhodes[23] and in that year the situation was so grave that it was almost impossible to pay the Hospital's mercenaries or to bring in essential grain imports.[24] These difficulties must have encouraged the Hospital as a whole and certain brethren as individuals to seek profit from certain forms of piracy. For example, at the end of 1411 the *galiota* from the Order's mainland castle at Bodrum, the ancient Halikarnassos just north of Kos, seized from two *barche* of Chios the goods of certain Turks from the jurisdiction of Altoluogo who were in *pax* or truce with the Hospital; however, following complaints from Chios, the Order had to disavow these activities and promise to return the goods. Early in

20. Text in Luttrell, *The Hospitallers of Rhodes*, No. X, pp. 200-201.
21. Text in P. Lemerle *et al.* (eds.), *Actes de Lavra*, Vol. III: *de 1329 à 1500* (Paris, 1979), p. 216.
22. Luttrell, *The Hospitallers of Rhodes*, No. XI, p. 110.
23. Valletta, National Library of Malta, Archives of the Order of St. John, Cod. 336, fol. 13v (kindly communicated by Anne-Marie Legras).
24. Malta, Cod. 339, fols. 204v-205v, 212, 214-216v, 217v-220; cf. J. Delaville le Roulx, *Les Hospitaliers à Rhodes jusqu'à la mort de Philibert de Naillac: 1310-1421* (Paris, 1913), pp. 316, 324, and A. Luttrell, 'Rhodes: base militaire, Colonie, Metropole de 1306 à 1440' (forthcoming).

1412 Fr. Louis Asiner, *miles*, and two other Hospitaller *fratres* of noble birth, together with the *consocii* and *marinarii* of Bodrum, sailed in their *galiotta* armed at Bodrum and attacked a Turkish *galiotta* somewhere near Mytilēnē; this they justified by the claim that Hospitaller galleys could attack Turkish shipping outside the Dardanelles: 'cum notorium sit quod galee nostre armate quando reperiuntur in marj extra strictum Romanum cum aliquibus lignis turchorum armatis iuste posce capere et lucrarj'. The defeated Turkish ship transferred its goods to a *galleota* from Mytilini; furthermore, the Hospitaller vessel was wrecked by the men of Mytilini and Jacopo Gattilusi, the ruler of that island, then seized, imprisoned, and tortured the Hospitallers and their crew. At about the same time the Hospitaller captain at Bodrum had to be excused when the Bodrum *galiotta* took cloth from a *grippum* of Chios, and the Hospitallers agreed to return the goods, declaring that Bodrum castle had been built to attack the Turks and not to rob Christians.[25]

In addition to the activities of shipping belonging to the Hospital as an order, there was a type of *corso* which involved individual Hospitaller brethren in arming vessels entirely at their own expense.[26] Thus on 14 April 1413 the Master's lieutenant at Rhodes licensed Fr. Jean de Pietris and Fr. Richard de Pontailler Commander of Ensigné in the Priory of Aquitaine, both of the *langue* of France, to sail against the shipping of the infidel enemy — 'contra infideles inimicos religionis nostre' — and that of their subjects, with the exception of the Orthodox monks of Mount Athos, and to seize their goods. These brethren were not to lose their seniority in the *langue* of France, an important consideration in the struggle for benefices, in consequence of their absence at sea on such ventures.[27] This formula apparently

25. Malta, Cod. 339, fols. 233v-234 [267v-268], 234 [268], 236v-237 [270v-271], 237 [271], 237v [271v]: these and other texts, some undated, are utilized, with some inaccuracies, in Delaville, *Les Hospitaliers*, pp. 327-8; Luttrell, *The Hospitallers of Rhodes*, No. II, pp. 103-4; id., *The Later History of the Maussolleion and its Utilization in the Hospitaller Castle at Bodrum = The Maussolleion at Halikarnassos: Reports of the Danish Archaeological Expedition to Bodrum*, Vol. II, Pt. 2 (Aarhus, 1986), pp. 147, 159.

26. There is no evidence before 1413, though licences were not copied into the surviving magistral registers; the texts of 1413 and 1416 published here were copied, quite exceptionally, into an unusual register which was kept, during the Master's absence in the West, by his lieutenants at Rhodes and which included documents of a type not normally found in the Master's 'Libri Bullarum'.

27. Document I below.

excluded attacks on friendly Muslims with whom there was a truce.[28] What it could mean in practice was shown when, on 25 August 1413, the Master and Convent issued a safe conduct allowing Anthonius Ruffin, *burgensis* of Rhodes, to bring a case in Rhodes against Fr. Richard de Pontailler who had, with an armed *galiocta*, attacked Ruffin's *gripparia* near Cyprus and seized his goods:

> quod te nuper cum quadam gripparia cum mercibus et mercimonijs tuis in bono proposito circa Insulam Cypri nauigante, Religiosus in Christo nobis carissimus frater Richardus de Pontailer, preceptor dAnsengue, lingue Francie grippariam merces et mercimonia tua, cum quadam sua galiocta armata, sine aliqua racione occasione uel justa causa vi cepit et spoliauit . . .[29]

Though all Hospitallers took vows of poverty and technically all property, goods, or money they had in their possession belonged to the Order and reverted to it on their death, there was no serious pretence that individual brethren could not hold lands and houses, accumulate and lend money, establish hospitals and other pious foundations, or otherwise dispose of capital; they were not, however, to indulge in trade.[30] An agreement of 1416 showed how Hospitaller brethren could themselves invest in and manage the *corso*. Again the protagonists were from the more northern parts of France. If these were predominantly from the *langues* of France and Auvergne rather than from those of Provence, Italy or Spain, that may have been because the former provided more numerous brethren interested in the *corso* not merely as an investment in wealth or as an expression of enthusiasm for holy war, but also perhaps because they came from a petty rural *noblesse* nourished on an ideology provided by a reading of chivalric romances which may have stimulated them to participate in piratical adventures against the infidel.[31] Material interests, however,

---

28. On truces valid on land but not at sea, see Luttrell, *The Later History*, pp. 147, 159; id., *The Hospitallers of Rhodes*, No. II, p. 104.
29. Cod. 339, fol. 255 [289].
30. These questions require a detailed examination of the statutes which are still largely unpublished.
31. This is the hypothesis of M. Fontenay, 'Les Chevaliers de Malte dans le *Corso* méditerranéen au XVIIe siècle', in *Las Ordenes Militares en el Mediterráneo Occidental (s. XII-XVII)* (Madrid, 1989), pp. 393-5 and Table 1, who documents a French predominance in the seventeenth-century Hospitaller *corso*.

remained powerful. Fr. Hugues d'Arcy who was Commander of Chalon-sur-Saône, Pontaubert, Bellecroix, and Avalleur, belonged to the Priory of Champagne. Fr. Hugues d'Arcy, *alias la caille*, was repeatedly involved in litigation to secure seniority, preferment, and financial advantage within the Hospital; eventually he secured the Priory of Champagne.[32] On 27 March 1416 he appeared before the Master's lieutenant at Rhodes together with Fr. Guidot de *Rauta*. The latter recognized the receipt from Fr. Hugues d'Arcy of 150 Venetian ducats which had been invested in the purchase of a fourth part of a *galeota*; if the vessel captured booty, Fr. Hugues was to receive a fourth of the profit calculated after expenses had been deducted, and if Fr. Hugues had to return to the West his proctor was to collect both the 150 ducats and a quarter of any profit.[33] Though the manner in which expenses were calculated was not specified, Fr. Hugues d'Arcy, a passive partner who was not involved in any personal risk or time at sea, seems none the less to have stood to gain a quarter of the booty.

After 1416 the Rhodian *corso* evolved in various complex ways[34] and rules to cover it were gradually established.[35] The *corso* acquired

32. Eg., Malta, Cod. 335, fols. 27-8v; Cod. 336, fols. 41v, 42-3; Cod. 338, fol. 81v; Cod. 339, fols. 20v-21, 128v, 164-164v (*bis*), 192; Cod. 346, fol. 25; Cod. 351, fol. 23v.
33. Document II below.
34. This topic awaits study for the period following 1416; for later years, see N. Vatin, *L'Ordre de Saint-Jean-de-Jérusalem, l'Empire ottoman et la Méditerranée orientale entre les deux sièges de Rhodes: 1480-1522* (Louvain–Paris, 1994), pp. 60-63, 85-129, 294-310.
35. A statute of 1462, which insisted that Hospitallers should not arm vessels without written licence, read:
Item pero chauemo visto perli tempi passati succeder molti dampnj, et inco[n]uenienti per casone darmar Nauilij allordine nostro, empero chel çe sono molti freri de nostra Religione che se dillectano et studiano di armar de molte, et uarie factione de Nauilij, Il perche volendo, Nuy de opportuno remedio prouedere per obuiar ad cotali dampnj, Statuymo, et ordinamo chel non sian freri de qualunche stato e condictione che se siano che ardiscono ne presuma darmar Nauilio alcuno, zoe come sono carauelle, o, Naue, balloneri, gallee, ne fuste, ne altri nauilij sença spicial liçentia del M[aestr]e la qual liçentia Volem che sia facta inscripto col termino preciso et speçificato del tempo che doura star armato tal Nauilio saluo se alcun armasse Imponente per uenire ad Rhodi perli seccorsj dellordine nostro et qualunche contrafara presumendo nauigar, Nuy absolute et Iudicamo et hauemo per Inobediente, et anche proybimo et non volemo chel sia frere alcuno che arma fuste, ne gallee al modo de pirrati, overo corsari, ne anche volemo chessi vadeno per patron, o, capitaney de cotali Nauilij sel nonli sera concesso de gratia speçial, soto

186

great importance as a form of state-controlled sea brigandage which became vital to the Hospitallers' prestige and image as holy warriors and also to their economy and that of their port; furthermore, it provided extra naval forces in time of emergency. A traveller of 1521 put the Hospital's total expenses on Rhodes at 97,977 gold ducats and its income at 47,000, remarking that the very considerable difference of some 50,000 ducats was made up from profits made by attacking the Hospital's enemies at sea.[36] In 1503 a *barca* armed by a Hospitaller was to pay on any prizes 'el diritto di nove per cento acostumato pagarsi da corsari'; the text did not clarify whether this nine per cent of booty went to the Master or to the Rhodian treasury.[37] After 1530, when the Hospital moved to Malta, the system which had emerged at Rhodes continued to function as an important element in the Order's activities until Malta was lost in 1798.[38]

DOCUMENT I

Malta, Cod. 339, fol. 179v [213v] (14 April 1413)

[Margin] pro f. Johanne de Pietris [(*et*) *al.*]

Fr. Lucius de Vallinis [sacre domus hospitalis sanctj Johannis Jherosolimitani humilis marescallus et locumtenens Reverendissimj in Christo patris et domini domini fratris Philibertj de Nahlhaco dei gratia eiusdem sacre domus magistri dignissimi pauperum Christi custodis] [39]

---

penna della priuaçione dellabito, et dognj officio et beneficio chauessero, o, che fusser per hauere. Et se al presente sa retrouano alcunj freri Incotali armamenti de fuste, et de gallee, Iudicamo quelli douere essere priuati dellabito de offiçij et benefiçij et donori, selloro non desarmano et lassano In termino duno anno lor fuste et lor gallee et cossi hauemo per declarato.
(Valletta, National Library of Malta, Biblioteca Ms. 501, fols. 329v-330v.)

36. Text in R. Röhricht and H. Meisner, *Deutsche Pilgerreisen nach dem Heiligen Lande* (Berlin, 1880), pp. 372-5.
37. Malta, Cod. 80, fols. 61-2. Some evidence suggests a tax of ten per cent: Vatin, *L'Empire ottoman*, p. 91, n. 39.
38. The best recent studies are those of M. Fontenay; see also S. Bono, 'Naval Exploits and Privateering', in V. Mallia-Milanes (ed.), *Hospitaller Malta 1530-1798: Studies on Early Modern Malta and the Order of St. John of Jerusalem* (Malta, 1993), with bibliography.
39. The full title is taken from fol. 179.

Religiosis in Christo nobis carissimis fratribus Johannj de Pietris et Richardo de Pontaillier preceptorj Dansigny [40] lingue nostre Francie Salutem in domino. Sperantes quod per strenuitates vestras Dej et patronj nostrj juvamine mediante viriliter gerere debeatis contra Infideles Inimicos Religionis nostre, aduersus quos magnj feruore affectu adire pro honore sancte fidei Orthodoxe et nostre Religionis, Idcirco licentiam vobis assensum pariter et consensum, armandj quandam galiottam vestram, et cum ea nauigandj et remigandj ac guerram contra Infideles Jnimicos Religionis nostre ac eorum subiectos et subditos, detractis calogeris montis sanctj,[41] et eorum bonis quibus in aliquo non jntendimus agrauare seu dampnificare per vos seu aliquem vestrum, et quidquid de ipsis seu eorum Rebus ceperitis ad vestrum beneplacitum faciendj de voluntate consilio et assensu Religiosorum in Cristo nobis carissimorum dominorum fratrum baliuorum et procerum[42] nostrj conuentus Rodj concedimus et Impertimur Cum tali prerogatiua ut in consequendo muneribus et beneficijs nostre Religionis habeaminj ac si essetis personaliter in conuentu Rodj residentes de voluntate et assensu pillerij ceterorumque fratrum lingue Francie in conuentu Rodj degentium,[43] mandantes vniuersis et singulis subditis nostris, ac non subditos sed amicos nostros obsecremus, ut in hijs vobis nostrj [44] contemplatione, auxilium consilium prebeatis et iuvamen. datum Rodj sub sigillo nostro quo in talibus vtimur.[45] die xiiij mensis aprilis. Anno a natiuitate dominj m⁰· iiijᶜ· xiijᵒ·

DOCUMENT II

Malta, Cod. 339, fol. 264v [298v] (27 March 1416)

die vigesimaseptima marcii anno incarnationis dominj millesimo quadringentesimo decimosexto comparuerunt in lobia coram domino locumtenente[46] fratres Hugo Darsi de Chalon, et Guidotus de Rauta,[47] quiquidem Guidotus confessus fuit debere predicto de Chalon Darsi,

40. Ensigné, Priory of Aquitaine (Diocesis of Sèvres).
41. *Mons Sanctus*: Mount Athos.
42. *dicti* crossed out.
43. *residentes* crossed out.
44. *Sic*.
45. In the Master's absence, his lieutenant is using his own personal seal.
46. The Master was in the West; his lieutenant at Rhodes was Fr. Luce de Vallins.
47. Or *Rarita*: unidentified.

VIII

summam centum et quinquaginta ducatorum venetorum per dictum Darsi eidem Guidonj traditorum pro empcione quarte partis eorum galiote,[48] de quaquidem parte quarta fuit contentus predictus frater Guido . . .[49] quod si jpse lucrum inde consequeretur quod predictus Darsi expensis deductis consequeretur, quartam partem ratione quarte partis galiotte. Et si contingetur quod predictus Darsi rediret ad partes occidentales ante auentum et regressum dictj G[uidoti] et galiote quod procurator dictj Darsj posset securare a dicto G[uidoto] dictos centum et quinquaginta ducatos uenetos cum quarte parte lucrj si quod in viagio sequeret.[50]

48. This implies that a *galiota* could be purchased for 600 ducats.
49. A line covers the erasure of several words.
50. This text was not a sealed bull but simply an official note or record copied into the lieutenant Master's register.

IX

The Spiritual Life of the Hospitallers of Rhodes

The spiritual life of a group of professed religious whose concerns were seldom intellectual and who left little explicit indication of their vocational attitudes was difficult to gauge even for contemporaries [1], as was made evident in and after 1307 by the conflicting perplexities aroused by some of the accusations brought against the Templars [2]. The Hospitallers' rules and regulations, their style of dress and architecture, their relics and liturgical practices afforded indirect insights into their collective mentality, but the motives of particular individuals for entering a military order and their vision of such an institution and of their own role within it remained largely obscure. Some Hospitaller brethren may have perceived themselves as joining a prestigious and cosmopolitan organization in which the military element dictated the tone, while others perhaps envisaged an essentially pious and predominantly priestly brotherhood devoted to an apostolic life of service to the poor and sick. In practice, many brethren must have been ordinary people seeking not so much the good of their own souls as a secure and respectable career leading to a modest benefice.

In terms of canon law a Hospitaller became a professed religious, but in reality he was joining an order of which the degree of spiritual commitment was sometimes seen as being inferior to that of monks or friars, whose rules were regarded as stricter, and as akin perhaps to the level of canons or members of lay confraternities [3]. The Hospitallers' activities, including their most warlike functions, were undoubtedly spiritual ones in the same sense that crusading could be regarded as an act of charity or love, yet it was also true that even their most sacred liturgical duties brought them financial rewards. Furthermore, religious practices at the Hospitallers' Convent or headquarters on Rhodes, for which their statutes and other legislation seem primarily to have been intended, differed widely from those in their European priories, while in the West itself there was considerable variation between one region and another.

The brethren of the military orders were Latin religious of the Roman Church. They had no cloistered conventual life and they differed from monks who followed an enclosed regime of prayer and labour, from mendicant friars who were dedicated to teaching, preaching and conversion, and from members of exclusively hospitaller ordens. Like all these, however, the Hospitallers took the three vows of the religious: poverty, chastity and obedience. The Hospital was in origin a hospitaller order and juridically it always retained a mixed hospitaller-military character; its brethren took an extra vow to serve the *domini infirmi* while their unchanged twelfth-century Rule made no reference to military activity or to knighthood or nobility. The Hospitallers came closest to being canons, following a mixed but essentially Augustinian Rule approved by the papacy, to which they were ultimately subordinate. In the military orders, unlike most other orders, it was the lay rather than the priestly element which predominated. The Hospitallers were regular not secular clergy, even if the military brethren were often referred to as *laici*, and they were largely exempt from episcopal jurisdiction. The brethren lived in houses or commanderies and were bound to their *vita communis* and to their community's liturgical routine. Their statutes regulated food, sleep, property, discipline and other matters, and the brethren had to say fixed prayers at established hours and on particular days [4]. As in other orders, the ideal of poverty was partially, sometimes indeed blatantly, compromised [5]. The Hospitallers' obligation to the poor and sick constituted, at least in theory, the most novel and vital aspect of their spiritual life [6]. The vow of obedience was fundamental, and it prevented Hospitallers from taking other vows. In fact, brethren were explicitly prohibited both by papal bull and by their own legislation from becoming crusaders or from fighting against fellow Christians. The Hospitaller's war was a holy and perpetual struggle directed only at the infidel; it did not depend on papal crusading bulls [7]. His cross was not that of a crusader but was worn in memory of God, and of the holy cross and of Christ's suffering upon it [8].

Fully professed Hospitallers were either *milites* or knights, priests or chaplains, or sergeants; donats and *confratres* owed a measure of obedience but took no religious vows. Except at Rhodes, the priests were normally quite numerous. In 1338 there were 58 knights, 144 sergeants and 117 priests in Eastern Provence [9], and 34 knights, 48 sergeants and 34 priests in the Priory of England [10]. In 12 houses of the Archdiocese of Prague in 1373 there were 31 knights and 82 priests, but no sergeants [11]. The proportions evidently varied considerably, and in 1373 in 70 of the

106 commanderies of the Priory of France, that is in the area lying north of the Loire, there were 124 priests, 49 sergeants and only 5 knights, though there must have been some 25 or 30 further knights from the priory who were on Rhodes or elsewhere. This was a notable statistic but it reflected an exceptional moment in which the population had been drastically reduced by war, plague and economic depression. The Priory of France had received from the Temple a large number of churches, amounting to 80 out of the 123 churches in 70 of its commanderies, and these could not be disposed of in the same way as other Templar properties, which meant that priests had to be provided for them [12]. Such churches could be served by non-Hospitaller priests provided they did not belong to another order, but these had to be paid. The situation at Dôle illustrated this crisis: in 1373 there were no liturgical books and where once there had been three or four Hospitaller priests together with a number of resident secular priests, there was just one daily low mass without music and a sung mass only on Sundays and feast days [13].

There were at any one time several hundred Hospitaller sisters living in more than twenty houses under a regime not unlike that of an enclosed nunnery. These *sorores* were fully professed religious and members of a military order, though their version of the Rule varied a little from that of the male brethren; they seldom if ever undertook medical or nursing duties in hospices or hospitals, their main function ostensibly being that of prayer [14]. The sisters were under obedience to the prior of their priory, they were supposed to pay responsions and occasionally, in Aragon for example, they attended prioral chapters. They were largely of noble or wealthy origin and were required to be literate. Their confessors were often Hospitallers and their worldly affairs were managed by a male Hospitaller. Especially important was the house at Sigena in Aragon which was a major royal foundation, a retreat for noblewomen which twice had a royal princess as its prioress in the fourteenth century [15]. The women's houses varied: a foundation of 1324 at Perugia saw a prosperous merchant securing a former Templar *domus* which he endowed for his family to hold in *jus patronatus* [16], while the convent at Beaulieu near Cahors received a noble sister who became a saint [17].

The Hospitaller Rule discouraged female contacts for the brethren, who were not allowed to have their hair or feet washed or their beds made by women [18]. Hospitaller attitudes were set somewhere between those of the Hispanic Order of Santiago, which accepted married brethren who took vows of conjugal chastity with consequent arrangements for childen's nurseries and the maintenance of widows [19], and the strict antifeminist position of the Templars; even the latter occasionally accepted women associates, particularly when property donations were involved [20].

Hospitaller commanderies quite normally housed women as servants, pensioners and married donats [21]. In 1373 the house at Arbois in the Diocese of Besançon was occupied by the commander who was a priest-brother aged sixty, his twenty-year-old nephew who was also a Hospitaller, a female servant aged fifty and a girl of ten [22]. Occasionally, as in 1319 at Bertaignemont in France, a Hospitaller *soror* actually resided in a male house [23]. Segregation was seldom complete and in any case Hospitallers were able, with permission, to travel, to visit their families and to go on pilgrimage; some had illegitimate children [24]. There was a serious case of adultery involving the Admiral of the Order at Rhodes in 1411 [25]. Such difficulties were recognized late in the fourteenth century by Philippe de Mézières who advocated that the brethren of his ideal military order should be married and live in the East with their wives [26].

Though the Hospital's priests formed the most numerous class, they were socially inferior to the *milites* who held the highest offices and who were predominant in the Convent. Hospitaller priests had the same general status and obligations as any others, while they also enjoyed the special privileges and exemptions of the Order. They administered the sacraments to the brethren and to the poor and sick; they could hold various offices within the Order and they participated in chapters. Those who wished to become priest-brethren had to prove that they were in minor orders before they could enter the Hospital and to spend one year in a *domus* before receiving full orders; they could not become a subdeacon until they were 18, a deacon before 22 or a priest before 28 [27]. In France boys were sometimes received *cum condicione* to live in a commandery as novices until they were old enough to take full vows and become a Hospitaller priest [28]. At Rhodes the Prior of the Convent controlled the Conventual church which had its complement of priests; other priest-brethren served the dependent chapels of the Conventual church and other chapels, while the Master had his own chapel and chaplains [29]. Hospitaller priests were generally subject only to their own Order and to the pope. In the West candidates for parishes and dependent churches had to be presented for induction to the local bishop, but normally he could not veto their appointment [30]. In Bohemia parish priests could be ranked as a commander, a *plebanus seu preceptor domus parrochialis*, even though the main function of their house was to take care of the parish; some Bohemian commanderies had a priest-brother with the title of preacher [31]. The Order's priests might hope to secure a reasonable safe, if often modest, benefice. Many became commanders and thus responsible for disciplining other brethren, supervising their houses' estates and managing their finances. In the Priory of France in 1373 some 64 percent of commanders were priests [32].

Certain large commanderies housed many priests and functioned as collegiate chantries. Thus the collegiate „priory" at Corbeil in the Île-de--France had been founded in 1224 by the King of France to maintain 13 Hospitaller priests who would pray for his father [33]; in 1373 it was fulfilling this condition by maintaining 11 Hospitaller priests and 4 donats, two of them also priests [34]. The Hospitaller church at Aix-en-Provence had been a burial place for the Counts of Provence and 12 priest-brethren were saying masses for some of them there in 1338 [35]. At Avalterre in Flanders the main house, the *domus sive preceptoria principalis*, had 33 dependent *maisons* or *domus*, 24 of them *cum capella* and 17 of them leased to seculars; it counted 31 *fratres*, 25 of them priests, two of them parish priests, 6 sergeants, one priest-donat and 7 lay donats; 9 of the priests, 4 of the sergeants and one donat acted as *rectores* of a *maison*; 17 houses were leased and two other houses which had no rector apparently had neither brethren nor priests in residence, and many of the priest-brethren may have lived at Avalterre [36]. The house at Glatz in the Priory of Bohemia had 13 priests and just one *miles* in 1373, at which time 3 secular priests and 2 other clerics were being paid to sing masses there daily [37]. The absence of military brethren from any particular house did not mean that they were excluded from it [38]. Spiritual life was naturally stronger where the community was reasonably large. An illuminated initial in a gradual made at Zittau in the Priory of Bohemia in 1435 showed 11 tonsured Hospitallers chanting from a single book [39], while another illumination of 1440/50 from Burgsteinfurt depicted a group of tonsured brethren dressed in black mantles with white eight-pointed crosses who were watching over a funeral bier [40]. A painting done in about 1470 by Geertgen tot Sint Jans, who though not a Hospitaller lived in the commandery at Utrecht, showed the burning of the bones of John the Baptist with five Hospitallers, whose faces were painted as real portraits, in solemn procession wearing black mantles with bonnets and white eight-pointed crosses; they carried two red banners each with a simple white cross on it [41]. Large priestly communities seem to have flourished mainly in the Priories of France, *Alamania* and Bohemia.

The Hospitallers' liturgical regime was regulated in detail. New statutes repeatedly insisted on the maintenance, furnishing and illumination of chapels and churches, on fasts and feasts and on dress, genuflexions, processions, services in the hospitals and communion for the sick. Divine service supposedly occupied a considerable part of the Hospitallers' day, being celebrated in their own chapels with their own priests reciting the offices. The senior priest of each house, sometimes known as its prior, was in charge of its church, ornaments, vestments and books; every church was to be lit night and day. Each night five priests were to read from the psalter on behalf of the Order's benefactors. The chaplains officiated at daily services, matins being preceded by 15 psalms. Brethren who were not priests had, if they could not read, to say a total of 150 paternosters daily at 10 different times instead of reciting the hours; alternatively, they could say all 150 at once. Brethren who failed to rise for matins were condemned to bread and water. A statute of 1262 listed 16 days with special masses of obligation and it referred to others unnamed. The Order's calendars indicated special offices for the feasts of John the Baptist, the Conception of the Virgin and so on [42]. The Hospital followed not the monastic hours with twelve lessons at matins but the less onerous canonical *ordo* with three nocturns and therefore only nine lessons; this might indicate that the Hospitallers were more like canons than monks, though two military orders, Alcantara and Calatrava, observed the Cistercian rule with the monastic *ordo* [43]. In the West where many houses were reduced to a complement of only one or two brethren, neither necessarily a priest, the whole liturgical regime must have suffered and the quality of religious life was inevitably diminished. In fact as early as 1262 there were complaints that some houses had no chaplain [44]. Of 70 commanderies in the Priory of France as many as 29 had only one *frater* of any type in residence in 1373, and in 11 houses there was no Hospitaller at all [45].

Brethren had to make their communion at three fixed times in the year, Christmas, Easter and Pentecost [46]. Hospitaller priests heard confession from the brethren, and a statute of 1262 stated that „a *frater* shall not confess his sins to anyone other than his prior or some other priest-brother of the house, except with permission from his superior" [47]. This regulation may have been intended to keep secrets within the Order, but there was little indication within the Hospital of the damaging misunderstandings which the Templar trials after 1307 showed to be current among some Templars who failed to distinguish between sacerdotal absolution and the lifting of penances by their non-priestly superiors following the confession of faults made in chapter. This capitular confession went back to the markedly different doctrinal climate of the twelfth century when pardon granted had not implied absolution from sin. The non-priestly lay brethren of the military orders had been accused of usurping the sacerdotal office by imposing penances and relaxing sins, and in about 1272 the *Collectio de Scandalis Ecclesie* suggested to the pope that the remedy lay in sending literate brethren to study theology. However, John of Freiburg stated that the Hospitallers had solved the problem by requiring brethren to be absolved by their prior, that is by the senior priest in their house. Brethren presumably found that confession to a priest in secret was preferable to communal judgement and scourging or some other punishment in chapter [48].

Some commanderies had a chapel within the house, while others had a separate church building; the ecclesiastical furnishings were mostly conventional. The Hospitallers obviously needed liturgical manuscripts. 20 Templar and 60 Hospitaller inventories mentioned over 350 books from France alone. In some cases the Hospital's books included works inherited from the Temple, and some large commanderies were well supplied. At Arles the Templars had had over 60 books, some 40 of them liturgical. At Toulouse between 1347 and 1428 the Hospital had about 25 manuscripts including a bible, a breviary and a *Flores Sanctorum* which were kept chained in the choir. There were 28 books at Mas Deu in Roussillon in 1377. Some small rural houses had only a single liturgical manuscript, always the missal; thus in 1398 Noirlieu, a dependent *membrum* of the Commandery of Neuville-au-Temple, had just *un bon messel*. The number of copies of the Order's statutes seems to have been small. Apart from breviaries and psalters for individual use, there were sometimes rituals for baptisms, marriages and the other sacraments. Certain volumes included the Hospital's calendar which showed special offices such as the nine weekly lessons for John the Baptist, the nine lessons of the holy cross to be read every Friday as laid down in 1354, and the feast of the Conception of the Virgin introduced in 1358. Luxurious illuminated books of hours seem not to have been commissioned before the late fifteenth century. Those possessions which brethren were permitted to hold for their lifetime included liturgical manuscripts which were supposed to pass to the Treasury on their death but books for personal use in prayer, for example breviaries and unglossed psalters, and books for general reading, such as chronicles and romances, were exempted from this regulation and most of them probably remained in the house where their possessor died. Others were lost: in about 1440 Fr. Bertrand Blanqui, chaplain at Roquebillière in the Commandery of Nice, sold his chapel's breviary and pawned both a sacramentary and a ritual [49].

There was naturally a concern for death and burial. The Master constituted a special case and his demise involved a ceremonial funeral with orations and some military pomp, followed by burial in a tomb with an inscribed slab; the tomb was often in the Conventual church within a chapel founded by the deceased, who had sometimes endowed chaplains to commemorate him there [50]. Masters were to be remembered in an annual mass [51] and they were recorded briefly in the so-called Chronicle of the Deceased Masters which developed from a list kept and continued for that purpose [52]. Dying brethren could make a *dispropriamentum*, which was not a will since they had in theory no property of which to dispose; in it they declared their minor possessions and petty debts. The deceased was to be buried in his mantle. Those brethren present were to pray for him and each was to offer a candle and a denier for the poor to whom the dead man's clothes were also given. The corpse, surrounded by candles, was to be watched in church by the priest-brethren singing psalms, attendance being compulsory for the non-clerical brethren who had to recite 150 paternosters. Some of the Order's liturgical books contained the Hospital's special office for the dead. After burial there were 30 masses and an annual anniversary office for the deceased, whose name was to be entered at the relevant day in the obit book of the house where he was buried. If a Hospitaller or anyone else died after the hour of vespers, the corpse was to be left on a bier with a lamp. There was no special provision for those killed in battle, but there were regulations concerning the burial of pilgrims and of those who died in the Order's hospital [53]. An illumination in the obituary book or necrology from Burgsteinfurt near Münster, datable circa 1445, showed tonsured Hospitaller priests seated with service books near a banner bearing a cross with a fleur-de-lys at each of its four points; the banner presumably covered the corpse and had a candle burning at each of its four corners. Another illumination in the same manuscript depicted an open tomb containing the body of a Hospitaller [54]. One of the earliest surviving obituary books is that from Eskilstuna near Stockholm which was begun late in the thirteenth century; most other known examples also belonged to Province of *Alamania*. These books showed the deceased's name on the anniversary of his death when he was to be commemorated with a mass. Donats, *confratres* and others who had made a payment or donation in return for prayer were also inscribed. Sometimes the names were entered in one of the Hospital's liturgical calendars [55].

There seems to have been no obituary book at the Convent where, by some time well before 1480, brethren were being buried just outside the city walls in the cemetery by Saint Anthony's church where the remains of some Masters and of senior officers, priors and ordinary brethren were interred and where commemorative services for them were held [56]. Just as some brethren began to use seals showing their family arms [57], so anonymous burial was gradually abandoned. The Masters apart, the earliest surviving tomb slab for an individual Hospitaller at Rhodes dates to the early or mid fifteenth century [58]. In the West, individual tomb slabs and personal monuments not directly connected to an actual burial place began to appear in the late thirteenth century, many of them commemorating rulers of priories [59]. At Freiburg-im-Breisgau the exact places within the Order's church in which certain Hospitaller brethren and sisters, as also various lay men and women, had been buried were being indicated in some way at least as early as 1308 [60]. The relevant accounts for 1386/87 recorded expenditures for the tomb of the Prior of France, Fr. Gérard de Vienne, and for three painted stone sculptures in his chapel, all paid for from the personal wealth he left on his death; the same accounts also included funeral expenses for two commanders [61]. Such payments were evidently permitted, despite prohibitions against personal wealth. Yet at Würzburg in 1330 an inscription actually recorded that a house had been purchased by Fr. Heinrich von Grünsfelt at his own expense — *comparavit domum istam propriis expensis* [62].

The Hospitallers' books included martyrologies and lives of saints [63]. Their Rule, prayers and diplomatic formulae invoked God, the Trinity, Christ and so on, and there were special references to the poor, to serve whom was a spiritual activity [64]; in fact the Master entitled himself *pauperum Christi custos*. The Rule explicitly enjoined brethren to dedicate themselves to God, the Virgin, the Baptist and the poor [65]. The Hospital's patron, Saint John, appeared in documents and on seals and coins, and his feasts were specially commemorated, while the Virgin appeared throughout the liturgy [66]. The Assumption of the Virgin on 15 August, the day on which Rhodes was taken, was made a special feast in 1311 [67] as was the Conception of the Virgin, in thanks for deliverance from plague, in 1358 [68]. At least one of the *langues*, that of Italy, had its own patron in Saint Catherine of Alexandria to whom were dedicated the hospices founded at Venice in about 1359 and at Rhodes in 1391 [69].

The Hospital's liturgical calendars naturally included days assigned to a number of saints directly connected with Jerusalem [70]. In Italy, and sometimes elsewhere, commanderies were dedicated to a particular patron, often John the Baptist or a local saint. In Northern and Central Italy San Giovanni del Tempio was a common Hospitaller dedication; it did not indicate a former Templar house [71]. There were a number of Hospitaller saints or *beati;* none were military in character and some had devoted themselves to the poor and sick, as for example had Santa Ubaldesca of Calcinaia, who died in 1206, and Santa Toscana of Verona, who was probably not a professed Hospitaller. Other Hospitaller saints included Ugo of Genoa. These all died well before 1310, and none appeared in the Order's medieval liturgy [72]. Saint Flor was one of four noble sisters who entered the Hospital's house at Beaulieu-en-Quercy; she was received at the age of twelve and died in 1347, after which her life was written by her confessor who was quite probably a Hospitaller priest. An extremely pious virgin, Flor spent time reading the liturgical hours; she confessed daily, complained that her house — in which she had a chamber — was too comfortable, suffered temptations, displayed the stigmata, experienced many visions, and repeatedly effected miraculous cures. She was visited by Franciscans, by a cousin who was a Benedictine and by a master in theology. A Hospitaller priest who contradicted one of her visions was punished by illness. Her sanctity was established in 1360 when her corpse was moved; many miracles followed, and during subsequent decades the cult was developed and brought pilgrims to her tomb at Beaulieu [73]. All this was, however, entirely exceptional for a Hospitaller.

The cult of relics was more spectacular and more lucrative. The Hospital lost its Conventual relics with the fall of Acre in 1291, except apparently for the body of its founder Gérard which seems to have been sent away, probably together with that part of the Syrian archives which survived, very possibly to Manosque in Provence. After 1312 the Hospitallers inherited the Templar relics which had been saved from Syria, and to them they added many items which were much venerated on Rhodes, including in 1484 the right hand of John the Baptist [74]. The acquisition of relics and the encouragement of pilgrimages to visit them through the organization of liturgical feasts and processions, initiatives evidently designed to bring some profit to the Order, were especially widespread in the Province of *Alamania* [75]. At Rhodes, the Hospitallers' architecture expressed Western styles and it reflected their military function, but the churches, the hospital, the *auberges* and a number of sculptured saints and inscriptions on the walls and buildings of the town demonstrated few explicit spiritual messages [76]. The Western commanderies and churches, and the frescoes and paintings which sometimes decorated them, were mostly in a local regional style, and while they displayed devotion to John the Baptist, to the Virgin or to some local patron saint, they seldom exhibited any specifically Hospitaller iconography [77]. The Hospital built or sometimes inherited a few round churches, and occasionally its churches had an upper storey with rooms to accommodate pilgrims or the sick [78].

Undoubtedly a spiritual matter was the celebration of personal offices, not merely for brethren, donats and *confratres* who were all entitled to burial and other sacraments in time of interdict, but also for others who in various ways purchased prayer for themselves, their families and others. Sometimes it was a Hospitaller himself who endowed such commemoration. People who pledged or invested monies or property to earn themselves a life-pension in a commandery could also arrange that on their death the capital, or sometimes just the income from it, was devoted to payment for prayers for the dead. Such requiem masses were especially popular in Germany and Bohemia. There the considerable revenues, sometimes from yearly rents, and the relevant documents were often kept in a separate fund held under key by the *pitanciarius* or *magister pitanciarie* of the house, who paid out the fee, technically a meal or *pitancia*, earned by the priests who said masses [79]. The commander could not use these funds for other purposes, though there was a major exception when the representatives of the *Ballei* of Franconia decided to raid *pitancia* funds to extinguish major debts in 1362 [80]. The economic aspect of this practice was important and the arrangements were sometimes complicated. An exceptional bequest made at Prague in 1405 created endowments for an altar, for wax, candles and other church ornaments, for brethren to say masses *pro pitancia* for the donor, for servants male and female, for a sacristan for masses, for a dinner for the brethren, for the brethren's infirmary and for a subsacristan, some bellringers, a cantor, a schoolmaster, a choirmaster, three choristers, a deacon, a subdeacon, lampbearers and resident paupers [81].

Assistance to the poor and sick was the Hospital's founding function [82]. It was upheld at Rhodes both in symbolic gestures, notably the ritual washing of the feet of the poor by the Master, and in the maintenance of a great hospital, for which a large new building was begun in 1440 [83]. Care for the inmates' spiritual life was reflected in special prayers recited for the patients every night, at least in the Conventual hospital, by priest-orethren who went in procession to the wards [84]. The Order's hospitals in the West most often sheltered pilgrims and travellers, the aged and the poor [85]. By the fourteenth century control of such hospitals was generally passing into secular municipal hands and many of the Hospital's foundations fell into decline or disuse; thus by 1338 the once flourishing hospital at Arles did no more than feed two paupers [86]. Almost everywhere almsgiving was much diminished, but arrangements which provided board and lodging for life to laymen and laywomen who had purchased or contracted for a life pension were common in many priories. These newer forms of welfare generated funds which did not support poor and sick people through donations from the wealthier, but catered rather for individual members of the middle and upper middle elements in society who invested capital or incomes in the Hospital, often according to precisely formulated contracts, in return for their material upkeep as residential pensioners. In 1338 there were 50 such *corrodarii* as against 119 *fratres* in England, white the situation at Skirbeck in Lincolnshire, where the infirmary housed 20 poor and where a further 40 paupers were fed daily, was unique [87]. In the Priory of France the 8 poor who were sheltered nightly at Douai were equally exceptional [88]. New foundations were a rarity, and an attempt made by the Order in 1402/3 to secure control of the lucrative pilgrim traffic to Jerusalem proved abortive [89].

In many priories the Hospital was responsible for a number of parishes and provided the parish priest, who was often a Hospitaller. There were 30 Hospitaller parishes in 15 of the 26 dioceses covering the Priory of France [90]. At Poznań in Poland the Hospitaller parish priest held a stall as a cathedral canon, a situation which led to complaints from the bishop when he met the Master of the Hospital at the Council of Constance in 1417 [91]. An extraordinary case was that of Treviso where, as a consequence of the Templar inheritance, the Hospital had three commanderies and three parishes within the city and a fourth parish just outside it. Together these constituted an exempt enclave within the diocese which encouraged the bishop to make occasional visitations when he was able to do so as an apostolic visitor. In 1373 he found that the parish of San Giovanni, which had once had two salaried secular priests, had only one; two non-Hospitaller priests were paid to officiate in the parish at San Martino; while at San Tommaso the commander was a priest-brother but no longer had a secular priest to help him. In about 1400 the townsfolk were complaining that mass was not being celebrated in two of these parish churches, and by 1437 all three lacked any resident Hospitaller of any type, each having just a single secular priest who was struggling on an insufficient salary; clearly there was no Hospitaller liturgical life of any kind [92].

The Hospitallers did occasionally support boys at school and university [93], but the situation in the Priory of Bohemia, where in the fourteenth century they had at least twelve schools, was in no way typical [94]. In 1373 there were 35 scholars at Strakonice while at Prague there were 27 scholars who ruled the schools, sang in choir, served at altar, rang bells, carried candles and so on, and „many others" who were maintained in the house [95]. A few individual Hospitallers had a university training and a degree, often in canon or civil law. In 1356 the Hospitallers secured a papal bull which enabled them to set up a college for their brethren to study canon law at the University of Paris. Lay lawyers were extremely costly, and in increasingly bureaucratic and legalistic times it was convenient for the Order to have its own experts; the Hospitallers may have remembered the disadvantages the Templars faced after their arrest in 1307 when it was partly through their own lack of legal understanding that the Templar brethren mismanaged their defence [96]. Occasionally there were Hospitallers such as Fr. Pietro de Imola, the Master's chancellor and secretary from 1323 to 1327, who had been lawyers before entering the Order [97]. On the other hand, Fr. Bertran de Tarragona was already a member of the Order when he graduated as a doctor of canon law in about 1349 [98]. By 1370 the Hospital had its own brethren acting as its procurators in the papal curia, and Hospitaller lawyers were active elsewhere. A distinguistihed Hospitaller, Fr. Gautier le Gras, who had been dean of the canon law faculty at Paris in 1389, became Prior of the Convent at Rhodes and was one of the three electors who represented the French nation in the election of Pope Martin V at the Council of Constance in 1417 [99].

Certain Hospitallers were cultural figures of some stature; thus the Master Fr. Juan Fernández de Heredia collected Greek manuscripts and compiled historical works [100], and Fr. Jean de Hesdin, a rare example of a Hospitaller master of theology, translated Valerius Maximus and wrote in opposition to Petrarch in defence of Avignon and France, as well as composing a series of prolix sermons [101]. In 1300 Fr. Johann von Frankenstein, a *capellanus* at Vienna, composed a poem on Christ's Passion [102]. Other German Hospitallers wrote sermons and theological tracts [103]. Some brethren could not read or did not know Latin, yet there were Hospitaller libraries whose contents went beyond mere liturgical works and lives of the saints or the crusading chronicle possessed by a Hospitaller at Douai in 1424 [104]. In 1349 Fr. Konrad of Glatz gave the Commandery of Zittau some 13 liturgical and theological works, including a Bible in two volumes [105]. In 1384 the Strasbourg commandery purchased books, including a Bible, an Aquinas and a book of sermons from the *domus* at Freiburg-im-Breisgau, and two years later the Commander of Strasbourg accepted from Fr. Heinrich Wolfach a legacy of some 10 books; further purchases at Strasbourg, including various sermons and Biblical commentaries, came in 1396 and 1398 [106]. An earlier Hospitaller priest Fr. Francon, Commander of Cologne, was the author of the late thirteenth century *Ars Cantus Mensurabilis* which was extremely important in the development of musical theory [107]. On the practical side, in 1396 Fr. Jean Bouteiller, a priest from the Priory of France, was called to Rhodes „to play the organ in the church" in 1396, when three *manestrely* were sent there as well [108]. As for the Hospitaller women, Sister Isabel de Aragón of Sigena, who died in 1424, appeared in a portrait reading a book with a monocle in one eye [109].

The Hospitallers made no effective attempt before about 1480 to compose or maintain any extensive chronological account of the Order's history. However, some manuscripts of the Rule and statutes did contain materials of a historical or pseudo-historical nature, most notably the *miracula,* the mythical account of the Jerusalem hospice which had been fabricated in the twelfth century in order to provide Biblical origins for the Order. These stories went on to describe the emergence of the Hospital at the time of the first crusade, while the so-called Chronicle of the Deceased Masters, to which additions were made as Masters died, provided a varied if extremely abbreviated chronological outline of the

Order's development through a series of brief comments on successive Masters. A few manuscripts compiled by Fr. Guglielmo di Santo Stefano between about 1287 and 1303 collected various legal writings and *esgarts*, the judgements made in chapter general, together with early statutes and other texts [110]. The Hospital's official language was French, but in 1357 the Master had the statutes themselves translated into Latin since some Italian brethren could not understand the French text [111]. On the other hand, the Rule had been turned from Latin into Anglo-Norman verse before 1187 and into German in 1253 [112]. These translations may have been intended to allow readings to be made to brethren at table, as was the practice in the Teutonic Order [113]. A crude translation of the psalter into French made on Cyprus between 1299 and 1309 was dedicated to Fr. Simon le Rat, who was Marshal of the Hospital and who succeeded Fr. Guglielmo di Santo Stefano as Commander of Cyprus [114].

Many Hospitallers were priests, few of whom were intellectuals, while some of the military brethren were illiterate. They were mostly ordinary men who had adopted an unusual vocation. Their motives and spiritual attitudes must have been rather varied but, with strong regional differences, they shared a common mentality and way of life. As the Order's original hospitable and charitable characteristics became largely symbolic the military element grew more dominant and more aristocratic; demands that knight-brethren produce written proof of birth and nobility became insistent during the fifteenth century [115]. That minority of Hospitallers who served at Rhodes were occasionally involved in battle and brutality [116], though they faced nothing comparable to the sustained harshness of the military experience of the Teutonic brethren in Prussia and Livonia. The confrontation with the infidel had the spiritual character of a holy war. The *milites* were knighted before entering the Order, and all brethren were received in the same way. Unusually, some Latin fragments of the statutes written at Cologne in the late fourteenth century included forms of blessing for sword and shield on the reception of knight-brethren [117]; this exceptional text was probably influenced by such typically German practices in the Teutonic Order [118], but these rites were not technically an integral part of the reception ceremony. Sword and spurs were buried with the Master at least in the case of Fr. Antoni Fluviá in 1437 [119].

Most priest-brethren were occupied with prayers and services, with the management of their commanderies if they were commanders and, in some cases, with parish concerns. Despite the written rules, those who adopted a primarily spiritual approach to these activities, who thought in terms of a life of service and poverty, were probably few. Priestly life was apparently strongest in the German and Bohemian priories, but this was also the area where the proportion of knight-brethren was very high and where the monetary aspects of requiem masses, entrance fees and life pensions were most developed. The Germans and Bohemians seldom went to serve on Rhodes and their religious activities may to some extent have been a form of compensation for that failure [120]. Collaboration with the laity could bring useful support and incomes. In the mid-thirteenth century the Spanish confraternity of Saint James at Acre linked itself to the Hospital, its priors swearing fealty to the Order and its members becoming *confratres,* while another confraternity at Acre, that of Saint George of Lydda and Bethlehem whose members were Greek Orthodox Melchites, was also attached to the Hospital [121]. Later, and especially from about the middle of the fifteenth century, other lay confraternities were attached to the Hospital, mainly in Germany but also in Northern Italy. Contemporary texts themselves confused *donati* and *confratres* who differed from each other but were all under obedience to the Hospital as non-professed affiliates of the Order. Pensioners, *corrodarii* and others who made contracts with the Hospital for their own material or spiritual advantage were associated with the Order but were not members of it; the poor and sick in hospital were also associated with the Order, especially through their prayers. It was important to the Hospitallers that all such people were personally attached to the Order in a relation of ,,brotherhood", but they were not necessarily related to each other within any kind of corporate confraternity [122]. There was also the apparently unique case of the Commandery of Strasbourg, founded in 1371, which became the centre of a movement, both lay and mystical, similar to the *devotio moderna* [123].

The individual Hospitaller's spiritual life, a personal and intangible matter, was seldom austere, ascetic or intense. A measure of scandal and complaint was inevitable. The Hospital's moral state and its abuse of its papal exemptions met some rather mild general criticism at the time of the dissolution of the Temple, and thereafter popes continued to complain, sometimes strongly and perhaps rather unfairly, of luxurious living, moral laxities and alleged charitable and military inactivity [124]. In 1338 Benedict XII initiated a series of inquests with a view to reforming the Hospital. Benedict fell ill before anything was achieved, but two very detailed anonymous projects, at least one of which was the work of a Hospitaller, were prepared for presentation to the pope, and some of their particular proposals appeared in statutes passed in subsequent chapters general; these included measures for the maintenance of Hospitaller churches and the improvement of liturgical practices [125]. That there was no fundamental reform of the Order, no movement or serious impulse to return to the primitive values of the Hospital's Rule such as those reform movements which prospered in various other religious orders, did not necessarily indicate that the Order was corrupt or decadent. For the Hospitallers, any revival of a Rule which made no mention of military activity or of noble qualifications would, of course, have been difficult, as a reading of the *miracula* recounting the origins of their Order must have reminded them.

Some kind of decay or decline was present throughout the Roman Church during the fourteenth century, and at the same time spiritual endeavour was moving away from established ecclesiastical institutions towards new forms of religious enthusiasm. A new papal inquest launched in 1373 demonstrated statistically that the Hospital's affairs, including its religious functions, were in dramatic crisis, but it showed that the problems were above all practical ones resulting from a general demographic and economic depression of universal proportions [126]. There was always a tendency for discipline to be relaxed. Following the papal schism and the demoralization it brought to the Order, statutes passed at Rhodes in 1420 sought to improve standards of divine service, to provide repairs and books for churches and chapels, to restore the practice of almsgiving and to ensure that *milites* made confession and knelt during services [127]. The Hospitallers continued to maintain their functions, military, charitable and liturgical, in East and West, but their spiritual life, often cramped by the decline in the size of the communities resident in individual commanderies, was naturally conditioned, often disadvantageously, by general changes in the society within which they operated.

Notes

[1] This paper concentrates on the earlier period from 1310 to 1421, omitting certain important topics for reasons of space. The legislation previous to 1310 is published in *Cartulaire général de l'Ordre des Hospitaliers de St.-Jean de Jérusalem: 1100—1310*, ed. J. Delaville le Roulx, 4 vols., Paris 1894—1906, and it is surveyed in J. Riley-Smith, *The Knights of St. John in Jerusalem and Cyprus: c. 1050—1310*, London 1967; the post-1310 statutes remain unpublished. The recent study of the Rule in G. Lagleder, *Die Ordensregel der Johanniter/Malteser*, St. Ottilien 1983, covers various spiritual topics but is notably incomplete; it is based, not on the Latin Rule, but on the German translation of 1253 which was occasionally defective; it ignores the Anglo-Norman translation which is datable before 1187 and is thus the earliest surviving version: *The Hospitallers' „Riwle"*, ed. K. Sinclair, London 1984. The chapter on „Die Spiritualität der Priesterbrüder" in B. Waldstein-Wartenberg, *Die Vasallen Christi: Kulturgeschichte der Johanniterordens im Mittelalter*, Vienna 1988, pp. 75—94, lacks precise documentation and largely describes the wholly atypical situation in the German and Bohemian priories of the Province of *Alamania*.

[2] A. Wildermann, *Die Beurteilung des Templerprozesses bis zum 17. Jahrhundert*, Freiburg-im-Breisgau 1971.

[3] A. Forey, *The Emergence of the Military Order in the Twelfth Century*, Journal of Ecclesiastical History, 36, 1985; idem, *The Military Orders from the Twelfth to the Early Fourteenth Centuries*, London 1992, pp. 16—17, 138, 143—144.

[4] A. Luttrell, *The Hospitallers of Rhodes and their Mediterranean World*, London 1992, I, pp. 1—4.

[5] Eg. ibid., XV, pp. 107—110.

[6] I agleder, pp. 76—78; this author emphasizes the novelty of concern for the poor for their sake rather than for the salvation of the agent of good works.

[7] Luttrell (1992), I, pp. 2—3.

[8] Riley-Smith (1967), pp. 254—255. The Rule stated that the cross was worn in honour of God and the holy cross (*Cartulaire*, 70, 19) while the *Usances* (ibid., 2213, 121) said it was in remembrance of Christ.

[9] B. Beaucage, *Visites générales des Commanderies de l'Ordre des Hospitaliers dépendantes du Grand Prieuré de Saint-Gilles: 1338*, Aix-en-Provence 1982, p. VII.

[10] L. Larking, *The Knights Hospitallers in England being the Report of Prior Philip de Thame to the Grand Master Elyan de Villanova for A.D. 1338*, London 1857, pp. LXI—LXIII.

[11] V. Novotný, *Inquisitio Domorum Hospitalis S. Johannis Hierosolimitani per Pragensem Archidiocesim facta anno 1373*, Historický Archiv 19, 1900.

[12] A.-M. Legras, *Les Effectives de l'Ordre des Hospitaliers de Saint-Jean de Jérusalem dans le Prieuré de France en 1373*, Revue Mabillon, 60, 1984, pp. 357——358, 365, 366 n. 54, 369; idem, *L'Enquête pontificale de 1373 sur l'Ordre des Hospitaliers de Saint-Jean de Jérusalem, I: L'nquête dans le Prieuré de France*, Paris 1987, pp. 103—106.

[13] Fundamental study, with much detail not here repeated, in A.-M. Legras — J.-L. Lemaître, *La Pratique liturgique des Templiers et des Hospitaliers de Saint--Jean-de-Jérusalem*, in: *L'Écrit dans la Société médiévale, Texts en hommage à Lucie Fossier*, Paris 1991, p. 106.

[14] Riley-Smith (1967), pp. 240—242; general information and bibliography in A. Forey, *Women and the Military Orders in the Twelfth and Thirteenth Centuries*, Studia Monastica, 29, 1987, and F. Tommasi, *Il Monasterio femminile di San Bevignate dell'Ordine di San Giovanni Gerosolimitano (Secoli XIV—XVI)*, in: *Templari e Ospitalieri in Italia: La Chiesa di San Bevignate a Perugia*, ed. M. Roncetti et al., Perugia 1987.

[15] A. Luttrell, *The Structure of the Aragonese Hospital: 1349—1352*, forthcoming.

[16] Text in Tommasi (1987), pp. 69—77.

[17] Infra.

[18] *Cartulaire*, 70, 4, 9; 2213, 30, 57, 64; cf. K. Sinclair, *New Light on Early Hospitaller Practices*, Revue Bénédictine 96, 1986, p. 120.

[19] M. Ferrer-Vidal Díaz del Riguero, *La Mujer en la Orden militar de Santiago*, in: *Las Mujeres y su Ámbito jurídico = Actas de las Segundas Jornadas de Investigación interdisciplinaria*, Madrid 1983.

[20] H. Nicholson, *Templar Attitudes towards Women*, Medieval History 1, 1991.

[21] Eg. Forey (1987), pp. 64, 69; Luttrell (1989), p. 106.

[22] G. Moyse, *Les Hospitaliers de Saint-Jean de Jérusalem dans le Diocèse de Besançon en 1373*, Mélanges de l'École française de Rome: Moyen Age — Temps Modernes 85, 1973, p. 484.

[23] Legras (1984), p. 361.

[24] Eg. A. Luttrell, *The Hospitallers of Rhodes between Tuscany and Jerusalem: 1310—1431*, Revue Mabillon, forthcoming; Nicholson (1991) discusses the military orders' attitudes to women.

[25] Valletta, *National Library of Malta*, Archives of the Order of Saint John, Cod. 333, f. 149, 229v-230.

[26] Cited in A. Luttrell, *Papauté et Hôpital: l'Enquête de 1373*, in Legras (1987), p. 42.

[27] Riley-Smith (1967), pp. 231—236 et passim; Legras — Lemaître, pp. 77—78.

[28] Legras (1984), p. 377; cf. Riley-Smith (1967), p. 234; Luttrell (1989), p. 104.

[29] Riley-Smith (1967), pp. 338—340; scattered details in G. Sommi-Picenardi, *Itinéraire d'un Chevalier de Saint-Jean de Jérusalem dans l'Ile de Rhodes*, Lille 1900.

[30] Riley-Smith (1967), p. 233; Luttrell (1989), pp. 110—111; much detail in F. Tingl — J. Emler, *Liber primus Confirmationum ad Beneficia Ecclesiastica Pragensem*, 8 vols, Prague 1867—1886.

[31] Novotný, pp. 61—62 et passim.

[32] Legras (1984), p. 371.

[33] *Cartulaire*, 1785, 1788, 1807, 1817, 1836.

[34] Legras (1987), pp. 79, 358—359. A collegiate house was founded at Caspe in 1394; other cases require investigation.

[35] J.-M. Roux, *Saint-Jean-de-Malte: une Église de l'Ordre de Malte à Aix-en--Provence*, Aix-en-Provence 1987, pp. 18—37.

[36] Legras (1987), pp. 148—158, 348—355.

[37] Novotný, pp. 67—68.

[38] The „priest commanderies" of which some scholars write do not seem to have existed in the fourteenth century.

[39] Reproduced in B. Waldstein-Wartenberg, *Die kulturellen Leistungen des Grosspriorates Böhmen — Österreich im Mittelalter*, Annales de l'Ordre Souverain Militaire de Malte, 33, 1975, p. 38.

[40] *The Order of St. John in Malta*, ed. Council of Europe, Malta 1970, plate 42; an example from a tomb slab of 1380 in Legras (1984), p. 393. The rules for tonsure are in the constitutions of 1495 for Hospitaller priests at Rhodes: text in P. M. Paciaudi, *De Cultu S. Johannis Baptistae Antiquitates Christianae...*, Rome 1755, pp. 366—369.

[41] A. Châtelet, *Early Dutch Painting: Painting in the Northern Netherlands in the Fifteenth Century*, trans: Oxford 1988, pp. 104, 220, and plates 88—89; plates 202—203 show two commanders painted by Geertgen tot Sint Jans.

[42] Riley-Smith (1967), pp. 235—236, 250—252; Sinclair (1986), pp. 120—122; Legras — Lemaître, pp. 83—94 et passim; on relevant fourteenth-century statutes, Legras (1984), pp. 366—368, and J. Delaville le Roulx, *Les Hospitaliers à Rhodes jusqu'à la mort de Philibert de Naillac: 1310—1421*, Paris 1913, passim.

[43] Legras — Lemaître, pp. 80—83.

[44] Riley-Smith (1967), p. 236.

[45] Legras (1984), pp. 359—361, 388—392.

[46] *Cartulaire*, 2213, 100.

[47] *Cartulaire*, 3039, 38.

[48] H. Lea, *The Absolution Formula of the Templars*, in his: *Minor Historical Writings and other Essays*, ed. A. Howland, Philadelphia 1942.

[49] Legras — Lemaître provides a general study with much detail from France; a Hospitaller breviary survives from the thirteenth century and other works, including the breviary printed in 1480, from the fifteenth. Waldstein-Wartenberg (1975) gives details for Germany and Bohemia; see also idem, *Beiträge zur mittelalterlichen Liturgie des Johanniterordens*, I: *Der Festkalender;* II: *Das Totengedächtnis*, Annales de l'Ordre Souverain Militaire de Malte 30, 1972, and K. Ulshöfer, *Ein Kalenderfragment des Johanniterhauses in Hall?*, Würtembergisch Franken, 62, 1978.

[50] J. Sarnowsky, *Der Tod des Grossmeisters der Johanniter*, infra.

[51] *Cartulaire*, 4612, 1.

[52] Luttrell (1992), IV, pp. 75, 88 n. 7 et passim.

[53] Paciaudi, pp. 430—435; Riley-Smith (1967), pp. 258—259; Legras — Lemaître, pp. 94—99, 108—109.

[54] *The Order of St. John*, p. 290 and plate 42; the body was to be covered with *un drap rouge au croiz blanche* (*Cartulaire*, 627, 6).

[55] Facsimile in I. Collijn, *Ett Nekrologium från Johanniterklostret i Eskilstuna*, Uppsala 1929, analysed in T. Nyberg, *Zur Rolle der Johanniter in Skandinavien: Erstes Auftreten und Aufbau der Institutionem*, in: *Die Rolle der Ritterorden in der Mittelalterlichen Kultur*, ed. Z. Nowak, Toruń 1985, pp. 138—142; see also Waldstein-Wartenberg (1972), with illustrations, and Legras — Lemaître, pp. 78, 107. For a female house, M.-M. Costa, *Els Necrologis del Convent d'Alguaire*, in: *Martínez Ferrando, Archivero: Miscelánea de Estudios dedicados a su Memoria*, Madrid 1968.

[56] Sarnowsky, infra, p. 208 n. 27; text of 1480 in K. Setton, *The Papacy and the Levant: 1204—1571*, II, Philadelphia 1978, p. 361, n. 45.

[57] The chronology of this development awaits study.

[58] S. Düll, *Drei Johanniter in Istanbul: Neue Untersuchungen zu den rhodischen Grabsteinen im Archäologischen Museum*, Istanbuler Mitteilungen 39, 1989.

[59] Some occasional fourteenth-century examples in Paciaudi, pp. 292, 296—298, 302; Legras (1984), p. 393; A. Luttrell, *The Hospitallers in Cyprus, Rhodes, Greece and the West: 1291—1440*, London 1978, XV, pp. 419—420; idem (1992), XV, p. 112; S. Düll, *Das Grabmal des Johanniter Pietro da Imola in S. Jacopo in Campo Corbolini in Florenz zur Renaissance-Kapitalis in erneuerten Inschriften des Trecento*, Mitteilungen des Kunsthistorischen Institutes in Florenz, 34, 1990. These and other early examples deserve further study. Compare a German example of 1330 with two others of 1504 and about 1512 in *Der Johanniterorden / Der Malteserorden*, ed. A. Wienand, 3rd ed: Cologne 1988, pp. 293, 294, 314.

[60] Text of 1617 circa in Karlsruhe, General Landesarchiv, Abt. 64 no. 13; for similar indications of burial locations at Strasbourg in a text of ca. 1465, J.-L. Lemaître, *Répertoire des Documents nécrologiques français*, Paris 1980, p. 918.

[61] Malta, Cod. 48, f. 131, 132, 132v.

[62] *Die Würzburger Inschriften bis 1525*, ed. K. Borchardt, Wiesbaden 1988, p. 32. 55, plate 32.

[63] Legras — Lemaître, pp. 107, 121—136.

[64] Lagleder, pp. 53—54, 56—58.

[65] *Cartulaire*, 70, 15.

[66] Lagleder, pp. 60—63; Legras — Lemaître, pp. 87—88, et passim.

[67] Riley-Smith (1967), p. 215, n. 4.

[68] Legras — Lemaître, pp. 91—92.

[69] Luttrell (1978), IX, pp. 374—375.

[70] Legras — Lemaître, pp. 90—94.

[71] F. Tommasi, „Templari" e „Templari Sancti Johannis": una Precisazione metodologica, Studi Medievali 24, 3 ser., 1983.

[72] Paciaudi, pp. 428—429; Riley-Smith (1967), pp. 271—272. The details in Proprium Missarum una cum Lectionario Ordinis Sancti Johannis Hierosolymitani, Rome 1987, are not all historically reliable.

[73] C. Brunel, Vida et Miracles de Sancta Flor, Analecta Bollandiana 64, 1946; Riley-Smith (1967), p. 272, incorrectly places Flor's death in 1299.

[74] Many relics are illustrated and discussed in The Order's Early Legacy in Malta, ed. J. Azzopardi, Malta 1989, in which, however, Luttrell's article [reprinted as Luttrell (1992), XVIII] fails to record the Templar origin of various Hospitaller relics, as established in F. Tommasi, I Templari e il Culto delle Reliquie, in: I Templari: Mito e Storia, ed. G. Minucci — F. Sardi, Sinalunga—Siena 1989. Luttrell (1992), XVIII, p. 9, n. 57, wrongly speaks of Gérard as appearing in an illumination in a Hospitaller choral book of 1521.

[75] Waldstein-Wartenberg (1988), pp. 82—86; The Order of St. John, p. 256, describes an illuminated indulgence of 1343 for Burgsteinfurt.

[76] A large and separate subject; see most recently E. Kollias, The City of Rhodes and the Palace of the Grand Master, Athens 1988; idem, The Knights of Rhodes, the Palace and the City, Athens 1991.

[77] The collection of Western examples is a desideratum: see Luttrell (1978), X; Legras (1987); and E. Schermerhorn, On the Trail of the Eight-Pointed Cross: a Study of the Heritage of the Knights Hospitallers in Feudal Europe, New York 1940.

[78] E. Grunsky, Doppelgeschossige Johanniterkirchen und verwandte Bauten, Düsseldorf 1970; illustrations in A. Wienand, Die Hospitalkirche der Johanniter als Bautypus, in Wienand, pp. 409—421.

[79] The various archives of the Province of Alamania are full of such documents; general remarks in Waldstein-Wartenberg (1972), pp. 86—91; (1988), pp. 79—81. The overall economic implications of the Pitanz system remain to be studied in detail.

[80] Text in W. Engel, Die Krise der Ballei Franken des Johanniterordens zur Mitte des 14. Jahrhunderts, Zeitschrift für Bayerische Landesgeschichte 18, 1955, pp. 285.

[81] Prague, Státní Ustrední Archiv, Archives of the Hospitaller Priory of Bohemia, no. 2298.

[82] Riley-Smith (1967), pp. 331—338 et passim; T. Miller, The Knights of Saint John and the Hospitals of the Latin West, Speculum 53, 1978. The later period is studied in A. Luttrell, The Hospitallers' Medical Tradition: 1291—1530, forthcoming.

[83] Texts and materials in I. Pappalardo, Storia sanitaria dell'Ordine Gerosolimitano di Malta dalle Origini al Presente, Rome 1958.

[84] E. Le Grand, La Prière des Malades dans les Hôpitaux de l'Ordre de Saint-Jean de Jérusalem, Bibliothèque de l'École des Chartes 57, 1896; K. Sinclair, The French Prayer for the Sick in the Hospital of the Knights of Saint John of Jerusalem at Acre, Medieval Studies 40, 1978.

[85] Luttrell (1978), IX, pp. 369—373; Waldstein-Wartenberg (1975), pp. 26—29; idem, Donaten — Confratres — Pfründner: Die Bruderschaften des Ordens, Annales de l'Ordre Souverain Militaire de Malte 31, 1973, pp. 14—15.

[86] G. Giordanengo, Les Hôpitaux arlésiens du XIIe au XIVe siècle, in: Assi-

stance et Charité = Cahiers de Fanjeux, XIII, Toulouse 1978.

[87] Larking, pp. 61, 214; Waldstein-Wartenberg (1973), pp. 16—18.

[88] Legras (1987), p. 288.

[89] Luttrell (1978), IX; idem (1992), X.

[90] Legras (1987), p. 99.

[91] Prague, no. 3071.

[92] Luttrell (1992), XIV, pp. 762—768.

[93] Ibid., XVII, pp. 239—242.

[94] Waldstein-Wartenberg (1975), pp. 29—32.

[95] Novotný, pp. 22, 50.

[96] Luttrell (1978), XVI; a list of graduate brethren is a desideratum.

[97] Ibid., XV, pp. 410—413.

[98] Madrid, Archivo Histórico Nacional, Sección de Ordenes Militares, San Juan, Llengua de Aragón, Carpeta 694 no. 21.

[99] Luttrell (1978), XVI, pp. 453—454.

[100] Luttrell (1978), XX—XXI.

[101] Ibid., XVIII, XXV; E. Beltran, *Seis Sermones desconocidos de Juan de Hesdin* († *1378—79),* Ciudad de Dios 192, 1979. An apparently different Hospitaller also named Fr. Jean de Hesdin wrote a long allegorical poem, the *L'Amoureuse Prise* completed in 1332: A. Thomas, *Frère Jean Acart, Poète français,* in: *Histoire littéraire de la France,* XXXVII, Paris 1938, pp. 412—418.

[102] *The Order of St. John,* p. 286; Waldstein-Wartenberg (1975), pp. 33—34.

[103] Eg. Waldstein-Wartenberg (1975), pp. 33—34; idem, (1988), pp. 337—397. Julian Plante of St. Johns University, Minnesota, kindly provided references to the Hospitallers Fr. Wenceslaus, *Tractatus de Septem Donis Spiritus Sancti* (as Seitenstetten, Ms. 173, f. 76—133, and Vienna, Schottenkloster, Ms. 296, f. 114v—200v) and Fr. Thomas de Stregonia (Strahovia), *Sermones* (as Schägl, Ms. 196 [820.122], and Seitenstetten, Ms. 255, f. 145—269).

[104] Legras — Lemaître, pp. 121—122, 126—127.

[105] *Regesta Diplomatica nec non Epistolaria Bohemiae et Moraviae,* ed. J. Emler et al., V fasc. 2, Prague 1960, p. 370.

[106] Legras — Lemaître, p. 99. Soon after 1500 the Breslau commandery possessed over 1000 manuscripts: M. Starnawska, *Die mittelalterliche Bibliothek der Johanniter in Breslau,* infra. These examples are all from the Province of Alamania.

[107] M. Huglo, *De Francon de Cologne à Jacques de Liège,* Revue belge de Musicologie 34—35, 1980—1981; cf. Franco of Cologne, *Ars Cantus Mensurabilis,* ed. G. Ragney — A. Gilles, Stuttgart 1974, dating it to 1280 circa.

[108] Malta, Cod. 329, f. 69; Bouteiller is documented in Paris, Archives Nationales, MM. 31, f. 119; 32, f. 38v, 50v, 53, 203 (references kindly provided by Anne-Marie Legras).

[109] Luttrell (1992), XVII p. 243.

[110] Riley-Smith (1967), pp. 32—38, 272—273; Luttrell (1978), XVII, pp. 2—4, 14; idem, introduction to A. Calvet, *Légendes d'Oc de la Fondation de l'Hôpital de Saint Jean de Jérusalem: XIV Siècle* [provisional title], forthcoming.

[111] Text in R. Valentini, *Redazioni italiane quattrocentesche di Statuti della Religione Gioannita,* Archivum Melitense 9, 1933, pp. 80—81.

[112] Supra, p. 75 n. 1.

[113] W. Potkowski, *Spirituality and Reading: Book Collections of the Teutonic Order in Prussia,* infra.

[114] M. Roques, *Traductions françaises de la „Consolatio Philosophia" de Boèce,* in: *Histoire littéraire de la France,* XXXVII, Paris 1938, pp. 441—443.

[115] A. Luttrell, *Latin Greece, the Hospitallers and the Crusades: 1291—1440,* I, London 1982, pp. 264—265.

[116] Idem (1992), II pp. 87, 111 nn. 25—27 et passim.

[117] Cologne, Historisches Archiv der Stadt Köln, Geistlich. Abt. 129A, f. 5v—8.

[118] Undated text in *Die Statuten des Deutschen Ordens nach den ältesten Handschriften,* ed. M. Perlbach, Halle 1890, p. 129.

[119] Sarnowsky, infra.

[120] Cf. undocumented survey in A. Luttrell, *The Hospitallers in Fouteenth-Century Germany,* St. John Historical Society Proceedings 2, 1988—1990.

[121] J. Riley-Smith, *A Note on Confraternities in the Latin Kingdom of Jerusalem,* Bulletin of the Institute of Historical Research 44, 1971, pp. 302—303.

[122] Waldstein- Wartenberg (1973); idem, (1988), pp. 76—78. Waldstein-Wartenberg's assumption that donats, *confratres* and other persons entered into obituary books belonged to a *Bruderschaft* seems to involve ambiguities. Medieval *donati* did not join a corporate confraternity: texts in L. Tacchella, *I „Donati" nella Storia del Sovrano Militare Ordine di Malta,* Verona 1986. The English *fraria* or *confraria* did not involve a corporate confraternity but a voluntary financial contribution: Larking, pp. XXX, 4, and W. Rees, *A History of the Order of St. John of Jerusalem in Wales and on the Welsh Border,* Cardiff 1947, pp. 22—24.

[123] Waldstein-Wartenberg (1988), pp. 76—78, 88—90; the Strasbourg commandery requires further examination.

[124] Luttrell (1978), XXIV; Forey (1992), pp. 204—220.

[125] Luttrell (1987), pp. 11—12.

[126] Ibid., pp. 31—42.

[127] Delaville le Roulx (1913), pp. 351—352.

X

The Hospitallers' Medical Tradition:
1291–1530

When the Hospitallers moved their Convent or headquarters to Cyprus after the loss of Acre and the final collapse of Latin Syria in 1291 they took with them a medical tradition which had earlier been transferred to Acre following the fall of Jerusalem in 1187. The Order of St John had grown out of a hospice in Jerusalem, and its Rule said nothing of military activities or of knighthood or nobility. It had gradually become a predominantly military institution, but even when the poor and sick were no longer of paramount concern the maintenance of its medical and charitable tradition was still of spiritual and moral significance, especially for opinion in the West. This divergence between declining tradition and active practice resulted in ambiguities. Many of the medical, liturgical and other regulations concerning hospital matters contained in the Order's statutes were applicable only in the main conventual hospital, while there was considerable terminological confusion between the poor, the sick and the sick poor; between pilgrims and other travellers; between charity and hospitality; and between medical hospitals, various types of hospice and the *infirmaria fratrum* reserved for the Hospitaller brethren. There was also a distinction between donats, who were members of the Hospital and under obedience to it, and those pensioners who could purchase or contract for board and lodging in retirement and old age.[1] The Hospitallers' original concern, reflected in their Rule, was with the poor, an involvement which was directed

---

[1] The bibliography is extensive but frequently second-hand and repetitive. Many statutes and other texts are published, with chaotic inaccuracy, in I. Pappalardo, *Storia Sanitaria dell'Ordine Gerosolimitano di Malta dalle Origini al Presente* (Rome, 1958); bibliography in W. von Ballestrem, 'Die Hospitalität des Ordens', in *Der Johanniterorden/Der Malteserorden: Der ritterliche Orden des hl. Johannes vom Spital zu Jerusalem, seine Geschichte, seine Aufgaben*, ed. A. Wienand, 3rd edn (Cologne, 1988), and B. Waldstein-Wartenberg, *Die Vasallen Christi: Kulturgeschichte des Johanniterordens im Mittelalter* (Vienna, 1988), pp. 422–3.

increasingly to those poor or pilgrims who became ill. This expressed a contemporary urge to give practical help to the suffering as an end in itself rather
than as a means through which the agent of the good works might hope to secure
salvation.[2]

Every religious order had some general charitable obligations, and the
different military orders undertook various hospitaller functions.[3] After 1291
the Hospital's brethren were aware of their Order's Benedictine origins in
Jerusalem on the eve of the First Crusade of 1099, and of the way in which
some sort of association or confraternity of lay brethren had developed into a
religious order serving the poor, the sick and the pilgrims. They knew of the
enlargement or rebuilding, before 1156, of a true medical hospital in the
Convent of which it was said, presumably with some exaggeration, that it housed
2,000 patients and that over fifty dead were sometimes carried out of it in a
single day. The Hospital had a tradition of extensive alms-giving to the poor,
of doctors and surgeons, of nightly prayers in the hospital for benefactors and
others led by the Order's priests, of provisions for orphans and lepers, of
maternity wards, and of financial support, medicines and diet, burial arrangements and the treatment of those wounded in battle.[4] The Hospitallers'
medical buildings and practices in the East may well have drawn on Islamic
and Byzantine models; they were less likely to have been responsible for
introducing Oriental medical methods to the Latin West.[5] However, the
diffusion of the texts regulating the sick, their confession, beds and food, and
their treatment as lords – *quasi domini*, matters which were indeed all found
in the Hospital's Rule, did not necessarily result directly from the Order's own
activities, since the prayer containing them was adapted from *ritualia* long in
use in the West.[6]

The Order's Jerusalem legacy included the history of the Amalfitan hospice
which functioned there before 1099 and the carefully concocted legends or
miracula which were reinterpreted after 1291 by the talented Hospitaller,
William of Santo Stefano.[7] These legends invested the Hospital with the

[2] Cf. G. Lagleder, *Die Ordensregel der Johanniter/Malteser* (Saint Ottilien, 1983), pp. 76–8.

[3] Cf. C. Probst, *Der Deutsche Orden und sein Medizinalwesen in Preussen: Hospital, Firmarie und Artz bis 1525* (Bad Godesberg, 1969). The Templars took over a major hospital in Constantinople after 1204: T. Miller, 'The Sampson Hospital of Constantinople', *Byzantinische Forschungen*,
15 (1990), pp. 128–30.

[4] J. Riley-Smith, *The Knights of St John of Jerusalem and Cyprus: c. 1050-1310* (London, 1967),
pp. 247–9, 332–8 *et passim*; H. Buschhausen, *Die italienische Bauplastik im Königsreich Jerusalem von
König Wilhem II. bis Kaiser Friedrich II.* (Vienna, 1978), pp. 240–3/ figs 27–31; R. Hiestand, 'Die
Anfänge der Johanniter', in *Die geistlichen Ritterorden Europas*, ed. J. Fleckenstein and M. Hellmann
(Sigmaringen, 1980). The Jerusalem building is also known from nineteenth-century plans.

[5] The proposals in T. Miller, 'The Knights of Saint John and the Hospitals of the Latin West',
Speculum, **53** (1978), with bibliography, should be treated with considerable caution.

[6] K. Sinclair, 'The French Prayer for the Sick in the Hospital of the Knights of Saint John of
Jerusalem at Acre', *Medieval Studies*, **40** (1978).

[7] Riley-Smith, pp. 32–7.

prestige of a bogus continuity stretching back into ancient times, placing many New Testament events in its Jerusalem building and even corrupting Old Testament stories of Melchior and Judas Maccabeus in order to take the tradition of alms and service to the poor back before Christian times.[8] A rhymed Anglo-Norman translation of the Rule, possibly made at Clerkenwell in London, contained these legends which, in that version, preceded the Rule and were evidently invented before 1187, possibly between 1140 and 1160; the Anglo-Norman version was copied in England between about 1300 and 1310.[9] The *miracula*, which were also used to facilitate fund-raising in the West,[10] were being copied and translated, often in manuscripts of the Rule and statutes, during the fourteenth and fifteenth centuries.[11] A Latin version was copied at Rhodes in about 1366 into a chancery formulary in which it served as an introduction to a long list of papal privileges granted to the Hospital.[12]

Well into the fifteenth century the main hospital at Jerusalem excited the admiration of pilgrims who continued to use the enormous building; in 1395, for example, Niccolò da Martoni mentioned the great hall and separate rooms used by pilgrims.[13] Another hospital which sheltered German-speaking pilgrims and others in Jerusalem was under German management but subordinate to the Master of the Order of St John at least after 1143; it had two storeys with halls one above another and a separate church.[14] In Acre, where the Order had a hospital by 1155,[15] there was possibly a large pilgrim hospice on the east side of the Hospitallers' central courtyard and apparently a hospital for the sick a little way south of the main Hospitaller complex.[16] The Order had a number

---

[8] Selected texts, discussion and bibliography in *RHC Occid*, 5 (Paris, 1895), pp. cix–xxviii, 401–35.

[9] *The Hospitallers' 'Riwle'*, ed. K. Sinclair (London, 1984); cf. idem, 'New Light on Early Hospitaller Practices', *Revue Bénédictine*, 96 (1986).

[10] K. Borchardt, 'Two Forged Thirteenth-Century Letters for Hospitallers in Franconia', Chapter 6 above, pp. 52–6.

[11] The present author has prepared a chronological list of mss to be published in a forthcoming work on the *Miracula* by Antoine Calvet.

[12] Arxiu de la Corona d'Aragó, Barcelona, Gran Priorato de Catalunya, Armari 24, vol. 13, fols 135v–136v.

[13] S. Schein, 'Latin Hospices in Jerusalem in the Late Middle Ages', *Zeitschrift des Deutschen Palästina-Vereins*, 101 (1985).

[14] Excavation evidence in A. Ovadiah, 'A Restored Complex of the Twelfth Century in Jerusalem', in *Actes du XVe Congrès International d'Etudes byzantines*, 2 (Athens, 1981); N. von Holst, *Der Deutsche Ritterorden und seine Bauten von Jerusalem bis Sevilla von Thorn bis Narva* (Berlin, 1981), pp. 27–9, 218–19; discussion in H. Kluger, *Hochmeister Hermann von Salza und Kaiser Friedrich II.* (Marburg, 1987), pp. 126–34.

[15] *CH*, 237, 471; cf. Riley-Smith, pp. 247–8.

[16] Excavation and other data, still debatable in interpretation, in B. Dichter, *The Orders and Churches of Crusader Acre* (Acre, 1979), p. 51; Z. Goldmann, *Akko in the Time of the Crusades: the Convent of the Order of St John* (Acre, 1987), pp. 22–5 (figs 3, 11). Cf. Goldmann's plans in Wienand, pp. 107, 115; cf. Riley-Smith, pp. 247–9, and D. Jacoby, 'Les Communes italiennes et les Ordres militaires à Acre: Aspects juridiques, territoriaux et militaires (1104–1187), 1191–1291', in *Etat et*

of hospitals elsewhere in the East[17] and there was possibly an infirmary for Hospitaller brethren in the Syrian countryside;[18] they seem to have held the pilgrim hospice at Abu Gosh on the road to Jerusalem, a pilgrimage site thought to be the biblical Emmaus, where a church was added to a square Muslim courtyard building which had once been a *caravanserai*.[19] The Hospital's chapel just outside the castle entrance at Crac des Chevaliers was decorated with frescoes showing the medical saint, Pantaleon, and his miracles.[20]

The Anglo-Norman *Riwle*, possibly datable between 1140 and 1160, elaborated on the brief medical provisions in the original Rule which had probably been written by about 1140; for example, it laid down that new-born babies were to sleep in cots apart from their mothers, a provision reappearing in the medical statutes of 1182.[21] A statute of 1176 allocated the produce of the two *casalia* of *Sainte Marie* and *Caphaer* north of Jerusalem for the provision of white bread for the Jerusalem hospital.[22] Six later statutes spoke of white bread and many other foods and fruits given on medical advice, of syrups, of urine tests, of staff numbers and night duty, and of finance, and they also listed six *casalia* devoted to the production of grain, meat and other supplies for the Conventual hospital; in addition to the two mentioned in 1176, these were Mount Gabriel and Cotquinanti both unidentified, *Sareth* or *Saarethe* and *Cole* or Chola, which the Hospital acquired in 1189 and which certainly had a warehouse.[23]

Colonisation au moyen âge et à la Renaissance, ed. M. Balard (Lyon, 1989), pp. 200–4, 210–11, fig. 2 (showing side rooms?). The Hospitaller church clearly lay to the south of the main complex and the *domus infirmorum* south of that. Possibly the large vaulted building east of the main courtyard was originally the brethren's residence which became a pilgrim hospice (*hospitale*) when the brethren's residence or *auberge* (*hospitium, alberge* or *herbaxium* on the maps) was moved nearer to the new walls in the suburb of Montmusard. Goldmann, p. 25, pl. XI (3), compares the facade of this presumed *domus infirmorum* with its upper and lower doorways and its staircases to those of the presumed fourteenth-century hospital at Rhodes (below, pp. 222–3) thus suggesting a continuity, but A. Gabriel, *La Cité de Rhodes: MCCCX-MDCCII*, 2 vols (Paris, 1921–1923), 2, pp. 9–10, and E. Kollias, *The Knights of Rhodes: the Palace and the City* (Athens, 1991), pp. 136–7, show that the Rhodian doorways and staircase were sixteenth-century alterations.

[17] For example, *CH*, 59, 244, 355 (Nablus); 79, 82 (Mont Pèlerin); 104 (*casale* of Turbessel); 258 (Toron); 665 (Antioch). Cf. J. Richard, 'Hospitals and Hospital Congregations in the Latin Kingdom during the First Period of the Frankish Conquest', in *Outremer: Studies in the History of the Crusading Kingdom of Jerusalem presented to J. Prawer*, ed. B. Kedar et al. (Jerusalem, 1982), pp. 90–91.

[18] For example, D. Pringle, 'Aqua Bella: the Interpretation of a Crusader Courtyard Building', in *The Horns of Hattin*, ed. B. Kedar (Jerusalem, 1992), pp. 163–7; idem, *The Churches of the Crusader Kingdom of Jerusalem: a Corpus*, 1 (Cambridge, 1993), p. 250.

[19] R. de Vaux and A-M. Steve, *Fouilles à Qaryet el- 'Enab, Abu Gôsh Palestine* (Paris, 1950), pp. 92–104; Pringle, *Churches*, 1, pp. 7–17.

[20] J. Folda, 'Crusader Frescoes at Crac des Chevaliers and Marqab Castle', *Dumbarton Oaks Papers*, 36, 1982, pp. 192–6.

[21] '*Riwle*', pp. 23–4, 57; *CH*, 627.

[22] *CH*, 494.

[23] A hitherto unnoticed fragment containing unknown statutes in Latin, probably datable post-1206, in Archives départementales des Bouches-du-Rhône, Marseilles, 56 H 4055; on Chola, see Riley-Smith, pp. 427 n. 2, 457.

The prayers of the sick in the Conventual hospital, which were to be recited by Hospitaller priests who came there every evening to pray for its benefactors and for the sick themselves, were probably composed at Acre in about 1197, but the text, in French, survives in only two manuscripts, of which the later is datable *c.* 1315; it may not have been used on Rhodes.[24] A Latin treatise, which was probably copied in about 1300 and bound with a group of Hospitaller materials including the Rule and statutes in German, the *miracula* in Latin and other documents such as papal bulls and imperial acts, discussed all sorts of matters concerning hospitals, doctors and patients. It was presumably used by Hospitallers, probably in Syria, although nothing in it indicated that it was describing the Hospitallers' hospital.[25]

When the Hospitallers established their Convent at Limassol in southern Cyprus in 1291, their resources were so low that in 1292 the complement there was fixed at a mere forty Hospitaller knights and ten sergeants-at-arms, each with two mounts, a squire and a page.[26] In March 1306 the Master explained to the Aragonese king that the Order lacked the resources to maintain the sick without borrowing at usury.[27] The military orders badly needed to present their Western public with a convincing role, and during their trials after 1307 the Templars were at pains to emphasize the extent of their alms-giving.[28] In 1297 the Hospitallers were said to be intending to build a new hospital for the sick and the poor at Limassol, and it was explicitly described as a replacement for the hospital in Acre which had formerly served needy pilgrims and the poor.[29] Statutes dating from 1300 to 1304 subsequently mentioned the Conventual hospital, the sick, the oaths of the resident doctors and surgeons, and the brethren's infirmary at Limassol.[30]

In about 1310 the Convent moved to Rhodes, and a Conventual hospital was apparently set up in an existing building somewhere near the sea walls.[31]

---

[24] L. Le Grand, 'La Prière des Malades dans les Hôpitaux de l'Ordre de Saint-Jean de Jérusalem', *Bibliothèque de l'Ecole des Chartes*, 57 (1896).

[25] An unnoticed item once in the Benedictine abbey of Bendickburen south of Munich, in Bayerische Staatsbibliothek, Munich, ms. Lat. 1245, fols 135–139; cf. *Catalogus Codicum Latinorum Bibliothecae Regiae Monacensis*, 1/2, 2nd edn (Munich, 1894), p. 218, with inaccuracies. The text awaits detailed investigation.

[26] Unpublished statutes in Marseilles, 56 H 4055; various mss of the statutes contain important and unpublished variations.

[27] Text in H. Finke, *Acta Aragonensia*, 3 (Berlin, 1922), p. 146.

[28] A. Demurger, *Vie et Mort de l'Ordre du Temple: 1118–1314*, 2nd edn (Paris, 1989), pp. 282–3.

[29] *CH*, 4336; this hospital may never have been built.

[30] *CH*, 4515 #5, 18, 4549 #19, 4612 #2, 4672 #1-4, 7, 11. The *Ospitel* and *ostel* of the *saiens* at Limassol of 1301 (ibid., 4549 #1, 10) did not refer to a hospital, the Latin translation as *in hospitio* being made at Rhodes in 1357: K. Sinclair, 'The Hospital, Hospice and Church of the Healthy belonging to the Knights of St John of Jerusalem on Cyprus', *Medium Aevum*, 49 (1980).

[31] In 1440 a *turrim que vulgariter dicebatur Turris Infirmarie Veteris* was near the walls of the *collachium* and the tower overlooking the port: Malta, Cod. 354, fol. 268, kindly communicated by Fotini Karassava-Tsilingiri and requiring further consideration.

As early as 1311 statutes referred to the *hospital dels seignors malades* at Rhodes and to a separate *enfermerie* for the brethren.[32] In 1314 the chapter general decreed the building of a proper hospital, allocating it 30,000 besants or about 6,750 florins per year from the two Rhodian *casalia* of Salakos and Apollona, with further incomes from Phileremos if those of the other two should prove insufficient.[33] An English visitor of 1345 wrote 'below the castle is the house of the hospital, mother, nurse, doctor, protector and servant to all the infirm'.[34] This may have been the two-storeyed building in the area of the arsenal close to the port on which were apparently placed the arms of Masters who ruled between 1319 and 1355, while on the adjacent building were those of Fr. Roger de Pins, Master from 1355 to 1365; with its vaulted upper floor and a chapel, it could well have been designed as a hospital.[35] In fact, a statute of 1357 decreed that the hospital, to serve both pilgrims and the 'poor sick', should continue to do so, as was the custom.[36] This task must have been accomplished, since in about 1420 Cristoforo Buondelmonti wrote of an area occupied by the *munitio* or arsenal which included the hospital which sheltered pilgrims.[37] The Conventual hospital lay within the *castrum* or *collachium* which was that part of the city reserved, in theory at least, to the Hospitaller brethren; there was no indication that it was available to the Greeks or other non-Latins.

Visitors continued to remark on the Conventual hospital. In 1395 Niccolò da Martoni reported that the Rhodian hospital had beds for pilgrims and the sick with doctors always on duty and the giving of great alms, *magna helemosina*; a few paupers were served meat and bread by the brethren and many others were given bread at the hospital.[38] In the same year the Lord of Anglure remarked that both sick and poor were received in it when ill.[39] In about 1420 Emmanuele Piloti wrote of ruined Rhodian merchants, presumably Latins, who ended their lives there in poverty.[40] More noble pilgrims also stayed in a hospice founded in 1391 outside the *collachium* but within the *borgo* by the Italian

---

[32] Biblioteca Vaticana, Vatican, ms. Vat. Lat. 3136, fols 66–68 ##2, 22.

[33] Text in Gabriel, **2**, p. 221.

[34] *Infra castrum est domus Hospitalis, mater, nutrix, medica, tutrix et ancilla infirmantibus cunctis*: text in G. Golubovich, *Biblioteca Bio-bibliografica della Terra Santa e dell'Oriente francescano*, **4** (Quaracchi, 1923), pp. 444–5.

[35] G. Jacopi, 'Monumenti di Arte Cavalleresca', *Clara Rhodos*, **1** (1923), p. 161; figs 134–6. Cf. Gabriel, **1**, pp. 9–11; **2**, pp. 34, 73; pl. XXII (i), and Kollias, pp. 136–9, pl. 115; there seems to be no published plan of this building which is now the archaeological institute.

[36] A. Luttrell, 'Rhodes Town: 1306–1350' (forthcoming).

[37] As cited in Gabriel, **2**, pp. 7, 9–10.

[38] 'Relation du Pèlerinage à Jérusalem de Nicolas de Martoni, notaire italien: 1394–1395', ed. E. Legrand, *ROL*, **3** (1895) pp. 584–5, 640.

[39] *La Saint Voyage de Jherusalem du Seigneur d'Anglure*, ed. F. Bonnardot and A. Longnon (Paris, 1878), p. 9.

[40] *Traité d'Emmanuel Piloti sur le Passage en Terre Sainte: 1420*, ed. P.-H. Dopp (Louvain and Paris, 1958), p.157.

Fr. Domenico de Alamania, and maintained by the Italian brethren who provided masses but not food.[41] The tradition of assistance to pilgrims remained strong, and in 1402–3 the Order made a potentially profitable, but ultimately abortive, agreement with the Egyptian sultan for concessions which would have allowed the Hospitallers to take pilgrims to the Syrian ports and to the holy places in and around Jerusalem.[42] In 1413 Fr. Pierre Pausedieu, Castellan of Afandou some 20 km south of Rhodes city, founded and endowed a hospice there to shelter travellers of all nations.[43] The Order's assistance was a reality to many pilgrims in the East, and on Cyprus in 1418 Nompar of Caumont stayed first in a Hospitaller house between Famagusta and Nicosia and then in the Order's 'great hostel' in Nicosia.[44] As late as the 1480s the Master of Rhodes was furnishing the old Jerusalem hospital.[45]

The Catalan Master, Fr. Antoni Fluvià, died in 1437 bequeathing 10,000 florins for a new Conventual hospital. Land was purchased and work began in 1440; after many financial difficulties the complex was finished sufficiently for the hospital to be transferred to it in 1483. On the ground level of this impressive courtyard building were stores and, facing outwards on to the street, shops to be let out for income. Medical matters were concentrated upstairs in a great open two-aisled ward with an altar or chapel in it and with curious cubicles built into the thicknesses of the walls: there was a smaller hall, refectory, kitchens, separate rooms and so on.[46] The hospital was described by the Czech pilgrim John Lord of Lobkowicz in 1493 when he and his servant were lodged there and were fed on white bread and wine:

That house, the Infirmary, is all built of cut stone and the inside is a straight square. And windows great and broad all around, that there is little wall between these windows: but one window next to the other, so that one may look into the house, and all of it is finely painted. Now the Master of Rhodes has endowed that house, that any man being Christian, of whatever lowly or great rank, who shall come there, if he be sick and ask for it for God's sake, should at once be taken in; and there he is at once provided with medicine and other necessities, to wit food and drink and bedclothes. If an important person, he is given a room of his own; and if any lesser man, then there is a fine hall, very long, and in it made beds in double

---

[41] A. Luttrell, *The Hospitallers of Rhodes and their Mediterranean World* (London, 1992), X, pp. 192–3, 199–200; described in *Andanças e viajes de un hidalgo español: Pero Tafur (1436–1439)*, ed. M. Jiménez de la Espada et al., rev. edn (Barcelona, 1982), p. 49.

[42] Texts and discussion in Luttrell, *Mediterranean World*, X, pp. 194–207.

[43] Malta, Cod. 339, fols 72v–73v.

[44] A. Luttrell, 'The Hospitallers of Rhodes between Tuscany and Jerusalem: 1306–1431', *Revue Mabillon*, 64 (1992), pp. 130 *et passim*; the systematic analysis of accounts of visitors to Rhodes is an important *desideratum*.

[45] Schein, 'Latin Hospices', p. 91.

[46] Gabriel, 2, pp. 14–36, and F. Karassava-Tsilingiri, 'The Fifteenth-century Hospital of Rhodes', Chapter 10 below; this paper has profited greatly from the unpublished work of Fotini Karassava-Tsilingiri.

row, and on some of them sick people are lying. And these beds are well made with clean white bedclothes, and on each bed there is a red cloth blanket, for there it is not as cold as [in Bohemia]. And near each of these beds a door opens upon the balcony, so that any of these sick can go out to take the air, whenever he chooses, upon that balcony; and there too he has a privy. Also in that house is a great kitchen, and in it several cooks, that prepare food for the sick. Also it is ordained, that each of these sick has a servant, that looks after him and serves him, whatever he needs. Also two doctors are ordained for this, sworn leeches, who look after the sick twice each day: once in the morning and once again in the evening. And there these doctors having in the morning examined his water, if anything from the Pharmacy be needed for him for his illness, they at once put to paper what he needs; there is next a Pharmacy endowed by the same Master. The officials appointed for this at once take this at the Pharmacy, though it be several florins' worth. And for that medicine the sick need pay nothing. Further the same doctors write a paper, what sort of dish should be given him, and when; and there the officials appointed for this must so provide this, what time these doctors write and order it. And these things are entrusted to three men: one Knight of the Order and two clerks, all of them being on oath for this. Also at that time I saw how the sick were served their meals in silver dishes, and they drink too from silver spoons. And none need pay anything for his stay there, except he freely of his goodwill gives anything to the servant that has waited upon him.[47]

Behind this activity lay a carefully organized administration. In 1440, the year in which the new building was begun, a detailed set of statutes provided probably the first major revisions of the Hospital's medical regulations since those of 1182. This and subsequent legislation controlled the inspection of stores, the oaths of officials, appointments of chaplains, confession and prayer, diet and clothing, precautions against fraud, burial, alms and bequests. The Hospitaller, a brother of the Order, remained in overall charge. There was some discussion of problems such as those arising when incurable Hospitallers occupied rooms for many months while there was no space for those who might be saved. Attention continued to be paid to symbolic matters and the maintenance of tradition. Every year on Maundy Thursday the Master's seneschal was to wash the feet of the poor, 'our lords the sick', while the Master entitled himself as 'guardian of the poor of Christ' – *pauperum Christi custos*.[48] The Master himself and his twelve companions were reported to feed twelve

---

[47] As translated in [C. von Schwarzenberg], 'What a Pilgrim saw at Rhodes', *Annales de l'Ordre Souverain Militaire de Malte*, 26 (1968), p. 104.

[48] Texts and details in Gabriel, 2, pp. 29–32, 35–6, 221–6; Pappalardo, pp. 80–81 126–7, 133–50, 162–4, 166–77, 218–23; and H. von Zwehl, *Nachrichten über die Armen- und Kranken Fürsorge des Ordens von Hospital des heil. Johannes von Jerusalem oder Souveränen Malteser-Ritterordens* (Rome, 1911), pp. 13–24. Gabriel, 2, p. 34, judges that the new hospital was exclusively reserved to the sick, but certainly there were exceptions. The *infirmarius* and the brethren's infirmary are not studied here. There seems to be no evidence for isolation wards on Rhodes.

paupers with their own hands every day.[49] It had been the custom that the responsions and other dues arriving from the West were carried before the sick in the Conventual hospital and only taken thereafter to the Treasury,[50] but that observance was in disuse by about 1340.[51]

The Conventual hospital also treated war casualties. In 1445, following Mamluk attacks on Rhodes, certificates of mutilation in war were issued so that those who, for example, had had a hand amputated in the hospital would not be regarded as criminals. In the same year the Master, somewhat exceptionally, conferred a medical degree, following lengthy examination, allowing a Jewish doctor, Jacuda Gratiano, *fisicus et professor artis medicine* who was the son of another Jewish doctor, to practise in the Conventual hospital after taking an oath on the Jewish holy scriptures. The doctors were to visit the wards twice a day, and one was to be on duty at night; there were to be two physicians paid 250 florins a year and two surgeons at 120 florins yearly. A scribe was to write down all prescriptions, and there were strict rules for the pharmacy where poisons were to be kept under lock and key.[52] The personnel included women, such as the slave Helena from Hungary who was freed in 1414 in recognition of her services to the sick, while in 1421 another slave, Jacobinus Armenus, was given his freedom in return for three years' work which he was to complete in the hospital.[53] In the fifteenth century, at least, the brethren's infirmary seems to have been within the main Conventual hospital where individual Hospitallers could have a private room.[54] In 1391 it was enacted that the commander of the lesser island of Kos was to have a garrison of twenty-

---

[49] Pero Tafur, *Andanças*, p. 49: probably written in about 1454.

[50] Riley-Smith, p. 331.

[51] Bibliothèque Nationale, Paris, ms. Lat. 4191, fol. 131v.

[52] Texts of 1440, 1445 and 1446 in Papparlardo, pp. 134–7, 142–3, 152–4, 156–7, and in R. Valentini, 'L'Infermeria degli Ospitalieri di S. Giovanni e i Minorati di Guerra', *Atti e Memorie della Accademia di Storia dell'Arte Sanitaria*, ser. 2, **16** (1950). The salaries seem low. Physicians from the West were promised a salary which, between 1385 and 1402, rose from 200 to 400 florins plus board, while in 1414 a surgeon was to be given 150 florins: Malta, Cod. 323, fol. 205; Cod. 325, fol. 174; Cod. 332, fol. 164v; Cod. 338, fol. 211v. In 1427 the Jewish doctor Vitale Gratiano received a papal licence to practise for the Hospital on Christian patients: text in *Pontificia Commissio ad Redigendum Codicem Iuris Canonici Orientalis: Fontes*, series III, 14 part 2: *Acta Martini PP. V (1417–1431)*, ed. A. Taūtu (Rome, 1980), pp. 846–7.

[53] A. Luttrell, *Latin Greece, the Hospitallers and the Crusades: 1291–1440* (London, 1982), **V**, pp. 98–9. Nicoleta Cibo, *religionis nostre soror*, held a Rhodian vineyard before 1436, but she was of a leading Rhodian family and her case was evidently an exception: Malta, Cod. 352, fols 140–140v. The Hospitaller *soror* Margarita de Nigroponte had her own house and dispensed bread and alms in Rhodes before 1347: text in A. Luttrell, 'Emphyteutic Grants in Rhodes Town: 1347–1348', *Papers in European Legal History: Trabajos de Derecho Histórico Europeo en Homenaje a Ferran Valls i Taberner*, 5 (Barcelona, 1992), pp. 1414–15.

[54] For example, Pappalardo, pp. 146–7. From the fifteenth century the Conventual hospital was often termed the *infermaria*.

five brethren with a doctor, an apothecary and medical supplies.[55] Attention given to public health in the *borgo* included detailed regulations for doctors and apothecaries; by 1441 there was a Latin hospice of Saint Mary to maintain paupers, and by 1442 there was a Greek hospice, also for paupers. Legislation of 1509 concerned two *domini sanitatis* or health commissioners, one Latin and one Greek, who were elected annually to impose strict measures against plague which included control of landings from shipping and on occasion, forty days of isolation; there were licences for burials, segregation arrangements for lepers, and measures to keep rubbish out of the sea.[56] When a major earthquake hit Kos in 1493, the government of Rhodes immediately sent doctors, medicines and supplies in a well-organized example of sustained disaster relief.[57] The introduction of printing facilitated the dissemination of information about the Hospital's medical and charitable roles, for example through the Vice Chancellor Guillaume Caoursin's popular illustrated works and the famous *Ricordi* of Fr. Sabba da Castiglione.[58]

Overall costs would have been virtually incalculable. Roughly 6,750 florins were allocated to the Conventual hospital from incomes on Rhodes in 1314.[59] When 5,000 ducats reached Rhodes at a moment of financial crisis in 1409 some 1,450 ducats, or 29 per cent of the total, were allotted to the hospital, the pharmacy and medical salaries.[60] A very incomplete budget for the Convent's expenses, paid mainly out of European rather than Rhodian incomes, was drawn up in about 1478 and showed expenses at Rhodes on the church, the hospital, the food and pay of Hospitallers and mercenaries, the stores and so on at a total cost of 92,060 florins per year. Of this sum, 7,000 florins, or roughly 7.5 per cent, almost the same proportion as in 1314, was allotted to the Conventual hospital, its pharmacy, its doctors and surgeons, while an overall sum for expenses on grain included further unspecified expenditures on lepers, nurses, orphans and foundlings.[61] Such figures reflected the importance to the Order of its hospital on Rhodes, which constituted not only a religious obligation and a source of ideological strength, but also a show-piece to impress a visiting public which would transmit the resulting image throughout Latin Europe, thereby helping to justify the Hospitallers' extensive possessions and privileges in the West; the Conventual hospital was to some extent a public relations exercise.

---

[55] J. Delaville le Roulx, *Les Hospitaliers à Rhodes jusqu'à la mort de Philibert de Naillac: 1310–1421* (Paris, 1913), pp. 230–31.

[56] Archivio Vaticano, Reg. Lat. 384, fol. 82v; 390, fols 173–173v. On public health, see National Library of Malta, Biblioteca, ms. 740 part 1, fols 3v, 26v–28, 34v, 36v–39, 55v–56v, 57v–59v, partly published in Pappalardo, pp. 166–7, 170–72, 175–7.

[57] Malta, Cod. 77, fols 110v–115.

[58] References in Luttrell, *Latin Greece*, II, pp. 146–50; cf. Waldstein-Wartenberg, *Vasallen*, pl. 11.

[59] Above, p. 64.

[60] Malta, Cod. 339, fols 206v–207.

[61] Paris, ms. Lat. 13, 824, fols 95v–96v.

The astonishing initial success of the Order in Jerusalem after 1099 produced a great wave of donations in the West, and that involved the acquisition of property and its organization into communities of brethren grouped in priories and commanderies, as well as the sending of men and responsions to the East. These brethren had a general hospitaller obligation to the poor and sick and, more specifically, to the maintenance of hospices for pilgrims and travellers, particularly in the many places where houses were located along major routes. That development took place within a wider context. The late eleventh century had been a time of religious enthusiasm which was reflected in the reformed papacy, in new monastic movements, in the earliest crusades and in other developments which came together in the emergence of the Order of St John at Jerusalem. In the West, on the other hand, many small groupings, confraternities and individuals founded hospitals, occasionally entrusting them to the Hospitallers. Often such small hospitals and hospices had no significant endowment and little permanent organization; while founders died and enthusiasms dwindled. Thus local bishops sometimes faced a dilemma which they might solve by transferring institutions in difficulty to a well-established body such as the Hospital. By 1300, however, times were changing. While donations and testamentary bequests to the Order decreased, the loss by 1291 of all its Syrian possessions and incomes forced the Hospital to concentrate on exporting its Western resources to the East. Furthermore, welfare institutions and responsibilities were increasingly becoming the concern of municipal authorities and lay confraternities.[62] There was a particular example of this process at Hall in Swabia, where in 1249 the town council united its hospital to that of the Hospitallers, who were not however bound to receive the seriously ill, but in 1319 the authorities took the hospital back because the Hospitallers were serving the poor so badly.[63]

Strangely, none of the Hospital's medieval saints or *beati* was connected with military activity or, the founder apart, with the Convent in the East; some were holy women. There was no sign of any such medieval tradition in the Hospital's liturgical calendars, although there were genuine local cults. The professed Hospitaller sisters were often of more noble birth than the men, but they seldom, if ever, did hospital work. The crusaders found a separate female hospice attached to the Benedictines in Jerusalem in 1099, but apparently it did not depend on the men's hospital. A fourteenth-century Western chronicler made the unlikely claim that there had also been a female hospital associated with the Order's German hospital in Jerusalem. The Hospitallers had a female house of St Mary Magdalene at Acre in 1219, but there is no evidence that professed sisters did medical work there or in Jerusalem. Pious Hospitaller saints such as St Toscana, a widow who wore the Hospitaller habit and had a cell near the Order's hospital in Verona probably late in the twelfth century, and St

---

[62] S. Reicke, *Das deutsche Spital und sein Recht im Mittelalter*, 1 (Stuttgart, 1932), pp. 93–111.

[63] Ibid., pp. 104–5, 110–11; W. Rödel, *Das Grosspriorat Deutschland des Johanniter-Ordens im Übergang vom Mittelalter zur Reformation*, 2nd edn. (Cologne, 1972), pp. 140–41.

Ubaldescha at Pisa, who died in about 1206, did tend the Order's sick and poor, but were probably donats rather than professed Hospitaller sisters. St Flor of Beaulieu near Cahors, who died in 1347, was of noble birth and a fully professed Hospitaller; she lived a saintly life but it was not that of a medical nurse.[64]

The Order of St John did play a leading hospitaller role in some places in the West. For example, in and near Arles, which was situated on the routes along the Rhône and where there was an early Hospitaller establishment, there were in the thirteenth century some twenty hospitals or leprosies for about 6,000 people, most of them caring for travellers or the poor rather than the sick. Easily the first and by far the largest foundation there, that of St Thomas in Trinquetaille the suburb across the Rhône, was made by the archbishop who granted it to the Hospitallers in about 1116–19; other hospitals at Arles came only after 1172. By 1338 this house at Trinquetaille was no longer functioning as a hospital but merely fed two paupers and gave some weekly alms; its buildings were destroyed by war in 1358. Yet it was not poor; in 1338 it housed two Hospitaller *milites*, two priests, four sergeants and six donats, five of them noble donats, while the former Templar house in Arles sustained six Hospitallers, one *miles*, one priest and four sergeants, plus six donats, four of them noble. The crisis had, however, come by 1373 when the two houses supported only eight Hospitaller brethren.[65]

The situation varied greatly from priory to priory and from commandery to commandery. A number of houses were situated on roads across the Alpine passes and along the Via Emilia and other routes leading to Rome or to Italian ports and embarkation points for the East; others were located along the pilgrim roads to Santiago in Galicia.[66] Hospice buildings, sometimes just a hall

---

[64] A. Luttrell, 'The Spiritual Life of the Hospitallers of Rhodes', in *Die Spiritualität der Ritterorden im Mittelalter*, ed. Z. Nowak (Toruń, 1993). F. Tommasi, 'Uomini e donne negli ordini militari di Terrasanta: per il problema delle case doppie e miste negli ordini giovannita, templare e teutonico (secc. XII–XIV)', in *Doppelklöster und andere Formen der Symbiose männlicher und weiblicher Religiosen im Mittelalter*, ed. K. Elm and M. Parisse (Berlin, 1992), p. 182, considers that the 1181 statutes and Johannes of Würzburg implied women nurses in Jerusalem; however, those texts mentioned women and maternity patients but not women nurses, let alone professed sisters. In 1219 there was a *domus Hospitalis in qua habitant sorores Hospitalis* at Acre; *CH*, 1656. L. Tacchella, *I Cavalieri di Malta in Liguria* (Genoa, 1977), p. 46, speaks of *consorelle* and *converse* serving in the Hospital at Genoa in 1251, but the document only mentions entry into the *religio* and the reception of its habit. Idem, *Le 'Donate' nella Storia del Sovrano Militare Ordine di Malta* (Verona, 1987), p. 14, claims that *donate claustrali* served the poor, the sick and pilgrims, but his source is a description (by Giacomo Bosio) of Sigena in the sixteenth century and it makes no reference to these categories.

[65] G. Giordanengo, 'Les Hôpitaux arlésiens du XIIe au XIVe siècle', in *Assistance et Charité = Cahiers de Fanjeaux*, 13 (Toulouse, 1978).

[66] Broad, if superficial, survey in E. Schermerhorn, *On the Trail of the Eight-Pointed Cross: a Study of the Heritage of the Knights Hospitaller in Feudal Europe* (New York, 1940), pp. 59–81; select details and bibliography, not here repeated, in Luttrell, *Latin Greece*, IX, pp. 369–77; idem, 'Tuscany and Jerusalem', pp. 118–21; Waldstein-Wartenberg, *Vasallen*, pp. 99–107, 128–34, 423; J. Matellanes Merchán and E. Rodríguez-Picavea Matilla, 'Las Ordenes militares en las Etapas castellanas del Camino de Santiago', in *El Camino de Santiago. la Hospitalidad monastica y las Peregrinaciones*, ed. H. Santiago-Otero (Salamanca, 1992), pp. 344–50.

and chapel, may often have been acquired rather than designed by the Hospitallers, or they may simply have been constructed in a local manner so that there was no specifically Hospitaller hospital style. Occasionally the hospice ward was built above the Hospitaller church as at Faenza, at Taufers in the Tirol, at Necharelz in Germany and at Torphichen in Scotland; however, this disposition was not limited exclusively to Hospitaller houses.[67] Other arrangements, also not exclusive to the Hospital, involved corridors, internal doors, windows and observation holes in the floor which permitted those in the wards or dormitories to pass into churches or chapels to assist at services or to attend mass without leaving their ward or bed.[68] The foundation text of 1298 for a hospice for the poor sick and pilgrims at Niederweisel in Hesse declared that it should allow those confined to the ward to see the host at mass, and the room, immediately above the church, did have three openings in its floor.[69] Hospices and wards were often located in buildings physically separate from the church or chapel. The placing of wards above, or immediately adjoining, the chapel was doubtless a matter of convenience, yet the hospice or ward was, in some sense, a religious place in which the inmates were associated with the liturgy. Indulgences had been given at the Hospital's *palais de malades* in Acre,[70] and both those who died in the hospital at Rhodes and those who visited it benefited from various indulgences.[71]

There were hospices and poorhouses in the West, their existence or survival often determined by local patterns of patronage and endowment. The Hospitallers occasionally maintained leprosies,[72] and in England they collected and buried the corpses of executed felons,[73] but by the thirteenth century there were increasingly problems with brethren dissipating charitable endowments and failing to provide hospitality.[74] The obituary book of the Order's house at Eskiltuna in Sweden recorded the death, probably in about 1310, of *frater magister Arnaldus medicus*, that is a Hospitaller with some type of medical qualification,[75] but genuine Hospitaller medical hospitals were rare. Some houses retained a doctor for a small annual fee to take some care either of the brethren or of the poor. At Naples in 1373 there was a hospice for paupers and a *medicus*

---

[67] E. Grunsky, *Doppelgeschossige Johanniterkirchen und verwandte Bauten* (Düsseldorf, 1970), partly repeated in Wienand, pp. 409–21.

[68] E. Ganter, 'Les Chapelles-Hôpitaux de l'Ordre de Saint-Jean de Jérusalem', *Annales de L'Ordre Souverain Militaire de Malte*, 19 (1961).

[69] Wienand, pp. 419–20, 639–40, with plans and section.

[70] H. Michelant and G. Raynaud, *Itinéraires à Jérusalem et Descriptions de Terre Sainte redigés en française au XIe, XIIe, et XIIIe siècles* (Geneva, 1882), p. 235.

[71] Pero Tafur, *Andanças*, p. 48.

[72] Schermerhorn, p. 67, without sources; on the Cologne leprosy; Rödel, pl. XIII–XIV.

[73] R. Pugh, 'The Knights Hospitallers of England as Undertakers', *Speculum*, 56 (1981).

[74] Examples in Le Grand, 325 n. 1; on alms, Schermerhorn, pp. 74–6; Waldstein-Wartenberg, *Vasallen*, pp. 138–9.

[75] I. Collijn, *Ete Nekrologium fran Johanniterklostret i Eskilstuna* (Uppsala, 1929), p. 17.

who looked after its sick.[76] At Toulouse, where the Order had long had a hospital in the bourg and another in the city, there was a steady tradition of donations, often quite humble ones, made by lay folk through wills, annual gifts and burial arrangements; sometimes such people became donats of the Hospital. Toulouse was exceptional in that the Hospitaller hospital founded in the Templar house in about 1408 had nearly a hundred beds for the poor and sick when destroyed by fire in 1446.[77] In 1373 the hospital by the sea at Genoa, a major travel centre, catered for the poor and for pilgrims who fell ill, with a surgeon and a physician retained to treat them; there were separate hospitals for men, with forty beds, a salaried manager and two male attendants, and for women, with thirty-two beds and a female servant caring for the poor, the sick and foundlings, each baby having a wet nurse and the Order providing dowries to marry off its girl foundlings.[78] The Hospitallers, who also had parishes and occasionally schools, were to some extent acting like other branches of the Church in their welfare concerns.[79]

Such charitable and welfare activities were badly affected by the Great Plague and the other crises of the fourteenth century. An English inquest of 1338 showed an *Infirmaria* then containing six sick brethren at Chippenham near Cambridge, while the commandery at Skirbeck in Lancaster had twenty paupers in its hospice and 40 at its gate every day, and Carbrook fed thirteen paupers daily; but little other charitable activity was recorded in that priory.[80] In 1418 the house at Cerisiers was a centre for brethren and donats of the Priory of France who contracted leprosy.[81] In 1338 a survey of houses west of the Rhône, in the very heartland of the Hospitaller West, showed limited expenditures on alms and on doctors and medicines for the brethren, although there was a small hospice for the sick poor and for maternity cases at Monteilh and a hospital at Aix-en-Provence also for the sick poor, which had just one female

---

[76] Luttrell, *Latin Greece*, **IX**, p. 372.

[77] J. Mundy, 'Charity and Social Work in Toulouse: 1100–1250', *Traditio*, **22** (1966), with many examples.

[78] Archivio Vaticano, Collectorie 431 A, fols 4 and 8 suggest that the women's hospital included nine Hospitaller sisters, but fol. 6v shows that they were in a *monasterium* next to the hospital: amend Tommasi, p. 197, on this point. Cf. V. Persoglio, *Sant'Ugo cavaliere ospitaliere gerosolimitano e la Commenda di S. Giovanni di Prè: cenni storicocritici* (Genoa, 1877), pp. 356–8. No document supports claims that Hospitaller *sorores* did medical work at Genoa. The hospital and its restoration are extensively documented: Tacchella, *Cavalieri*, pp. 11–73, 159–62, and *La Commenda di Prè: un Ospedale Genovese del Medioevo*, ed. G. Rossini (Rome, 1992), with full bibliography. A pauper hospital of San Leonardo di Bisanzio, with a lay *hospitalarius* and six or eight beds in 1373 (Collectorie 431 A, fols 3, 5v, 7v), was at Cavi di Lavagna on the coast road east of Genoa: Tacchella, *Cavalieri*, pp. 52, 105–7.

[79] The social security role is studied, but mainly before 1291, in J. von Steynitz, *Mittelalterliche Hospitäler der Orden und Städte als Einrichtungen der Sozialen Sicherung* (Berlin, 1970).

[80] L. Larking, *The Knights Hospitallers in England being the Report of Prior Philip de Thame to the Grand Master Elyan de Vilanova for A.D. 1338* (London, 1857), pp. 61, 78, 82.

[81] Malta, Cod. 342, fols 17–17v.

servant and a doctor available; furthermore, three paupers were fed daily at the very large house at Manosque and two daily at Trinquetaille across the Rhône from Arles.[82] By 1373 things were undoubtedly worse. Thus at Bersantino near Manfredonia in Puglia, where it was said that great sums had once been spent, the commander was in 1373 an absentee and nothing was being expended on *curialitas* or charity.[83] In the Priory of France eight poor were sheltered nightly at Douai and there was an expenditure on alms at Avesne-le-Sec, but there was no other sign of any hospice or hospital in that priory in 1373.[84] Of the thirty houses in the diocese of Besançon in 1373 many were ruined or abandoned and only two claimed to provide even minimum alms [85]

In some priories the commanderies were mostly small and poor; in the Priory of Pisa, for example, there were houses in 1373 with an annual profit of 25 florins or less, in some cases nil. Corneto was an exception, having a hospital with twenty beds and a doctor which was managed by a married couple who received 22 florins a year.[86] In the Priory of Bohemia, also in 1373, the poor were given bread three times a week in Prague, while at Strakonice fourteen paupers received bread and occasionally money as well; there were from six to–fourteen poor at Boleslava.[87] There were hospitals of some sort at Glatz, Zittau, Breslau and Lowenberg in Silesia, at Strakonice and Prague in Bohemia; at Laa, Enns, Vienna and Furstenfeld in Austria; and elsewhere.[88] Shortly before 1371 the prior provided for twelve poor and sick at Prague and he constructed and endowed a hospital at Svetla.[89] In the German priory there was also a considerable number of hospices, although there too there was little sign that they were genuine medical hospitals.[90]

While the most profound and unprecedented economic depression plunged welfare activity into a crisis in general, the older hospital tradition was maintained as a result of a new development within the Order itself in which leading Hospitallers, often utilizing personal wealth, despite their vows of poverty,

[82] B. Beaucage, *Visites générales des Commanderies de l'Ordre des Hospitaliers dépendantes du Grand Prieuré de Saint-Gilles: 1338* (Aix-en-Provence, 1982), pp. 68–9, 351, 354, 463–70, 595, 599 *et passim.*

[83] Luttrell, *Latin Greece*, IX, p. 373.

[84] A-M. Legras, *L'Enquête pontificale de 1373 sur l'Ordre des Hospitaliers de Saint-Jean de Jérusalem* (Paris, 1987), pp. 288, 311 *et passim.*

[85] G. Moyse, 'Les Hospitaliers de Saint-Jean de Jérusalem dans le diocèse de Besançon en 1373', *Mélanges de l'Ecole française de Rome: Moyen Age – Temps Modernes,* 85 (1973), 475, 486.

[86] Luttrell, 'Tuscany and Jerusalem', p. 120 *et passim;* further detail in idem, *Latin Greece,* IX, *passim.*

[87] V. Novotny, 'Inquisito Domorum Hospitalis S. Johannis Hierosolimitani per Pragensem Archidioecesim facta anno 1373', *Historicky Archiv,* 19 (1900), pp. 22, 45, 58.

[88] B. Waldstein-Wartenberg, 'Die kulturellen Leistungen des Grosspriorates Böhmen-Osterreich in Mittelalter', *Annales de l'Ordre Souverain Militaire de Malte,* 33 (1975), surveys a selection of the extensive evidence.

[89] Státní Ustredí Archiv, Prague, Archives of the Hospitaller Priory of Bohemia, no. 2386.

[90] Reicke, pp. 101–6; B. Waldstein-Wartenberg, 'Donaten – Confratres – Pfründner: Die Bruderschaften des Ordens', *Annales de l'Ordre Souverain Militaire de Malte,* 31 (1973), p. 15.

occasionally set up individual foundations. In 1325 the Master, Fr. Hélion de Villeneuve, founded and endowed a hospice and chapel for the poor sick which was documented at Aix-en-Provence in 1338.[91] Just before 1360 Fr. Napoleone de Tibertis, Prior of Venice, apparently acting in association with various laymen, founded the hospice of Santa Caterina next to the commandery in Venice, not for the sick and pilgrims but for the poor and aged; it was managed by a married couple and in 1414 there were eight downstairs beds and further beds upstairs, but after 1451 the local confraternity of San Giorgio gradually secured control of the building.[92] In about 1408 Fr. Raymond de Lescure, Prior of Toulouse, founded a hospital in the former Templar house there both for the sick and poor and for Santiago pilgrims, endowing it with the incomes of the Hospitaller house at Garidech.[93] Most spectacularly, in about 1445 Fr. Juan de Beaumont, Prior of Navarre, endowed and established a large hospice for the poor and sick at Puente la Reina, also on the Santiago route.[94] The most famous such foundation was that made by the Master Fr. Antoni Fluvià of the new hospital at Rhodes.

The Hospitallers had another function, not strictly medical, in the provision of board and lodging, death-care facilities and posthumous prayer to single persons or couples, secular people who purchased or contracted for various forms of life pension or annuity. These newer forms of welfare generated funds which did not support the poor and sick through donations from the wealthier, but catered for individuals of some means who invested their own capital or incomes, often according to precisely worded contracts. Such arrangements were already quite common in the Toulouse area in the thirteenth century.[95] There were many pensioners in England where the unrestricted sale of pensions, sometimes to quite wealthy people, could become a business affair, but while it initially produced income the resulting expenditures had by 1328 helped to provoke a financial crisis.[96] Comparable systems were widespread in the German priory.[97] Part of the Hospital's charitable function was thus 'privatized' by being made to pay for itself.

The Order's sick constituted not a brotherhood or a formal confraternity, but rather a spiritual community with its own liturgy, its obligations such as those

---

[91] J. Raybaud, *Histoire des Grands Prieurs et du Prieuré de Saint-Gilles*, 1 (Nîmes, 1904), p. 278.

[92] Text and details in Luttrell, *Latin Greece*, IX, pp. 373–80, 328–3.

[93] Text in M. du Bourg, *Histoire du Grand-Prieuré de Toulouse* (Toulouse, 1882), appendix pp. xvii–iii (correct the date given as 1413).

[94] Luttrell, *Latin Greece*, IX, p. 370, with further bibliography; cf. L. Romera Iruela, 'La Fundación del Monasterio del Crucifijo en Puente la Reina', *Anuario de Estudios Medievales*, 11, (1981).

[95] Examples in Mundy, 'Charity and Social Work', pp. 257–74.

[96] Larking, pp. xxxvi, lix–x, 215–20 *et passim*; W. Rees, *A History of the Order of Saint John of Jerusalem in Wales and on the Welsh Border* (Cardiff, 1947), pp. 20–21, 58–9.

[97] Waldstein-Wartenberg, 'Donaten', pp. 16–18.

of making confession and testament, and its rights, such as those to treatment, burial, posthumous commemoration in prayer and so forth. After about 1300 the general trend was, despite occasional individual foundations, towards an often dramatic decline in the wealth of individual commanderies and of the number of brethren within them, so that community life and liturgy became increasingly rare, as did charity, hospitality and medical care; the sick lost their central place in the Order's life and ideology. The establishment of the hospital wards at Acre and at Rhodes in a separate building with its own chapel seemed to exemplify this detachment of the hospitaller function from the main activity of the brethren; service to the sick performed by Hospitaller knights and sergeants was replaced by treatment provided by a medical staff who, together with the Conventual hospital's own priests, came to form a separate community.[98] Yet the Conventual hospitals at Rhodes, and later on Malta, retained their importance precisely because they conspicuously maintained the ancient tradition of service to the poor and sick.

The existence there of its hospital effectively defined the Convent. When Rhodes fell to the Turks in 1522, the Master and Convent left on a small fleet carrying, *inter alia*, the Order's most precious holy relics and part of its archives. With hundreds of refugee Rhodians to support and many sick aboard ship, the medical tradition was soon in evidence. Reaching Sicily in April 1523, the Order installed its Conventual hospital in the priory building at Messina where the Master, Fr. Philippe Villiers de l'Isle Adam, went daily to feed the sick. That building overflowed with the sick and plague-stricken, and in the summer of 1523 the Conventual hospital was transferred to the galleon of the Prior of Saint-Gilles. The Master and Convent then sailed northwards, but plague kept them out of Naples harbour and so the Conventual hospital was set up in isolation at a deserted malarial spot by the shore to the west of Naples, in that part of Baia which looks westwards. The sick and healthy were installed in some ancient vaulted buildings described as 'grottos' and known as the cave of the Sibyl at Cuma, which were furnished with hangings, planks, tables and mats, and defended by ditches and artillery. Subsequently the hospital moved with the Convent to Civitavecchia, to Viterbo, to Corneto, to Villefranche, to Nice where it was installed in the commandery, to Siracusa and finally, in 1530, to Malta.[99] There a Conventual hospital was at once set up in a house in Birgu and a new hospital building was begun in 1532 and completed in 1533; by 1538 it had been decided to enlarge it.[100] The tradition was maintained and indeed,

---

[98] As suggested ibid., pp. 14–15; that work leans heavily on the scarcely typical German–Bohemian documentation, and (cf. Luttrell, 'Spiritual Life', 89) it confuses *confratres*, donats, the sick and others with confraternities.

[99] Pappalardo, pp. 192–202; on the Baia interlude, see J. Bosio, *Dell'Istoria della Sacra Religione et Ill.ma Militia di San Giovanni Gierosolimitano*, 3 (Rome, 1602), p. 16.

[100] A. Critien, *The Borgo Holy Infirmary now the St Scholastica Convent* (Malta, 1950), pp. 10–21; P. Cassar, *Medical History of Malta* (London, 1964), pp. 39–44; idem, 'Medical Life at Birgu in the Past', in *Birgu – a Maltese Maritime City*, ed. L. Bugeja et al., I (Malta, 1993).

the Conventual hospital continued to be governed by many of the statutes passed on Rhodes.[101]

The new city of Valletta, built after 1565, included a Conventual *infermeria*. The hospital at Birgu had not catered for pilgrims, who seldom passed through Malta, or for the Maltese population which had its own hospital at Rabat,[102] but the great hospital at Valletta and its numerous subsidiary institutions formed part of an extensive welfare apparatus designed to help placate the Catholic Maltese people.[103] That was a departure from the situation on Rhodes where the Conventual hospital had not served the Greek population. When the Order's government moved to Rome in the nineteenth century a Conventual hospital was found for it there,[104] and the Hospital, having lost its military function, continued its existence by reverting to the original hospitaller activity it had never entirely abandoned. With the enormous expansion of medical activity, modern health services have evolved in which non-governmental forms of health care are backed by compulsory national health insurance. The Order of Malta and independent national institutions, such as the St John's Ambulance Association service in Britain, and the *Malteser Hilfdienst* and the *Johanniter* in Germany have all come to play a significant role in society, building on the Hospitallers' medical tradition kept alive across some nine centuries.

---

[101] Pappalardo, p. 83.

[102] S. Fiorini, *Santo Spirito Hospital at Rabat, Malta: the Early Years to 1575* (Malta, 1989). The Rhodian surgeon Leonardo Myriti received citizenship in Malta in 1534: ibid., pp. 63–4.

[103] A. Williams, '*Xenodocium* to Sacred Infirmary: the Changing Role of the Hospital of the Order of St John, 1522–1631', chapter 11 below, pp. 100–1.

[104] Pappalardo, pp. 240–66.

XI

THE HOSPITALLERS' WESTERN
ACCOUNTS, 1373/4 AND 1374/5[1]

1. This text was published in A. Luttrell, 'The Hospitallers' Accounts for 1373/4 and 1374/5: an Aragonese Text,' *Medievalia*, vii (1987), without my being able to see proofs or correct innumerable errors; the introduction is here expanded considerably and various amendments are made. A. Luttrell, 'Papauté et Hôpital: L'Enquête de 1373,' in A.-M. Legras, *L'Enquête pontificale de 1373 sur l'Ordre des Hospitaliers de Saint-Jean de Jérusalem*, i: *l'Enquête dans le prieuré de France* (Paris, 1987), 22–28, 35–37 *et passim*, contains preliminary information on the Hospital's finances.

INTRODUCTION

The military order of the Hospital of Saint John of Jerusalem had a Treasurer from the time of its early years in the mid-twelfth century; by 1268 he was employing two scribes at the Convent, the order's headquarters in Syria. A statute of 1283 provided for a monthly *computum* or audit to be held by the Master and a group of senior brethren. Fr Joseph Chauncey, who was Treasurer for some twenty-five years, was so competent that Edward I made him Treasurer of England in 1273.[2] At Rhodes during the fourteenth century the Treasury apparently kept no budget showing the overall state of the Hospital's finances, though by about 1478 there was a lengthy list of the incomes of the Western priories and commanderies, of receipts from Rhodes and Cyprus, and of the Convent's expenses in the East.[3] The dues or *responsiones* from the rich Commandery of Cyprus were received by the Treasurer at Rhodes and the Master issued a quittance for them.[4] The Master had separate incomes of his own, and by 1365 these were being managed by the Seneschal of his household; the Master gave a receipt for them.[5]

The bulk of the Convent's income came from the Western priories, the monies being collected and transferred to Rhodes by a Procurator-General in the West, alternatively known as Receiver-General in the West, who was based in Southern France. His accounts, usually presented in Latin, were normally inspected and approved by the Master and certain senior brethren at Rhodes, where a quittance was sealed; the document was sometimes copied into the Master's register.[6] The accounts for 1367/8 and 1368/9 were approved in Rhodes on 1 March 1371; they covered financial years which commenced on 26 March, the beginning of the Incarnation year, but they were complicated by the fact that priories owed their dues for a different year which ended on 24 June, the day of the Hospital's patron Saint John.

---

2. J. Riley-Smith, *The Knights of St. John in Jerusalem and Cyprus: c. 1050–1310* (London, 1967), 310–312; *Handbook of British Chronology*, ed. E. Fryde *et al.* (3rd ed: London, 1986), 104.

3. Paris, Bibliothèque Nationale, Ms. latin 13,824, fos. 75–96v, and London, British Library, Add. Ms. 17,319, fos. 20–38 (lacking the expenses); the date and contents await study. The archives of the Treasury at Rhodes do not survive.

4. The accounts for 1349/50 and 1350/1 are published in A. Luttrell, 'The Hospitallers in Cyprus: 1310–1378,' *Kypriakai Spondai*, 50 (1986), 178–179.

5. Valletta, National Library of Malta, Archives of the Order of St John, Cod. 319, fo. 265.

6. J. Nisbet, 'Treasury Records of the Knights of St. John in Rhodes,' *Melita Historica*, ii no. 2 (1957); Nisbet lists the accounts of Procurators-General in the West between 1364/5 and 1396/9, publishing those for 15 April 1364 to 26 May 1365. No other such accounts have been published.

The returns for 1369/70 were also quitted at Rhodes on 1 March 1371.[7] All these figures were presented by Fr Arnaud Bernard Ébrard, Commander of Bordeaux, who was already Procurator-General by 27 May 1362.[8] On 2 February 1372 the Master relieved him of his post, instructing him to hand over 15,000 florins to the Archbishop of Nicosia, who had deposited that sum in the Treasury at Rhodes, and 15,698 florins to the new Procurator-General, Fr Aimery de la Ribe, Commander of Raissac.[9]

In October 1374 Fr Aimery de la Ribe presented to the Master, then at Beaucaire, a detailed list of receipts and payments; this was in Latin and it mentioned that Ribe paid a notary to record Treasury business.[10] These accounts noted sums received from Ébrard, other monies which had been due for 1369/70 and 1370/1, and sums received by Ribe as recently as 23 December 1373; they referred to monies sent to Rhodes in 1372. The periods covered were not specified precisely though most of the transactions reported concerned the years 1371/2 and 1372/3. No total was given but the sums listed amounted to just over 37,955 florins. The parchment was written out in the form of a magistral bull approved, sealed and dated at Beaucaire on 18 October 1374, but it was not in fact sealed there, presumably because the approval of the brethren in the Convent at Rhodes was required. Not until 26 May 1376 at Rhodes, following an audit by the Master and certain associates who included the layman Giovanni Corsini, the Treasurer Fr Henri de Saint Trond, Fr Focauld de Conac and many others, was a quittance issued in a brief and separate new bull copied onto the foot of the original parchment; it had holes for two seals and was marked *Cor.ta* and *Reg.ta,* corrected and registered.[11] On 10 October 1374, just eight days before Ribe presented these accounts, the Master had appointed Fr Juan Fernández de Heredia as his lieutenant in the West and as *generalis negotiorum gestor* with powers over *responsiones* and other monies,[12] and it was he who presented the Western accounts for 1373/4 and 1374/5. Fr Aimery de la Ribe none the less remained *procurator generalis* in the West at least until September 1375.[13]

The parchment containing the Western accounts for the financial

---

7. Malta, Cod. 16, nos. 46, 48.

8. Malta, Cod. 16, no. 9; on Ébrard, see J. Delaville le Roulx, *Les Hospitaliers à Rhodes jusqu'à la Mort de Philibert de Naillac: 1310–1421* (Paris, 1913), 144 n. 2.

9. Malta, Cod. 16, no. 50.

10. *Item solui notario scriptori negociorum Thesauri mecum commoranti xxv flor' auri:* Malta, Cod. 16, no. 53.

11. Malta, Cod. 16, no. 53: total calculated in Nisbet, 102. How this text was registered cannot be established as the register for 1376 is lost.

12. Malta, Cod. 23, no. 3.

13. Document dated at Rhodes on 30 September 1375: Malta, Cod. 23, no. 1.

4

years 1373/4 and 1374/5 was written out for, and in the native tongue of, the Aragonese Hospitaller Fr Juan Fernández de Heredia, who was *Castellán de Amposta* as the prior in Aragon was confusingly entitled. Aragonese was little used, or at least seldom written, outside Aragon. The most notable exception was the series of translations and compilations produced at Avignon between about 1370 and 1396 for Fernández de Heredia, who in 1377 became Master of the Hospital. His personal letters and the documents in the registers of his Hospitaller priories were often in Aragonese and there were evidently one or more scribes in his household at Avignon who wrote in that language. In 1374 Fernández de Heredia was the papal Captain-General of Avignon and the unofficial representative there of the Aragonese king, while he was also the Hospitallers' prior in both Aragon and Catalunya and the Lieutenant in the West of the Master of Rhodes; until about 1369 he also held the Provençal priory known as the Priory of Saint Gilles.[14] The Hospital made use of Fernández de Heredia's financial capabilities. In 1373 an assembly of Hospitallers at Avignon agreed, somewhat unrealistically, to raise large sums by imposing extraordinary taxes in order to finance a *passagium* against the Turks. There was to be a special taille and efforts were to be made to collect debts, arrears, mortuaries and other sums due. Fernández de Heredia was appointed to manage these incomes many of which were to be transferred to Avignon by the papal bankers, the Alberti Antichi of Florence.[15]

Though the accounts for 1373/4 and 1374/5 were in Aragonese, the opening passage of the parchment on to which they were copied in the form of a quittance to be validated by the Master and Convent was in Latin, as were its closing clauses. The eventual date when the quittance would be sealed could not be determined when the parchment was written out at Avignon, and when it reached Rhodes the leaden bull of the Master and Convent was attached to it; however, the dating clause was not added, nor were the phrases *Cor.ta*, or corrected, and *Reg.ta*, or registered. Possibly another copy, subsequently lost, was sent back to Fernández de Heredia as a receipt while the undated parchment was retained at Rhodes. In general, the annual accounts kept in the West recorded the *responsiones*, that is the ordinary dues collected by the priors from the commanders for transfer to Rhodes; any arrears or *arrerages* which happened to have been paid; the *spolia* or *despullya*, the personal effects and monies of deceased brethren; the mortuaries or *mortuoria*, apparently the wealth and

14. See A. Luttrell, *The Hospitallers in Cyprus, Rhodes, Greece and the West: 1291–1440* (London, 1978), and *idem*, *Latin Greece, the Hospitallers and the Crusades: 1291–1440* (London, 1982).

15. Luttrell (1982), XV 404–406; in Legras, 21–25, 35–37.

revenues of offices from the time of their incumbent's death until the day of the following chapter, that is of the financial year in which the incumbent died;[16] and the vacancies or *vagantes*, probably the income of such offices for the year following the financial year in which the incumbent died.[17] Certain commanderies which were set aside as magistral *camere* or *cambras* also paid their income to the Master, and these payments were in some cases handled by the Procurator-General in the West. In 1373/4 and 1374/5 the special taille fixed at one third of the *responsiones* was also being collected. All these incomes were channelled through the priories except that, for special historical reasons, five large Southern Italian commanderies paid their dues directly. Non-payments were often noted and were so frequent that no individual annual account represented a complete or nearly-complete record for a given financial year. Payments in various currencies were translated into florins current at Avignon.[18] Expenses in the West were for the securing and writing of bulls, for couriers, and for pensions and retaining fees paid to the Hospital's Cardinal Protectors and to a number of Hospitaller and papal officials at the *curia*. In 1373/4 and 1374/5 there were expenditures on repaying monies advanced by the Alberti Antichi, on the papal mission of Hospitallers and theologians sent to Constantinople, and on repayments in the West of loans made by Latin merchants at Rhodes.

16. According to a statute of 1367: Delaville, 162 n. 5. All brethren owed *spolia*, while only those holding office paid mortuaries; numerous entries in the accounts for 1378/88 (Malta, Cod. 48) showed confusions between an officer's personal effects and liabilities, and the possessions and incomes of his office. Thus the commander's silver or animals could be paid as mortuaries after the deduction of his funeral expenses.

17. The Master and Convent could at moments of crisis temporarily be granted the revenues of vacant priories or commanderies, as in 1344 and 1357: texts in M. Barbaro di San Giorgio, *Storia della Costituzione del Sovrano Militare Ordine di Malta* (Rome, 1927), 221–223. Nisbet, 96, without sources, and B. Waldstein–Wartenberg, *Rechtsgeschichte des Malteserordens* (Vienna, 1969), 114, citing the text of 1357 in Barbaro, 223, state that the vacancy was the income of the office in the financial year following that of the mortuary year, that is of the year in which the officer died; that is not, however, what the 1357 text stated. The accounts for 1373/4 and 1374/5 show that mortuaries were referred to a commander, vacancies to a commandery. These questions await clarification.

18. In 1372/5 a florin *de camera* was worth 28 sous of Avignon; a florin *currens*, 24 sous; a florin *de sententia*, 27½ sous; 6 florins *correntes* were worth 5 francs; etc. Except that in 1373/4 the accounts calculated the florin *de sententia* at 27⅔ sous, the equivalencies in the 1373/5 accounts coincided with those in the papal documents: K. Schäfer, *Die Ausgaben der apostolischen Kammer unter Johann XXII. nebst der Jahresbilanzen von 1316–1378* (Paderborn, 1911), 54*, 59*. Florins *correntes* were apparently equivalent to, or identical with, those of Provence current in Avignon: H. Rolland, *Monnaies des Comtes de Provence: XII–XIV Siècles* (Paris, 1956), 153–154, 164. Twelve *denarii* made one sou; one groat or *grossus*, a silver coin, was apparently worth 2 sous. Sums in the tables are given correct to the nearest florin; brackets indicate calculated or corrected sums; in the notes *grossi* are converted into sous.

6

These transactions were set down with a variety of ambiguities. The totals which could be derived from the accounts gave a very incomplete impression of the Hospital's overall incomes, and they did not include other revenues collected in Rhodes and Cyprus; furthermore, the Master had personal incomes which were separate from those of the Convent. The payments recorded in the West for the years from 1367 to 1373 averaged about 22,700 florins annually, and those between 1378 and 1399 about 38,500 florins annually; the years 1367/9 brought in 50,412 florins, 6 *grossi* and 4 *denari,* at 25,206 florins a year, and the year 1369/70 brought in 23,044 florins 3½ *grossi.*[19] The marginally higher figures for 1373/4 and 1374/5 reflected the extraordinary measures agreed in 1373 for the *passagium* against the Turks. The totals were somewhat uncertain, and the accounts often contained mistakes.[20] In 1365 there were complaints that one Procurator-General in the West had omitted 4,000 florins which were missing *in cartularijs rationum thesauri,*[21] while a remark on the obverse of the accounts for 1367/9 noted an error which was corrected in the accounts for 1369/70.[22] Where the sums in the surviving copy of the 1373/4 and 1374/5 accounts did not add up to the totals given, this was apparently because the figures were transferred incorrectly from the original accounts rather than because the totals had been added wrongly in the first place in the records kept at Avignon.

Anyone in the Treasury at Rhodes who attempted to analyse these accounts would have found careless copyings and other difficulties. Fluctuations in exchange rates and the costs of exchanging monies must have caused discrepancies. The text for audit in Rhodes copied totals from individual pages of an account book being kept in Southern France.[23] Errors in the parchment sent to Rhodes would have frustrated calculations there but that particular text was a receipt, not the original accounting record. Nine priories were listed as paying nothing in 1373/4, though some of these paid their arrears in 1374/5; Portugal had paid nothing for nine years. No total was given for 1373/4 but incomes seem to have amounted to 42,230 florins and expenditures to 35,263, leaving a considerable unaccounted difference which may eventually have reached Rhodes. Of the expenditures, over 5,000 florins went to the Constantinople mission; other expenses in the West amounted to more than 3,000 florins; and over 26,000

19. Based on details in Nisbet, 102–104.
20. Luttrell, in Legras, 36–37, notes some accounting anomalies in these years.
21. Malta, Cod. 319, fos. 3v–4.
22. Malta, Cod. 16, nos. 46, 48.
23. An extremely detailed account book for the Western incomes and expenditures from 1378 to 1389 is in Malta, Cods. 48 and 55. In 1371/3 Fr Aimery de la Ribe, Procurator-General in the West, paid 4½ florins *pro uno libro empto ad copiandum ibidem bullas vel alia negotia Thesauri*: Malta, Cod. 16, no. 53.

florins were paid to the Master, who was then in the West and must have expended part of this sum before reaching Rhodes. The incomes from Italy seem to have arrived in Avignon en bloc, as suggested by the unlikely equalities in the figures given; they may have been transferred by the Alberti who regularly moved monies for the Hospital.[24] The English Hospitallers, whose returns were listed as nil in the accounts for 1373/4 and 1374/5, may have preferred to send their monies by way of Venice rather than through France.[25]

The returns for 1374/5 were presented less carefully than those for 1373/4. They included special payments imposed on 25 September 1374 in order to raise 10,000 florins for the journey or *passage* to Rhodes of the newly-elected Master, Fr Robert de Juilly.[26] 46,830 florins were apparently recorded as having been received while sums totalling perhaps 6,111 florins were said still to be owing from Italy together with 500 florins due from the Archbishop of Rhodes; these would, if eventually paid, have produced a grand total of 53,441 florins. Expenditures amounted to 34,278 florins of expenses detailed and a further 17,765 paid to the Grand Commander of the Hospital; these would have totalled 52,043 florins, a sum not unlike that of the expected total incomes. These figures were subject to various cautions and reservations, but they did indicate the general order of magnitude of the Convent's Western incomes.

The accounting methods employed by the Hospitallers in Southern France were capable of dealing with the collection of monies from the priories, with the transfer of funds to the East, with repayments in the West of sums advanced to the Treasury at Rhodes, and with a variety of payments and pensions in the West. A religious order could certainly handle the necessary calculations. The Templars had operated quite complex banking procedures in the thirteenth century,[27] and the Cistercians were keeping accounts of their central receipts by 1290; by about 1340 they had something like an overall budget of their incomes and expenses.[28] The Hospital faced the complication of having to integrate two separate operations, the collection of a surplus in the West and the management of receipts and expenditures in the East; its survival at Rhodes was heavily dependent on the efficient functioning of its Western financial organisation.

24. Luttrell (1978), VII 180; VIII 322, 325.
25. Luttrell (1978), V 199; (1982), I 259.
26. Malta, Cod. 320, fos. 32–32v.
27. J. Piquet, *Des Banquiers au Moyen Âge: Les Templiers* (Paris, 1939).
28. P. King, *The Finances of the Cistercian Order in the Fourteenth Century* (Kalamazoo, 1985).

THE HOSPITALLERS' WESTERN INCOMES FOR 1373/4

Priory or Commandery	Responsiones	Taille	Arrears	Mortuaries	Spolia	Vacancies	Total
England	—	—	—	—	—	—	—
France	6,000	2,000	—	600	1,928	—	[10,528]
Aquitaine	2,670	—	—	—	—	—	[2,670]
Champagne	1,000	312	—	—	—	—	[1,312]
Auvergne	2,180	250	—	70	--	—	[2,500]
S. Gilles	3,919	1,000	530	1,939	—	—	[7,387]
Toulouse	1,646	246	305	301	—	—	[2,498]
Catalunya	2,742	1,711	950	—	—	—	5,403
Amposta	917	—	1,500	—	—	—	2,417
Navarre	500	231	—	—	—	—	731
Castile	—	—	—	—	—	—	—
Portugal	—	—	—	—	—	—	—
Lombardy	—	—	41	—	217	—	258
Pisa	922	288	—	—	—	—	1,210
Rome	—	288	—	—	—	—	288
Messina	—	—	—	—	—	—	—
Naples	692	346	—	—	—	—	1,038
Alife	—	—	—	—	—	—	—
Capua	692	231	—	39	—	—	963
S. Eufemia	—	—	—	—	—	—	—
Venosa	346	115	—	—	—	—	461
Monopoli	—	—	—	—	—	—	—
Barletta	—	—	—	—	—	—	—
Venice	922	288	—	—	—	—	1,210
Hungary	—	—	—	—	—	—	—
Alamania	1,012	344	—	—	—	—	1,356
Bohemia	—	—	—	—	—	—	—
	[26,160]	[7,650]	[3,326]	[2,949]	[2,145]	[—]	[42,230]

THE HOSPITALLERS' WESTERN INCOMES FOR 1374/5

Priory or Commandery	Responsiones	Taille	Arrears	Mortuaries	Spolia	Vacancies	Total
England	—	—	—	—	—	—	—
Ireland	—	—	—	—	—	—	—
France	6,250	1,250	—	1,042	—	1,317	9,859
Champagne	1,042	312	—	—	—	—	[1,354]
Aquitaine	1,250	—	—	—	—	—	[1,250]
Auvergne	2,000	500	—	—	—	—	[2,500]
S. Gilles	4,548	852	646	650	—	893	7,589
Toulouse	817	178	380	—	—	—	1,375
Catalunya	2,900	1,769*	—	—	—	—	[4,668]
Amposta	916	1,327*	—	—	—	—	2,243
Navarre	500	337*	—	—	—	30	867
Rome	922	288	—	—	—	—	[1,210]
Venosa	342	114	—	—	—	—	[456]
Pisa	922	288	—	—	—	—	[1,210]
Alamania	1,000	459	100	—	—	—	[1,559]
Bohemia	1,200	612*	2,008	—	—	—	[3,820]
Hungary	300	—	—	—	—	—	[300]
Venice	800	382	—	—	—	—	[1,182]

Barletta	2,000	1,024*	—	—	—	—	[3,024]
Monopoli	400	229*	553	—	—	—	[1,182]
Messina	—	1,182*	—	—	—	—	[1,182]
Lombardy	—	—	—	—	—	—	—
Castile	—	—	—	—	—	—	—
Portugal	—	—	—	—	—	—	—
	[28,109]	[11,193]*	[3,687]	[1,692]	[—]	[2,240]	[46,830]

SUMS SAID TO BE OWING FOR 1374/5

Priory or Commandery	Responsiones	Taille	Arrears	Mortuaries	Spolia	Vacancies	Total
Venosa	300**	51*	—	—	—	—	[351]**
S. Eufemia	600	255*	804	—	—	—	[1,659]
Naples	600	459*	—	—	—	—	[1,059]
Alife	500	229*	653	—	—	—	[1,382]
Capua	600	306*	—	500	—	—	[1,406]
Rome	—	127*	—	—	—	—	[127]
Pisa	—	127*	—	—	—	—	[127]
	[2,600]	[1,554]*	[1,457]	[500]	[—]	[—]	[6,611]***

    * Includes sums paid or due for the Master's passage to Rhodes
   ** Incomplete sum
  *** Total given by the ms. plus 500 florins owed by the Archbishop of Rhodes

THE HOSPITALLERS' WESTERN ACCOUNTS, 1373/4 AND 1374/5

Valletta, National Library of Malta, Archives of the Order of St John, Cod. 16, no. 52: original parchment with seal.[1]

Nouerint Vniuersi, et singuli presentes inspecturj et auditurj. Quod Nos frater Robertus de Julliaco, dei gratia sacre domus hospitalis sancti Johannis Jerosolimitanj Magister humilis et pauperum Christi custos. Et Nos Conuentus Rodj domus eiusdem Confitemur et in uerbo ueritatis publice recognoscimus nos uidisse et recepisse computa et raciones per Religiosum in Christo nobis carissimum fratrem Johannem Ferdinandj de Heredia domus eiusdem Castellanum Emposte et priorem Cathalonie, ac locum nostrum tenentem in ultramarinis partibus generalem ad nos missa et missas videlicet de omnibus vniuersis et singulis pecunijs parcium ultramarinarum per eundem locum nostrum tenentem receptis datis solutis et assignatis ad nos et nostri Conuentus Thesaurum spectantibus, et alijs expensis missionibus et solucionibus per eum factis, scilicet de annjs dominj Millesimo, Trecentesimo Septuagesimo quarto, et Septuagesimo quinto prout infra sequitur. Primerament del Priorado d'Anglaterra por responsio del anyo suso escripto de lxxiiij nichil. Item por tallya nichil. Item por arrerages nichil. Item por mortuorum nichil. Item por vagantes nichil. Summa nichil. Item recebio de Francia los quales recebio el senyor maestro por responsion del priorado de Francia conptando v. francos por vj flor.', et tornan dellos a florines correntes que fazen por todos .vj.^{m} flor.' Item recebio por tallya del dito priorado, la qual tallya es ij^m. xxx flor.' de sentencia conptando los arazon de xxvij sol.' viij. drs.' por florin tornando los a florines correntes .ij.^{m} flor.'[2] Item por arrerages del dito anyo nichil. Item por mortuorum del anyo suso scripto conptando arazon de v. francos por vj flor.' et tornandolos a florines correntes vj^c flor.' Item por la despuylla de fray G. de Chaucony spitallero del Couent de Rodes,[3] el qual morio en Auinyo en lanyo suso scripto entre dineros et vaxella dargent .m. viiij^c. xxviij

---

1. In the transcription *flor.'*, *sol.'*, *drs.'* and *gros.'* are left in those forms, while "7" is normally transcribed as *et*, *n̄y* as *ny*, *an̄yo* as *anyo, nich'* as *nichil,* and *s. de p.* as *summa de priorado* or *pagina* spelling and punctuation follow the original, but proper names are capitalised.

2. Ms. "*m*", but "*ij*", making 2,000 florins, is almost precisely the equivalent of 2,030 florins *de sentencia*; furthermore, on 29 August, 11 September and 11 October 1374 the Master gave Fernández de Heredia quittances for 6,000 florins of *responsiones* and 2,000 florins of taille from the Priory of France which the Master had received directly from the collector of that priory: Malta, Cod. 23, no. 4; Cod. 320, fos. 2, 11v, 44v–45.

3. Fr Guillaume de Chauconnin, the Hospitaller of Rhodes, who apparently died in Avignon in June or July 1374: Legras, 417.

flor.' Item por Vagantes nichil. Summa de priorado .ix ꝫ vᶜ xxviij flor.⁴ Item recebio del priorado de Aquitania por responsion del dito priorado del anyo suso scrito conptando v. francos por vj florines et fagon flor.' correntes ij ꝫ vjᶜ lxx flor.' Item por tallya nichil. Item por arrerages nichil. Item por mortuor' nichil. Item por vagantes nichil. Item recebio del priorado de Champanya por responsion del dito priorado del anyo suso scripto mill.' flor.' Item por tallya del dito priorado del dito anyo es assaber a razon de v. francs per vj flor.' fazen de Correntes .iijᶜ xij. flor.' vj gros.' Summa de priorado .ij ꝫ dC. lxx flor.'⁵ Arrerages, mortuor' et vagantes nichil. Item recebio, del priorado de Aluernia por la responsion del dito priorado del anyo suso scripto, ij ꝫ Clxxx flor.' Item por tallya del dito priorado del dito anyo .ijᶜ l. flor.' Item per mortuor' del dito anyo lxx flor.' Summa del dito priorado. S(umma) de p(agina)⁶ ij ꝫ Vᶜ x. flor.'⁷ Item recebio del priorado de sant Gilj por responsion del dito priorado del anyo suso scripto .iij ꝫ viiijᶜ xviij flor.', sol.' xvj. Item por tallya del dito priorado del anyo suso scripto, M flor.' Item por arrerages Vᶜ xxix flor.' sol.' xvj. Item por mortuor' M. viiijᶜ xxxviij flor.' sol.' xv. Summa del priorado .vij ꝫ iijᶜ xcvj flor' xj gros.'⁸ Item recebio del priorado de Tholosa por responsion del dito priorado del anyo suso scripto .M. vjᶜ xlv. flor.', xxij sol.' Item por talha .ijᶜ xlvj flor.' .ij. sol.' x. Item por arrerages .iijᶜ iiij. flor.' xxvj sol.' Item por mortuor' iijᶜ flor.' xviij. sol.' x. drs.' Summa del priorado .ij ꝫ iijᶜ xcvij. flor.' x. gross. Summa de priorado .ix ꝫ viijᶜ xciij flor.' .x. gross.'⁹ Item recebio del priorado de Catalunya por la responsion del dito priorado del anyo suso scripto .ij ꝫ vijᶜ xlj flor.' .xiij sol.' ij dr.' Item por tallya del dito priorado, M .vjᶜ ij. flor.' xviij sol.' iiij. Item daltra part por tallya del dito priorado, C. viij. flor.' v. sol. xj. Item por arrerages viiijᶜ l. flor.' Summa del priorado vᵐ¹⁰ .iiijᶜ j. flor.' xxxvij sol.' v. dr.' correntes. Item recebio dela Castellania d'Amposta¹¹ por responsion dela dita Castellania¹² del anyo suso scripto es assaber xjᵐ torneses que fazen de flor.' correntes viiijᶜ xvj flor.' xvj. sol.' Item por tallya (nichil).¹³ Item por arrerages .m.d. flor.' Summa dela Castellania, ijᵐ iiijᶜ xvi. flor.' xvj

4. The correct total is 10,528 (not 9,528) florins.

5. The figures amount to 1,312 florins 12 sous (not 2,670 florins, which was the total for the previous entry for Aquitaine).

6. Total from the page in the account book being copied.

7. The figures amount to 2,500 (not 2,510) florins.

8. The figures amount to 7,385 florins 23 sous (not 7,396 florins 22 sous).

9. This entry of 9,893 florins 20 sous represents the combined totals for Saint Gilles and Toulouse.

10. Ms: vᶜ

11. *Castellania d'Amposta:* the Priory of Aragon.

12. Ms. repeats *dela dita Castellania.*

13. Ms. omits *nichil.*

sol.' correntes. Summa de priorado vij.ᵐ viijᶜ xix. flor.' iiij. gros.', v. drs.' correntes.[14] Item Recebio por responsion del priorado de Nauarra del anyo suso scripto Vᶜ flor.' Item por tallya del dito priorado .ijᶜ xxx. flor.' xiij sol.' iiij. dr.' Summa del priorado vijᶜ xxx flor.' xiij sol.' .iiij. dr.' Item recebio dei priorado de Castella por responsion del dito priorado del anyo suso scripto nichil. Item por tallya del dito priorado nichil. Item por arrerages nichil. Item por mortuoris nichil. Item por vagantes nichil. Summa de priorado vijᶜ xxx flor.' xiij sol.' iiij dr.'[15] Item recebio del priorado de Portugal por responsion del dito priorado del anyo suso scripto nichil. Item por tallya nichil. Item por arrerages nichil. Item por mortuor' nichil. Item por Vagantes nichil. Item Recebio por arrerages del priorado de Lombardia xlj flor.' .ij. sol.' i ij. Item por la despulla de fray Milan Farina[16] .ijᶜ xvij flor.' viij sol.' iij. Summa del priorado. S(umma) de p(agina) .ijᶜ lviij flor.' x sol,' vij drs.' Item recebio por responsion del priorado de Pisa del anyo suso scrito .viiijᶜ xxij. flor.' .v. sol.' viij. Item por la talha del dito priorado .ijᶜ lxxxviij. flor.' sol.' iiij. dr.' viij. Summa del priorado .m.ijᶜ x. flor.' .x. sol.' iiij dr.' Item Recebio del priorado de Roma por la tallya del dito priorado del anyo suso scrito .ijᶜ lxxxviij. flor.' .iiij. sol.' Summa de priorado m.iiijᶜ xcviij. flor.' correntes .xv. sol.'[17] Item recebio del priorado de Messina por responsion del dito priorado del anyo suso scripto nichil. Item por tallya nichil. Item por arrerages nichil. Item por mortuor' nichil. Item por vagantes nichil. Item Recebio del priorado de Napols por responsion del dito priorado del anyo suso scripto vjᶜ xcj. flor.' sol.' xvj. Item por tallya del dito priorado .iijᶜ xlv. flor.' xx sol.' Summa del priorado. S(umma) de p(agina). m.xxxvj flor.' correntes .xxvj sol.'[18] Item Recebio por responsion del Scambi d'Alif[19] delanyo suso scripto nichil. Item por tallya nichil. Item por arrerages nichil. Item por mortuor' nichil. Item por vagantes nichil. Item Recebio del priorado de Capua por responsion del dito priorado del anyo suso scripto vjᶜ xcj flor.' xv. sol.' xj dr.' Item por tallya del dito priorado .ijᶜ xxx flor.' xiij sol.' iiij. dr.' Item por mortuoris xxxix flor.' xiij sol.' .x. dr.' Summa del priorado S(umma) de p(agina). viiijᶜ lx flor.' xliij sol.' j. dr.' correntes. Item Recebio del Priorado de Sancta Eufemia[20] por responsion del anyo suso scripto nichil. Item por tallya nichil. Item por arrerages nichil. Item por mortuoris nichil. Item por vagantes nichil. Item recebio del

14. 7,819 florins 8 sous 5 *drs.'* is the total for Catalunya and Amposta.

15. This entry for Castile, which paid nothing, results from adding Castile and Navarre.

16. Fr Milano Farina: unindentified.

17. 1,498 florins 15 sous is the total for Rome and Pisa.

18. *xxvj sol.'* should read *xxxvj sol.'*

19. *Scambi d'Alif:* the Commandery of Alife in the Kingdom of Naples.

20. Naples and Santa Eufemia were Commanderies, not priories.

XI

priorado de Venosa[21] por la responsion del dito priorado del anyo suso scripto .iij.ͨ xlv. flor.' .xx. sol.' Item por tallya .C. xv. flor.' .vj. sol.' .viij. Summa de priorado .iiij.ͨ lx. flor.' xxvij. sol.' viij drs.' correntes. Primo Recebio del priorado de sant Esteue de Monopoly,[22] por la responsion del dito priorado del anyo suso scripto, nichil. Item por tallya nichil. Item por arrerages nichil. Item por mortuoris nichil. Item por vagantes nichil. Item recebio del Priorado de Barleta por la responsion del anyo suso scripto nichil. Item por tallya nichil. Item por arrerages nichil. Item por mortuoris nichil. Item por vagantes nichil.[23] Item recebio del priorado de Venecia por la responsion del dito priorado del anyo suso scripto .viiij.ͨ xxij flor.' Vᵒss.' iiij. dr.' Item por tallya del dito priorado .ij.ͨ lxxxviij. flor.' sol.' iiij. viij. dr.' Summa del priorado.[24] Item recebio del priorado d'Ongria por la responsion del dito priorado del anyo suso scripto nichil. Item por tallya nichil. Item por arrerages nichil. Item por mortuoris nichil. Item por vagantes nichil. Summa de priorado .m.ij.ͨ x, flor' x. sol.'[25] Item Recebio del priorado d'Alamanya por responsion del dito priorado del anyo suso scripto .m. xj. flor.' xij sol.' Item por tallya .iij.ͨ xliiij flor.' vj. sol.' Summa del priorado.[26] Item Recebio por responsion del dito priorado de Boemia del anyo suso scripto nichil. Item por tallya nichil. Item por arrerages nichil. Item por mortuoris nichil. Item por vagantes nichil. Summa de priorado m.iij.ͨ lv. flor.' xviij sol.' Pagamentos fechos enel anyo de lxx(i)v.ᵒ[27] Primerament fueron liurados por la companya de los Albertes antigos mercaderos de Florença, a xx. dies de octobre del anyo .m.ccc.lxxiiij. en Auinyo al senyor Maestro del Hospital, es assaber en florines doro de Cambra .xij ᵐ ij.ͨ l. Item en florines correntes doro .xij ᵐ ij.ͨ l. por las manes de Matheu de Vita dela dita companya conptando el flor.' de Cambra a xxviij sol.', e lo flor.' corrent a xxiiij sol.', fazen flor.' correns xxvj.ᵐ v.ͨ xlj flor.' xvj. sol.' correntes.[28] Item pago la dita Companya al Cardenal de Mende, al Cardenal de Thoroana, a monss. de Florença, a mons. de sant Eustati,[29] es assaber a cascuno dellos por la pension del anyo de lxxiiij. iij.ͨ flor.' doro correns a cascuno que fazen m.ij.ͨ flor.' correntes. Item pago la dita companya a fray R. Asam procurador en cort de Roma porel el dito

---

21. Santa Trinità di Venosa in Puglia: a commandery, not a priory.
22. San Stefano Monopoli in Puglia: a commandery not a priory.
23. The whole entry for Barletta is repeated.
24. The missing total is 1,210 florins 10 sous.
25. This sum of 1,210 florins 10 sous is the total for Venice.
26. The total for *Alamania* is 1,355 florins 18 sous.
27. Ms: *lxxṽ*.
28. 26,541 florins 16 sous were paid to the Master.
29. The Hospital's cardinal Protectors were Guillaume de Chanac (*Mende*), Aycelin de Montaigu (*Thoroana*), Pietro Corsini (*Florença*) and Pierre Flandrin (*S. Eustati*).

senyor Maestro[30] por la pension del anyo suso scripto, l. flor.' correntes. Item pago la dita companya e los quales fueron pagados enel palacio del papa, es assaber alos porteros dela primera puerta florins viij. Item a los dela .ij.ª porta flor.' xij. Item a los maceres[31] del papa flor.' xxv. Item a los maestres vxeros del papa flor.' l. et esto por pension del anyo de lxxiiij, que fazen en somma, xcv flor.' correntes. Item pago la dita Companya a miss' Alexandre Delantella,[32] et a miss. Francisco Bru,[33] et a miss. Jac(omo) Sona[34] por la pension del anyo de lxxiiij, es assaber a cascuno .l. flor.' correntes que fazen, Cl. flor' correntes. Item pago la dita companya a fray Pere Buxon[35] por la pension suya dela procuracion de la religion de lanyo de lxxiiij. iijᶜ flor.' correntes. Item pago la dita companya a maestro Feri Casinell procurador del senyor Maestro[36] por la pension del anyo lxxiiij. iijᶜ flor.' correntes. Item pago la dita companya a fray Aymeric dela Riba[37] por la pension del anyo lxxiiij. iiijᶜ flor.' correntes. Item pago la dita companya a miss. Ramon Bernat[38] por la pension del anyo suso scripto .l. flor.' correntes. Item pago la dita companya a Matheu Sobolinj[39] notario por scripturas xxv flor.' correntes.[40] Item fueron pagados a fray Thomas dela orden de los predicadores[41] por lo viage de Constantinoble .C. florins correntes. Item a el mismo por la dita razon, xlvj flor.' correntes xviij sol.' Item pago la dita companya a maestro Bartholomeu Cieras dela orden delos menores[42] por el viage de Costantinoble es assaber iijᶜ lxxx flor.' de sentencia conptando el flor.' a razon de xxvij. sol.' viij drs.' que fan flor.' correntes .iiijᶜ xxxviij flor.',

30. Fr Raymond Adizam, later styled *presbiter bacallarius in decretis*, who was here pensioned as the Master's procurator in the *curia*. He was possibly the earliest Hospitaller with legal qualifications to hold such a position: cf. Luttrell (1978), XVI 453. His pension was augmented on 20 October 1374: Malta, Cod. 320, fo. 50.

31. The *servientes armorum seu masserii*, the pope's sergeants-at-arms or noble guard: B. Guillemain, *La Cour pontificale d'Avignon, 1309-1376: Étude d'une Société* (Paris, 1962), 419-421.

32. Alessandro d'Antella, *advocatus* in the *curia*: ibid., 573 n. 69, 606-607.

33. Francesco Bruni, papal secretary: *ibid.*, 297-299, 568 n. 40, 571, 712.

34. Jacopo da Ceva, papal *advocatus* fiscal: *ibid.*, 607.

35. Fr Pierre Boysson, chaplain and *familiarius* of the Master, a procurator of the Hospital at the *curia* in 1370, and by 18 March 1379 Prior of the Convent at Rhodes: Delaville, 151, 164, 212, 214-215, 299; Luttrell (1978), XVI 453.

36. Ferry Cassinel, doctor in theology and professor of law, a kinsman of the new Master Fr Robert de Juilly, his procurator in the Priory of France, and in 1374 his procurator at the *curia*; Delaville, 197; Luttrell (1978), XVI 453.

37. Fr Aimery de la Ribe, Commander of Raissac, nominated Procurator-General in the West on or shortly before 2 February 1372: Delaville, 144 n. 2; *supra*, 3.

38. Ramon Bernat: unidentified.

39. Matteo Sobolini, notary: unidentified.

40. Pensions and 25 florins for *scripturas* amounted to 2,570 florins.

41. Tommaso de Bosolasco, OP: Luttrell (1982), XV 407 n. 68.

42. Bartolomeo Cherrazio, OFM: *ibid.*, XV 407 n. 68.

sol.' .j. dr.' .iiij. correntes. Item pago la dita companya a Maestro Thomas de Boço dela orden delos fraires predicadores por el viage de Costantinoble es assaber .iijͨ lxxx flor.' de sentencia conptando el flor.' a razon de xxvij sol.' .viij. dr.' por flor.', que fan .iiijͨ xxxviij flor.' sol.' .j. dr.' iiij correntes. Item pago la dita companya a fray Hesse d'Alamanya,[43] por la messageria de Costantinoble por paga de vj meses es assaber .iiijͨ lxj. flor.' ij. sol.', viij correntes. Item pago dotra parte la dita companya al dito fray Hesse por la paga de .v. meses por la dita missageria es assaber, vͨ xviij flor.', xviij sol.' correntes. Item pago la dita companya a fray Bertran Flota[44] por la paga de v. meses por la messageria de Costantinoble es assaber Vͨ xviij flor.' correntes xviij. sol.' Item pago dotra parte al dito fray Bertran Flota por paga de vj meses por la dita missageria es assaber .iiijͨ lxj flor.' correntes .ij. sol.' viij dr.' Item pago la dita companya a los de suso nombrados por nolit dela galea en que andaron es assaber Vͨ lxxvj flor.' correntes sol.' ix. drs.' iiij. Item pago la dita companya a Johan Corsin[45] por su prouision dela missatgeria que fizo en Jenoua et en Venecia por los afferes dela missageria de Costantinoble es assaber flor.' .vijͨ lxvij flor.' correntes. .xviij sol.' Item pago la dita companya a Michel de Rodulfo, et a Luys de Felipo Marin mercaderos de Jenoua, et a miss. Rafael Espindola[46] por cambio que fezieron alos missageros suso scripto, el qual cambio recebiron a Pera segunt que aparesce per vna scriptura seyellada con .iiij. seyellos delos ditos .iiij missatgeros et pagueren ne en flor.' correntes .M.Clij. flor.' correntes .xviij sol.' viij dr.'[47] Item posen en paga la dita companya los quales fezieron de messiones en los afferes dela religion es assaber por xviij processos apostolicals las quals fueron embiadas por los priorados dela religion et desto mostraren los jnstrumentes xxxviij flor.' Item por .j. correu, que embiaren en Anglaterra por afferes dela religion, vij flor.' .xij sol.' Item por correus que embiaron en Francia en Champanya, en Aluernia, en Aquitania por afferes dela religion xv flor.' Item por .j. correu que enbiaron en Portugal por los afferes dela religion xxx

43. Fr Hesso Schlegelholtz, Commander of Freibourg-im-Breisgau: Delaville, 185; Luttrell (1982), XV 407–408.

44. Fr Bertrand Flotte, Commander of Naples until December 1374 or a little later, who became Grand Commander of the Convent on 6 May 1375: Delaville, 150 n. 1; Luttrell (1982), XV 407–408.

45. Giovanni Corsini, brother of Cardinal Pietro Corsini, acted for the pope in crusading negotiations at this time: Luttrell (1982), XII 286; XV 400, 407, and A. Benvenuti Papi, 'Corsini, Giovanni,' *Dizionario Biografico degli Italiani*, xxix (Rome, 1983), 638–640.

46. Michele di Ridolfo, Luigi di Filippo Marino, Raffaele Spinola: Genoese.

47. The Constantinople mission expended 5,479 florins 12 sous plus 728 florins in the 1374/5 accounts, a total of 6,207 florins 12 sous; amend Luttrell (1982), XV 467 n. 68, which gives 6,677 florins. Pera was the Genoese suburb of Constantinople.

16

flor.' Item por .j. correu que embiaron en Pulha, et enel Regno[48] en Jenoua, et en Venecia, en Pisa, et en Florença .x. flor.' Item por .j. correu que embiaron en Alamanya et en Boemia xxx flor. Item por scripturas et processos en pargamin los quales se fueron delantes delos Cardenales .liiij. flor.' Item por bollas, et obliganças que fezieron en la Assembleya que se tuuo en Auinyo .Cxcv. flor.' xij sol.' Item por v. bollas las quales fueron por aferes dela religion .l. flor.' Item por vna bolla de franquesa dela Religion la qual bola preso M(aestr)o Ferri[49] C.xvj flor.' xvj sol.', Item por mession que fizo .j° dela companya como ando a Marselha por afferes del Maestro.[50] Item que fueron dados a Duran correu que ando al prior de Nauarra et de Castella por requerir los xxv. flor.' Item por .j. correu que aporto letras al valcho[51] .xx. sol.' Item por libros en que escriuron los comptos dela religion xvj flor.' Item por messiones que fizo Matheu de Vita como ando a Belcaire por aportar moneda al Maestro,[52] et por contar con el .vij. flor.' los quales messiones totas fazen en summa .vjᶜ j. flor.' correntes .xij sol.' Item posen en dat.'[53] los quales pagoron por cambio de los Mil ducados doro los quales fueron pagados alos (a)mbaxadores que fueron en Costantinoble a razon de vij flor.' por cento et son en Summa .lxx flor' correntes.[54] Reebudas fechas por parte del senyor Castellan d'Amposta prior de Cathalunya, lugartenient del senyor Maestro et Couent en todas las partidas daquamar delas monedas delos priorados daquamar[55] segunt que se sieguen .. Primerament Reebe del priorado d'Anglaterra por la responsion del dito priorado del anyo suso scripto nichil. Item por tallya nichil. Item por arrerages nichil. Item por mortuoris nichil. Item por Vagantes nichil. Item Recebio del priorado de Yrlanda por responsion del dito priorado del anyo suso scripto nichil. Item por tallya nichil. Item por arrerages nichil. Item por mortuoris nichil. Item por vagantes nichil. Summa de pagina nichil. Item recebio del priorado de Francia por responsion del dito priorado a razon de cinco francos por vj flor.' et fazen de

48. *enel Regno*: to the Kingdom of Naples.
49. Ferry Cassinel: *supra*, note 36.
50. Amount omitted.
51. *valcho?*
52. Matteo de Vita of the Alberti Antichi was received by the Master as a *confrater* of the Hospital at Beaucaire on 22 October 1374: Malta, Cod. 320, fo. 49v.
53. *en dat.'*: in credit.
54. Couriers, bulls and 70 florins in exchange expenses *apparently* amounted to 671 florins 12 sous, making an apparent total of expenses for 1374/5 of 35,263 florins 4 sous. A quittance issued by the Master on 11 October 1374 before he left Avignon showed he had received 35,500 florins for the year: Malta, Cod. 23, no. 4. The version registered in Cod. 320, fos. 44v–45, was full of errors with some figures being changed to match those in Cod. 23, no. 4, but with others being left unaltered so that the totals no longer added correctly. The 1374/5 accounts commence at this point.
55. Ms: *daquamas*.

florins correntes .vj.^{m} ij.^{c} l. florins correntes. Item recebio por la tallya del dito priorado de aquellos xij.^{m} xl[56] flor.' de sentencia que fazen de sentencia por tallya comptando a razon xxvij sol.' .viij drs.' por florin, et ha paga de correntes .M.ij.^{c} l. flor.' correntes. Item recebio por vagaciones del dito priorado comptando a razon de v. por vj .M.xl flor.' correntes gros.' viij. Item por vagacion dela baylia de Henaut .C.iiij flor.' correntes gros.' .ij. Item por vagacion dela baylia de Sant Baubure .C. xiiij flor.' correntes gros.' .vij. Item por vagacion dela baylia de Orliens xxxj flor.' correntes gros.' .iij. Item por la baylia que vago de Mont de Sisons xxvj flor.' sol.' .j.[57] Item por mortuoris fray G. de Huyllac[58] .M.xlj flor.' correntes viij gros.' Summa del priorado de Francia .jx.^{m} viij.^{c} lviiij flor.' iiij gros.' correntes, Item recebio del priorado de Champanya por la responsion del dito priorado del anyo suso scripto .M.xlj flor.' correntes gros.' viij. Item por la tallya del dito priorado .iij.^{c} xij flor.' et medio correntes. Item arrerages nichil. Item mortuoris nichil. Item vagantes nichil. Item recebio del Priorado de Aquitania por responsion del dito priorado del anyo suso scripto .m.ij.^{c} l. correntes. Item tallya nichil. Item arrerages nichil. Item mortuoris nichil. Item vagantes nichil. Item recebio del Priorado de Aluernia por responsion del dito priorado del anyo suso scripto .ij.^{m} flor.' correntes, Item por la tallya del dito priorado V.^{c} flor.' correntes. Item por arrerages nichil. Item por mortuoris nichil. Item por Vagantes nichil. . Item recebio del priorado de Sant Gili por responsion del dito priorado del anyo suso scripto .iiij.^{m} v.^{c} xlviij flor.' correntes. Item por la tallya viij.^{c} .lij. flor.' gros.' iij. Item por arrerages delos anyos lxxiij. lxxiiij. V.^{c} xxij. medio correntes. Items por arrerages delas tallyas delos anyos passados .C.xxiij. gros.' viij. Item por vagantes viij.^{c} xciij. flor.' Item por mortuoris vj.^{c} l. flor.' Summa del priorado de sant Gilj que ha pagado vij.^{m} v.^{c} lxxxviiij. flor.' gros.' v. correntes. Item Recebio del Priorado de Tholosa por responsion del dito priorado del anyo suso scripto .viij.^{c} xvij. flor.' correntes, gros' .ij. $\frac{1}{2}$. Item por la tallya del dito anyo .C.lxxviij. flor.' gros.' ij. Item por arrerages del anyo de lxxiiij .C.xxix flor.' gros' viij. Item pago mas por arrerages del anyo lxxiiij por las cambras del prior .ij.^{c} l. flor.' gros.' viij correntes. Summa que ha pagado el priorado de Tholosa segunt damunt, M. iij.^{c} lxxv flor.', gros' ij, drs.' xj correntes,[59] Item recebio del dito Priorado[60] por responsion

56. Ms: *aquellos xi^{m}xl*, perhaps for *Mii.^{c}xl*, but the arithmetic gives approximately 1,084 florins. After *aquellos* is a sign which is repeated in the margin, perhaps to indicate some doubt; the passage is evidently garbled.

57. Exceptionally, the accounts listed the vacancies of four French commanderies: Hainaut, Sainte Vaubourg, Orléans and Mont-de-Soissons.

58. Fr Guillaume de Huillac: unidentified.

59. The figure given amount to 1,296 florins 4 sous (not 1,375 florins 4 sous 11 *drs*'.).

60. ie. Priory of Catalunya.

del anyo suso scripto, ij^m viiij^c flor.' correntes, Item por la tallya del dito anyo, m.ij^c xxxiij flor.' xj sol.' drs.' iiij correntes, Item por el passage del senhor Maestre V^c xxxv. flor.' correntes .. Los delas Cambras de Cathalunya M(aestre)e Ferri lo ha preso del anyo lxxiiij.lxxv. Summa, que ha pagado Cathalunya .iiij^m vj^c lxviij flor.' xj sol.' drs.' iiij.[61] Item recebio dela Castellania d'Amposta por la responsion del anyo suso scripto viiij^c xvj flor.', gros.' iiij. correntes. Item ha pagado de tallya .V^c lxxvj flor.' gros.' iiij, drs.' xvj correntes. Item por el passage del senyor Maestre .ij^c l. flor.' correntes, Item por las cambras del senyor Maistre .V^c flor.' Summa que ha pagado lo Castellan d'Amposta entre todo .ij^m ij^c. xlij. flor.' correntes gros.' viij drs.' .xvj. Item recebio del priorado de Nauarra por responsion del dito priorado del anyo suso scripto .v^c flor.' correntes Item por la tallya .ij^c xxxv flor.' gros.' .j. drs.' xvj. Item por el passage del senyor Maestre .C.ij. flor.' correntes. Item por vagantes .xxx. flor.' correntes. Summa que ha pagado el priorado de Nauarra segunt que desuso viij^c lxvij flor.' correntes gros.' .j. drs.' xvj. Item fazo Reebuda los quales recebiron la companya delos Albertes del priorado de Roma por la responsion del dito priorado del anyo de lxxv^o viiij^c xxij. flor.' correntes sol' v. dr' .iiij. Item que Reebiron la dita companya por tallya del dito priorado de Roma .ij^c lxxxviij flor.' correntes sol' .iiij dr' viij. Item faze reebuda los quales reebiron los ditos Albertes del priorado de Venosa por la responsion del dito priorado del anyo de lxxv .iij^c xlij flor.' correntes, gros' iiij $\frac{1}{2}$. Item por la tallya del dito priorado .C. xiiij flor.' correntes gros.' j$\frac{1}{2}$. Item faze reebuda los quales recebiron la dita companya delos Albertes por la responsion del priorado de Pisa del anyo lxxv. Viiij^c xxij flor.' correntes, sol.' v. dr.' iiij. Item por la tallya del dito priorado .ij^c lxxxviij flor.' correntes gros.' ij. dr' .viij. .. Las quantitas suso scriptas son stadas assignadas porell Castellan d'Amposta al grant Comandador.[62] Primo por la responsion de Alamanya .M. flor.' Item por la tallya iij^c vj. flor.' Item por arrerages .C. flor'. Item por el passage del senyor Maestro .Cliij flor.' Item por la responsion del priorado de Boemia del anyo de lxxiiij. M.ij^c flor.' Item dela tallya .iiij^c viij flor.' Item la responsion del anyo de lxxv. M.ij^c flor.' Item dela tallya .iiij^c viij flor.' Item de arrerages .iiij^c flor.' Item del passage del senyor M(aestr)e .ij^c iiij. flor.' Item la responsion del priorado de Vngria los quales ha recebidos el prior de Venecia .iij^c flor.' Item la responsion del priorado de Venesia viij^c flor.' Item por la tallya .ij^c lv. flor.' Item del passage del senyor M(aestr)e .C.xxvij flor.' $\frac{1}{2}$. Item del priorado de Barleta por la

---

61. Ferry Casinell, the Master's procurator, took the incomes of the magistral *camere* which are not in the accounts.

62. The Grand Commander of the Convent was Fr Bertrand Flotte nominated on 6 May 1375: Delaville, 150 n. 1; *supra*, note 44.

responsion que non de ha pagado ren de todo el tiempo que ha tuuido lo priorado, et el grant comendador ha firmado porell .ij ꝫ flor.'[63] Item por la tallya del anyo de lxxiiij.lxxv. viijˢ xvj flor.' Item porel passage del senyor Maestro .ijˢ viij. flor.' Summa de pagina delas assignaciones fechas viiij ꝫ viiiˢ lxxxv flor' .½.[64] Sant Esteue de Monopolj la responsion del anyo de lxxiiij .iiijˢ flor.' Item por la tallya .C.liij. flor.' Item por la responsion del anyo de lxxv .iiijˢ flor.' Item por la tallya .C.liij flor.' Item porel passage del senyor M(aestr)e lxxvj flor.' ½. Venosa ha pagado responsion et tallya a los Albertes, et deue porel passage de mons. lo m(aestr)e .lj. flor.' Item deue dela responsion .iij. flor.' Item deue .iij. flor'[65] .. Santa Eufemia deue de .ij. anyos responsion et tallya, et faze por .ij. anyos la responsion .vjˢ flor.' Item por tallya .ijˢ iiij flor.'[66] Item porel passage del senyor M(aestre) .lj. flor.' Napol de Responsion vjˢ flor.' Item de tallya .iijˢ vj. flor. Item porel passage del senyor M(aestre) .Cliij flor.' Los Escambis d'Alif deue dela responsion del anyo de lxxiiij .vˢ flor.' Item por tallya .Cliiij. flor.' Item porel passage del senyor Maestro .lxxvj flor.' Item por la responsion del anyo de lxxv? Vˢ flor.' Item por la tallya .Cliij flor' .. Capua de responsion .vjˢ flor.' Item por tallya .ijˢ iiij. flor.' Item porel passage del senyor Maestre .C.ij. flor.' Roma ha pagado responsion, et tallya deue porel passage del senyor Maestre .C.xxvij flor.' ½. Pisa ha pagado responsion tallya alos Albertes, et deue solament porel passage del senyor M(aestre) .C.xxvij flor.' ½. Mescina no ha pagado res delos anyos de lxxiiij et lxxv, et por la tallia, et por lo passage del Maestre M.C lxxxij. flor.' ½. Lombardia no ha pagado res delos anyos de lxxv, lxxv mas esta hombre en sperança de auer ne alguna cosa. fray Richardo Caracho de Chichano tiene por mortuor' Vˢ flor.'[67] Item que son stados inprestados a larceuispo de Rodas lo quales deue pagar en Rodas .Vˢ flor.' Castiella non ha pagado res despues que esti prior[68]

63. The Prior of Barletta at least between 25 November 1373 and about 30 October 1375 was Fr Raymond de Sabran: *Lettres Secrètes et Curiales du pape Grégoire XI(1370–1378) relatives à la France*, ed. L. Mirot—H. Jassemin (5 fascs., Paris, 1935–57), nos. 3137, 3779. The Grand Commander apparently pledged to pay the 2,000 florins.

64. The *pagina* contained the 9,885½ florins (to be corrected to 9,732½ florins) for *Alamania*, Bohemia, Hungary, Venice and Barletta, which had been assigned to the Grand Commander, who was probably charged to collect them in Italy; the monies from *Alamania* and Bohemia were normally sent to Venice.

65. Venosa had paid its dues (*supra*) and can scarcely have owed two sets of only three florins; the copyist must have erred, and 300 florins may well have been the sum owed.

66. This perhaps meant that Santa Eufemia owed 600 plus 204 florins each year for two years.

67. Fr Riccardo Caracciolo, Commander of Cicciano in the Priory of Capua: Delaville, 249.

68. Fr Lop Sánchez de Somoza, destituted in 1375 for his refusal to pay: *ibid.*, 195–196.

tiene el priorado. Portugal deue de ix anyos que non ha pagado res
.. Aquestos son los pagamientos et assignaciones fechas porel senyor
Castellan delas monedas de suso scriptas del anyo de lxxv. Primerament ha pagado dela moneda de Francia ala cambra de nuestro
senyor el papa porel deudo que mons. el Maestre deuie ala cambra
del papa .V.ᵐ flor' de Cambra que ualen conptando v. francos por vj
flor', et ualen flor' correntes .V.ᵐ viijꟲ xxxiij flor.' Esti pagamento fue
fecho porque la cambra fizo arestar las monedas de Francia entroque
se pagoron delos ditos V.ᵐ flor' de Cambra. Item ha pagado ala
companya delos Albertes los quales fueron deuidos a ellos porel pre-
stamo que se fizo delos xxiiij.ᵐ v.ꟲ flor' que priso mons. el Maestro por
(ir) al Couent, et por otras expensas fachas porels ditos Albertes .iij.ᵐ
lxiiij flor.'⁶⁹ Item pago por mandamento de mons. lo M(aestre), et del
Couent segunt paresce por bulla de mons. el maestro, et del Couent,
la qual fue dada en Rodas los quales fueron pagados a algunos
mercaderos segunt aparesce por carta fecha por m(aestre) Antonj
not(ario),⁷⁰ florines de Cambra, iij.ᵐ que ualen a flor' correntes .iij.ᵐ
V.ꟲ flor.' Item por perdua de monedas .iij flor.' Item a pagado per
mandamiento de mons. lo m(aestre) et del Couent segunt paresce por
bulla de mons. el Maestro et Couent la qual fue dada en Rodas los
quales fueron pagados alos mercaderos segont paresce por carta
publica fecha por not(ario) flor' de Cambra .vj.ᵐ vijꟲ lxxxv. que fazen
flor' correntes vij.ᵐ ix.ꟲ xv flor' gros' .x. Item pago alos freres menores
et predicadores que fueron en Costantinoble por mandamiento de
nuestro senyor el papa, ultra la somma que les fue pagada en lanyo
de lxxiiij vijꟲ xxviij flor.' Item pago alos officiales de nuestre senyor el
papa xcv. flor.' Item pago a mons. Anchelet⁷¹ segunt paresce por la
bulla de mons. el M(aestre) .V.ꟲ flor.' Item pago por la pension de iiij
Cardenals m.ijꟲ flor.' Item pago alos officiales de nuestre senyor el
papa xcv. flor.' Item pago a iij aduocados, et a miss. Frances Bru,⁷² a
cascu .l. flor', fazen .ij.ꟲ flor.' Item pago a M(aestr)e Matheo procurador delas contradichas⁷³ xxv. flor.' Item pago al procurador
general de Cort de Roma, iijꟲ flor.'⁷⁴ Item pago por bollas processos
correus andantes por diuersas partidas por los negocios dela religion

---

69. These 24,500 florins appeared above as 26,541 florins 26 sous, and the 3,064
florins of charges listed here probably included interest on money loaned; the 'ir' is
supplied.

70. *Antonio notario:* unidentified.

71. *Mons. Anchelet*, possibly the papal scribe Ancelin Martin: Guillemain, 342, 366.

72. Francesco Bruni, papal secretary.

73. Matheo, *advocatus* in the *audientia litterarum contradictarum*.

74. One of the Hospital's procurators, *magister* Matteo de Lucha, was confirmed as
procurator in the *curia* on 10 October 1374: Malta, Cod. 320, fo. 45. The total for
pensions was 1,795 florins.

clvj flor.' gros' .j. Item pago a Loys Tallaborch[75] por la pension a el assignada por mons. lo maestre .xxx. flor.'[76] Item que ha pagado manualment al grant comendador segunt aparesce por carta f(act)a conptando v. francos, por vj flor' et fazen flor' correntes vj^m vj^c xxix flor.' Item pago al grant Comendador dotra parte por man de fray Aymeric dela Riba .m. v^c xcvij flor' gros' vj, drs' .iiij. Item pago al dito grant Comendador dotra part .ij^m v^c flor.' Summa que son las pagas fechas del anyo de lxxv a florines xxxiiij^m ij^c xxviij gros.'[77] Item las assignaciones fechas al grant comandador las quals son de suso scriptas .xvij^m vij^c lxv. flor' .. [78] Que quidem computa et rationes, ut premittitur sic uisa et recepta ipsa tenore presencium ratificamus aprobamus et omologamus et dictum fratrem Johannem Ferdinandj de Heredia nostrum locumtenentem, ac omnia bona sua et arnesia presentia et futura quitamus liberamus et absoluimus per presentes.

[a leaden bull attached with string is inscribed:]
BVLLA MAGISTRI ET CONVENTVS/
HOSPITALIS IHERVSALEM

75. Lodovicus Tailleburgui, inhabitant of Avignon, was granted a life pension of 30 florins a year by the Master on 22 October 1374: Malta, Cod. 320, fo. 50v. He was a *campsor* or moneychanger: Cod. 16, no. 53.

76. Couriers, bulls and Tailleburgui's pension amounted to 186 florins 2 sous.

77. These expenses included 4 florins lost, 11,415 florins in repayments of monies advanced at Rhodes, and 728 florins to the two friars who went on the Constantinople mission; the total of sums as given was 34,277 florins 22 sous (not 34,228 florins).

78. These 17,765 florins do not seem to be 'written above' (*suso scriptas*) since the three sums listed as having been advanced to the Grand Commander amounted to 10,726 florins, and this entry remains somewhat inexplicable; the 17,765 florins probably represented a hypothetical balance between incomes and expenses, since 34,278 plus 17,765 amounts to 52,043 florins while incomes would apparently have amounted to 53,441 florins if monies said to be owing were added to those paid.

XII

The Hospitaller Province of *Alamania* to 1428

This paper does not attempt to survey the earlier history of the Hospitallers in their vast German province, but rather to consider the limited theme of the relationships between the Order's central, provincial and local administrations. It is based on documents taken from a wide range of material scattered through many archives, though for the twelfth century the surviving documents are scarce and some must be rejected as forgeries; consequently, some of the earlier dates given are merely approximations. Many changes and developments in the Hospital's administrative arrangements were conditioned by political and other events but these cannot be considered here [1].

The bibliography of published work is enormous but extremely unequal [2]. Scholarly investigation into the German Hospital has been hindered by a concentration on German archives and on local affairs, which have not always properly been understood in terms of the Order's general and central institutions. There has also been a tendency to assume that technical terms used in the Teutonic Order had the same meaning for the Hospitallers. A further difficulty is that Joseph Delaville le Roulx in his great *Cartulaire*, though not in his latest works, consistently referred to priors and priories as „grand priors" and „grand priories", thus causing extensive confusions, especially in the published lists of priors. Given that the documents provide very little indication of the early administrative structure of the German Hospital, the titles of officials mentioned in the texts are extremely important, but many such documents were drawn up by papal or secular chancery officials or by others who had little need to understand the precise local arrangements of the Hospital in places as distant as Denmark or Moravia. The Hospitallers themselves were often equally imprecise. The difference between a *magister*, a *preceptor*, a *prior*, a *magnus preceptor* and so on was not always made clear, and often it can only be a matter of conjecture, with continual risk of error, through the inspection and interpretation of individual documents. The seals have seldom been published, though some Bohemian seals are excellently presented by Libor Jan [3].

It is important to establish definitions, however numerous the exceptions or alternatives. The Master of the Hospital, who did not call himself „grand", ruled the central headquarters or Convent in Syria and, after 1291, on Cyprus and Rhodes; his lieutenant in the East was the grand commander who was, confusingly, also called the grand preceptor. By the fourteenth century the Conventual brethren were divided into *langues,* that is tongues or nations, and each usually had its senior officer or *pillerius,* its *auberge* or residence and other separate arrangements. In the European provinces, which roughly corresponded to the Conventual *langues,* there were brethren or *fratres,* who in Central Europe were sometimes termed *cruciferi,* living in commanderies, which were also known as preceptories or *domus.* Normally each commandery had a commander responsible for paying the dues or *responsiones* for transmittal to the Convent; if there was a senior priest in the house who was not its commander he was the *prior* of that *domus.* It was not unusual for a priest to become a commander, but if at certain times a house contained no *milites* or knight-brethren, that did not make it a „priest commandery", a term not used in the early centuries. Commanderies were grouped in priories, which were not entitled „grand", ruled by priors, who were not „grand" either, or by lieutenants. Priories were in their turn grouped in provinces, though that was not always the term employed. Western provinces could from time to time be ruled by a centrally-appointed officer known as the grand preceptor of his province, who might however sometimes be known as grand commander. There was occasionally a grand preceptor with jurisdiction over all the provinces, who was in effect the master's lieutenant in the West. Confusingly, a grand preceptor might be styled merely as preceptor, with the result that those who mistakenly call priors „grand" cannot easily understand how a „grand prior" could be subject to a preceptor who is not called „grand". That problem is compounded when a grand preceptor who was also a prior called himself a prior and acted like a prior. Various forms of the term *bailivus* were employed to indicate almost any position in the Hospital as well as the particular office known in German as the *Ballei.* While the Priory of *Alamania* covered modern Germany and all or parts of Belgium, Holland, Poland and Scandinavia, and the Priory of Bohemia included Bohemia, much of Poland, Moravia, Austria and, at certain times, Hungary and *Esclavonia,* these two priories together formed a province which, confusingly again, was also known as *Alamania.* Furthermore, within the Priories of *Alamania* and Bohemia, there were also subordinate priories, such as those of *Dacia* and Poland, which were only occasionally independent.

*

*   *

The Hospital emerged as an independent order, at first with a purely charitable and hospitaller character, in the years following the capture of Jerusalem by the crusaders in 1099 [4]. German contingents took part in all the major twelfth-century crusades and many Germans went to Syria as pilgrims [5], so they and their neighbours certainly knew of the Hospital in Jerusalem and quite soon they were making donations to it [6]. It is possible that Germany was visited between 1119 and 1124 by an envoy sent by the second Master, Fr. Raymond du Puy, to seek charity in the West, since a papal letter of recommendation for this agent was copied into two twelfth-century Austrian manuscripts [7]. At some point before 1143 a separate German hospital was founded in Jerusalem; this two-storied hospice, which by about 1165 at the latest was flanked by its own church with a crypt, was situated at some distance from the Hospitallers' compound [8]. In 1143, following quarrels both within the Kingdom of Jerusalem and elsewhere in unspecified places *in aliis mundi partibus*, the pope instructed that the hospital of the *Teutonici* in Jerusalem and its endowments be subject to the Master of the Hospital who was, however, to appoint for it a prior and attendants who could speak to the sick German pilgrims in their own language. At the same time another papal letter commanded the *fratres Hospitalis Jerosolimitani per Alamaniam constituti*, who were presumably in Germany or nearby, to submit to the Hospital's jurisdiction [9]. The German hospice survived until the fall of Jerusalem in 1187 [10], but it is uncertain whether that hospice and its endowments and members, some of which could have been in Germany or elsewhere in the West, had passed completely or even partly under Hospitaller control. There is no other indication of any Hospitaller holdings in *Alamania* before about 1145, and only two Hospitallers from the area that was later to become the German province are recorded in Jerusalem before 1187: Fr. Martinus, *preceptor* of Bohemia, Hungary and other parts in 1186, had been sent from Jerusalem to Bohemia in about 1183, and the *nobilis vir P. miles de Boemia* was killed by the infidels in Jerusalem in or just before 1187 [11].

The Hospital's earliest foundations within the German province were apparently in Austria and Bohemia. Probably between 1145 and 1147 the Austrian noble Kadold de Harroz, on setting out for Jerusalem, gave the Hospital properties which later formed the nucleus of the Commandery of Mailberg north of Vienna [12]. Thereafter donations, privileges and confirmations from kings, bishops and nobles steadily accumulated: by 1156 at Duisburg just north of Cologne; in 1160 at Werben in Altmark in the east of Saxony; at Gran in Hungary by 1161; and by 1166 at Zagość in Poland; in 1169 at Prague; and at some time before 1187 at Poznań [13]. Many of these acquisitions were in the eastern borderlands whose rulers and bishops probably intended that the Hospital's priests, churches and settlements should reinforce the process of colonization and conversion. Neither the fall of Jerusalem and the loss of the original hospital there in 1187 nor the subsequent emergence of a separate Teutonic Order seriously interrupted the flow of donations throughout *Alamania*. These foundations were the result of many diverse local interests rather than of particular initiatives taken by the Order's central governing body, but once the Hospital had been given these properties it had an interest in exploiting them for the sustenance of its main purpose in the Kingdom of Jerusalem.

How the German brethren and possessions were at first organized within the confused overall European structure of the Hospital is not clear. In the East linguistic difficulties were evidently a serious drawback. Some German nobles may have spoken, or at least have understood, French which was the Hospital's official language, but as late as 1448 the senior German at Rhodes was unable to sit on a judicial committee because he spoke only German [14]. While Italian, Hispanic and even English brethren might to some extent communicate in some form of Romance speech, many Germans must have felt themselves excluded. In any case, there were apparently few German *fratres* in Syria. In Germany too there were problems. In 1253 the Master sent from Syria to the *preceptor*, presumably the grand preceptor, of *Alamania*, a Latin translation of the Hospital's rule with instructions that it was to be read aloud in the yearly chapter, while variant texts then in use in Germany were to be handed in to the prior [15]. There was at least one manuscript, datable perhaps to about 1288, which contained versions of the statutes, some in German, which were extremely garbled, and some in Latin; it also included a Latin version of the *Miracula*, the legendary stories concerning the Biblical origins of the Hospital [16]. Also circulating in Franconia, apparently in the first half of the thirteenth century, were various forged charters which rehearsed details of the *Miracula* while offering indulgences in return for financial contributions [17].

In *Alamania* the Hospital's houses and properties were organized in broadly the same manner as throughout the West, with much the same degree of continuing confusion over boundaries, jurisdictions and titles, matters inevitably complicated by political influences and divisions. As elsewhere, the basic local unit, centred on the *domus* in which most brethren resided, was the commandery; the commander was often entitled *magister* or *preceptor*. Thus the *domus* at Gran in Hungary had a *magister* in 1187, as did Gross Tinz in Silesia in 1203 [18]. Commanderies were grouped in priories ruled by a prior, and he too was sometimes called *magister* or *preceptor* or by some other phrase; occasionally more than one priory was ruled by the same officer, but such priories probably retained their individuality with separate finances and chapters. How commanders and priors were chosen is not clear but must often have depended on local circumstances [19]. In some areas, such as Bohemia and Hungary, royal favour was influential, and even when the Master and Convent exercized their theoretical powers of appointment, problems of time and distance could make it difficult for them to impose their choice in Western priories.

The extensive Province of *Alamania* was eventually divided into two major zones: the Priory of *Alamania* with the subordinate Priory of *Dacia* and the Priory of Bohemia which included Moravia, Poland, Austria and other groupings. From the late-twelfth century onwards a system of Hospitaller priories emerged in *Alamania*, as elsewhere in the West, apparently without any particular imposition from the East. In 1182 the pope addressed a confirmation of possessions in Prague and Manetin to *fratri Bernardo preceptori et aliis fratribus Hospitalis Jerosolimitani in Boemia, Polonia et Pomerania constitutis*, and in 1186 a Fr. Martinus was *preceptor* in Hungary, Bohemia and all adjacent lands to their south, east and north. Fr. Bernardus was probably an early Prior of Bohemia and Fr. Martinus a grand preceptor who may have had jurisdiction in Germany as well as in Hungary and Bohemia. Germany was evidently a separate area where in 1187 *Arleboldus, prior Alemannie et omnis conventus tam clericorum quam laicorum* held an annual chapter [20]. Between 1184 and 1247 papal, Hospitaller and princely documents gave Hospitaller officers a plethora of administrative titles. The Prior of *Alamania* or Germany was also termed *magister, summus magister, magister et provisor, summus procurator, procurator generalis, preceptor* and even *universalis magister*. In Hungary there was a *prior* in 1208 and a *procurator* in 1216. Austria had a *prior* in 1207; Poland a *magister* by 1201; Silesia a *magister* in 1205; Moravia an officer who had jurisdiction over a number of houses there in 1234, a *prior* in 1238 and a *magister* in 1254; Lorraine a *magister* in 1222; *Dacia* a prior in 1231; and other geographical circumscriptions and other combinations of titles were also employed [21].

A clearly autonomous priory within the province was that of Bohemia, where royal interest and power evidently acted as a unifying force. A Fr. Bernardus was *prior Boemie* in 1181 [22]. In 1182 he was *preceptor* in Bohemia, Poland and Pomerania, and he was Prior of Bohemia in 1188 and in 1194, in which year a Fr. Meinardus was *preceptor*, possibly grand preceptor. There was an unnamed Prior of Bohemia and Moravia in 1205; between about 1217 and 1240 a Fr. Hugo, who also governed in Poland and Moravia, was ruling in Bohemia, though not always with the title of *prior*; a Fr. Johannes was Prior of Bohemia in 1255 [23]. These developments concerned Bohemia in particular, since in 1205 there was a *magister* in Silesia and in 1207 a *magister* in Austria. In 1263 there was a separate Prior of Austria and Styria, and in 1244 and 1274 a separate Prior of Austria [24]. The Priory of Hungary, which also enjoyed extensive royal support, became independent in the time of Andreas II. In 1186 Hungary was being ruled jointly with Bohemia, apparently by a grand preceptor, but by 1208 it had its own prior. It had a *procurator* in 1216 and a *prior* in 1217, 1218 and 1226 [25]. From about 1232 to about 1254 the prior was the royal protegé Fr. Raimbaud de Voczon, whose origins are obscure. By the mid-thirteenth century the Hungarian priory was clearly an independent unit [26].

The Polish commanderies had a *magister* of Poland in 1201, a *preceptor domus sancti Johannis in Polonia* in 1230, and a *prior* in 1246; a Fr. Gelolfus was prior in 1252, when he attended a chapter of the whole Province of *Alamania* at Cologne, and in 1255 [27]. The boundaries of Hospitaller *Polonia* seem to have varied considerably. Pomerania, to the north of Poland, was grouped with Poland and Bohemia in 1182 and still in 1238 when the pope confirmed to the Prior and brethren of Moravia the donations of Schlawe, Jestin, Moizelin, Leibschau and Stargard in Pomerania [28]. There were a limited number of foundations and confirmations in Poland outside Silesia during the thirteenth century [29], but little evidence of Hospitaller life there survived. As a consequence of political changes various foundations in Silesia originally made by Polish dynasties passed more directly under the control of the Prior of Bohemia. Some Hospitallers possibly fought the Mongols at Legnica in Silesia in 1241 when they may, like the Templars, have suffered losses of men and destruction of properties [30]. In 1261 a joint Prior of Poland and Moravia, Fr. Mauritius, was at Gross Tinz in Silesia and concerned with Silesian and Moravian affairs, but Poland proper was becoming separate from the Hospital in Silesia, though the latter continued to be termed *Polonia*. In 1268 a Fr. Mauritius was lieutenant in the Commandery of Poznań, and in 1277 and 1283 a Fr. Mauritius was Commander of Mirow in Mecklenburg and of Werben in Saxony [31]. From about 1284 to about 1296 Poland was ruled jointly with Bohemia and Moravia by a prior in Bohemia, Fr. Hermann de Hohenlohe, who was German, but in 1309 Fr. Berthold de Henneberg was acting as lieutenant in Poland of the Prior of Germany when he confirmed an act of the Commander of Poznań [32].

Whereas in East Central Europe the Priories of Bohemia and Hungary developed in an independent way with their subordinate Priories of Poland, Moravia, Silesia, Austria and *Esclavonia* which included lands in Slovenia, Croatia and Dalmatia, there remained a separate and rather large area which became the Priory of Germany. This administrative unit apparently existed by 1187 when Fr. Arleboldus, *prior Alemannie*, was holding annual chapters [33]. His apparent successors were addressed by a variety of titles: Fr. Albert, *summus procurator*, from 1222 to 1225; Fr. Heinrich de Heimbach, *magister*, in 1207; Fr. Heinrich, *magister summus*, in 1215; Fr. Heinrich and Fr. Eginhard, jointly *magistri et provisores domorum* in Germany, in 1216; and Fr. Heinrich de Guntramshofen, *generalis procurator*, in 1218. Thenceforth similar titles for the German prior reappeared, with a *universalis magister* in 1228 [34].

In Scandinavia, but generally under the jurisdiction of the Prior of *Alamania*, were various isolated foundations, royal and otherwise, with houses at Vibourg and Antvorskov in Denmark by as early as about 1170. There was a church at Eskilstuna in Sweden probably before 1185 and lands at Verne in Norway by 1198 [35]. By 1231 there was a Hospitaller prior for all *Dacia*. The *prior* of Antvorskov was a Fr. Henricus de Housheit in 1266; in 1288 this *prior* was holding a chapter at Antvorskov; and in 1290 there was a *prior* named Fr. Ebbo at Eskilstuna. At a chapter-general held on Cyprus in 1294 *Dacia* was, like Poland, considered a separate priory [36], but apparently these *priores* were sometimes rulers of individual houses rather than of priories. They were in any case too distant for any close control by officers in Germany and in practice they were largely independent of them. In 1433 the Hospitallers' Scandinavian possessions were listed and valued as part of a projected exchange with lands of the Teutonic Order in Southern Italy and Sicily, a scheme resulting from the difficulties which both orders encountered in securing their revenues at long range [37].

*

* *

With the steady growth of the Hospital's military and administrative responsibilities in Syria and elsewhere in the East, the Order's establishment in the West and the development of priories there became more extensive and also more widely dispersed. The Convent in the East was naturally concerned to secure control over the Western provinces and there evolved a new official appointed theoretically by the Master and Convent, unlike the priors who were supposedly named in chapter-general but whose origins were normally more or less local. These new officers, often known as grand preceptors, usually enjoyed a jurisdiction corresponding to a Western province or to a group of Western priories. There was occasionally a Grand Preceptor of *Outremer*, that is of the whole West, while others for Spain, Italy and France began to appear between about 1170 and 1190. The complicated manner of their development was reflected by contemporaries and scribes who provided them with a bewildering variety of titles; frequently they failed to distinguish grand preceptors from priors, especially when the same person was both a prior of one or more priories and at the same time a grand preceptor controlling a group of priories. Thus in 1289 Fr. Berenger de Laufen issued a document as *magnus preceptor ... per Alemaniam* but sealed it with the *sigillum nostri prioratus* [38]. Grand preceptors were named only from time to time by the Master and chapter-general; sometimes they were appointed to carry out a specific task, and in 1296 it was emphasized that the office had an occasional character. As direct representatives of the Hospital's central government, grand preceptors, who had their own seal, could convoke a chapter of several priories or attend chapters of an individual priory. They received instructions from the Master and transmitted them to priors or directly to other brethren. In 1292 the Grand Preceptor in the West, whose office was superior to that of a provincial grand preceptor, was empowered to licence the creation of *milites* and *donati*. He could confirm appointments of commanders and, apparently, make temporary appointments when death caused vacancies. He and the grand preceptors of individual provinces exercized much of the power of the Master and Convent while also conducting some of the business of an ordinary prior [39].

Fr. Martinus, who as early as 1186 was *preceptor* of Hungary, Bohemia and all lands to their south, east and north, was probably Grand Preceptor of Bohemia and Hungary, but was clearly not in charge of *Alamania* to their west [40]. The first clear example of a grand preceptor for the Province of *Alamania* came much later between 1249 and 1252 with Fr. Clemens, *magnus preceptor* in Germany, Bohemia, Moravia and Poland, but not at that point in Austria or Hungary. In 1251 and 1252 Fr. Clemens held chapters of the whole province at Cologne; that of 1251 was termed a *capitulum generalis,* while that of 1252 was evidently not limited to Germany since it was attended by the Prior of Poland. In 1255 Fr. Heinrich de Fürstenberg, who was then Grand Preceptor in Germany, Bohemia, Poland and Moravia, was in Silesia and with him were the Priors of Poland and Bohemia [41]. Both Fr. Clemens and Fr. Heinrich de Fürstenberg may well also have been Priors of Germany, and indeed some of their acts concerned matters within that priory [42]. By 1250 at the latest the Hungarian Hospital had its own grand preceptor [43]. However, in 1258 Austria, and in 1266 *Dacia* and Hungary, were within the jurisdiction of the Grand Preceptor of *Alamania* [44]. The whole of *Alamania* had become a single province, and the appointment of a grand preceptor was presumably designed, at a comparatively late stage with respect to other provinces, to impose a measure of central control on a disparate, distant and politically disjointed region.

Fr. Heinrich de Fürstenberg was a German noble with an unusual career. From 1255 onwards he was, with interruptions, Grand Preceptor of Germany. In 1270 and 1272, but not in 1271, he was simply Prior of Germany, and in 1259 and 1262 he was in Syria as *magnus preceptor Hospitalis in Accon* or Grand Commander in the East [45]. His successors as grand preceptor were all Germans: Fr. Heinrich de Boxburg, Fr. Hermann de Brunshorn, Fr. Berenger de Laufen, Fr. Friedrich de Kindhausen, Fr. Gottfried de Klingenfels, Fr. Heinwich de Kindhausen, and Fr. Helfrich de Rüdigheim, this last from 1305 to 1310. Though there is no indication of how or why they were appointed, they seem to have held office in a more permanent way than grand preceptors in other provinces. Their jurisdictions varied, Austria and Styria sometimes being explicitly included [46].

The statutes passed in Cyprus in 1294 contained a list of Hospitaller grand preceptors and priors which included a Grand Preceptor of Germany, and Priors of Germany, Poland, Bohemia and Denmark but not of Hungary or *Esclavonia* [47]. Royal influence over the Hospital was strong in Hungary [48] and in 1247 King Bela IV made a grant to Fr. Raimbaud de Voczon, whom he described as Grand Preceptor *in partibus cismontanis* [49]. By it the Hospital was to populate much of the frontier regions of Severin, the western part of Wallachia north of the Danube, and of *Cumania,* and to defend them with up to 100 military *fratres* both against Mongols and Cumans and also against schismatic Bulgarians and others. This agreement to fight against fellow Christians was somewhat exceptional in early Hospitaller history, and equally exceptional was the papal grant made in 1248 to the Hungarian Hospitallers and to those fighting with them against the Mongols the same crusading indulgences as those conceded for Syria by the general council then in session at Lyons [50]. Had they been realistic, these arrangements, which envisaged an enormous force of brethren, might have led to developments similar to the very extensive operations of other military orders in Spain and Prussia, to the attempts to settle the Teutonic Order in Siebenbürgen north of Wallachia, or to the establishment of the Hospital itself in Cilician Armenia or, after 1204, in Latin Greece; but the agreement was never put into action [51].

Fr. Raimbaud de Voczon, who was Prior or at times Grand Preceptor of Hungary from 1237 onwards [52], was Grand Preceptor in Italy, Hungary and *Esclavonia* in 1250 and 1253, and in 1253 and 1254 in Austria as well [53]. Exceptionally, in 1266 and 1279 for example, Hungary was listed within the jurisdiction of the Grand Preceptor of Germany [54]. In 1259 Fr. Raimbaud de Voczon's successor Fr. Arnoldus was also described as *major preceptor* of Hungary and *Esclavonia* [55]. The Priory of Hungary and *Esclavonia* held its own chapter, in 1275 for example [56], and its independence was emphasized in 1280 when Fr. Hermann de Brunshorn entitled himself *magnus preceptor* in Germany, Bohemia, *Dacia*, Austria, Poland and Moravia, and also, but separately, as *gerens vices summi magistri per Ungariam* [57]. In 1267 the exiled Latin Emperor, Baudouin II, invited Fr. Pons de Fay, Prior of Hungary and *Esclavonia,* who was possibly a Frenchman from the Auvergne, to take troops to recapture Constantinople, offering to restore to the Hospital the lands it had once held in the Eastern empire [58]. The turning point came with the recognition in 1308 of a French Angevin as king of Hungary. The Angevins ruled in Naples and Provence and thereafter Hungary normally formed part of the Hospitaller Province of Italy or, sometimes, of Provence [59].

The Grand Preceptor of Germany received extraordinary offical recognition at the chapter-general of 1301 which passed special statutes, in French, for the Province of *Alamania*; these were confirmed in 1304. Hospitaller statutes designed to apply exclusively in a single province were otherwise unknown. These statutes of 1301 envisaged the Grand Preceptor of Germany as virtually the direct ruler of its priories. He might, with the counsel of his provincial chapter, replace a commander who was in debt or who could not pay his *responsiones* because his commandery was indebted; the new commander would have to promise to restore the commandery, and if he failed to do so the grand preceptor could take it over himself while the new commander would lose the commandery and be punished. There was considerable emphasis on debts. Commanders were not to construct new buildings or borrow money without the grand preceptor's licence. He would be able to employ for his own purposes pensions which had reverted to the Order and he might, with the counsel of his convent, sell pensions for up to 1000 marks, though these were to revert to the Hospital on their purchaser's death. He was empowered to employ as many Hospitaller priests and sergeants-of-labour as necessary, but he was not to create *milites*, sergeants or priests without the licence of the Master of the Hospital. The same chapter, in passing a general statute that no prior should hold two priories from the chapter-general, specifically excepted *Alamania* from that provision, evidently to cover the multiplicity of titles in the province [60]. The provision limiting the creation of new brethren and the existence of a provincial chapter implied a permanent organizational unit with regular functions more like that of a prior than that of a grand preceptor, whose appointment was normally a temporary one made in the Convent. Probably there were difficulties as well as debts in the province, so that the quite exceptional legislation of 1301 was intended to enable the Province of *Alamania* to be administered and reformed as a single unit [61]. The Convent may have been impelled to create a special kind of quasi-permanent Grand Preceptor of *Alamania* precisely because it was scarcely able to control that province's priors or their appointment.

The obvious general reasons for such special developments in *Alamania* were the province's remoteness from the Syrian Convent, the problems of language and the resulting scarcity of German representation in the Hospital's central government. Many parts of Germany were geographically no further from the East than were France or England, yet the sheer size of the province and the diversity of political regimes within it created real difficulties. In Bohemia the result was a tendency for Poland, Moravia and Austria to be governed as partially separate units; on occasions there were lieutenants in Austria and Styria, as also in Poland. The size of the German priory brought yet another confusing development, that of lieutenants for High or Southern Germany and for Low or Northern Germany; sometimes both posts were held by the same person. High Germany comprised parts of modern Switzerland, Baden, Alsace, Breisgau, Bavaria, Wurtemburg, Franconia and Thuringia, while Low Germany included the Lower Rhine, the Netherlands, Nassau, Hesse and apparently Brunswick and Hanover. From 1251 there was often a lieutenant in Low Germany of the Prior of Germany, and from 1253 a similar lieutenant in High Germany. In 1257 and from 1289 to 1310 there was actually a full Prior of High Germany whose priory had its own seal, and from 1296 to 1310 there was similarly a full Prior of Low Germany; in 1317 there was also a prior for Central *Alamania*. In 1302 there was a lieutenant of the Grand Preceptor of *Alamania* in High Germany. Sometimes the grand preceptor or the prior had a lieutenant for the whole Priory of *Alamania*. In 1259 and 1263 there was a lieutenant of the Master in High Germany. These developments were not necessarily caused merely by the priory's size, for Masters and grand preceptors were able, by naming lieutenants, to keep priories vacant and thus receive their incomes, as indeed occurred in other provinces as well [62].

Those who were merely lieutenants did not enjoy fully the incomes, patronage or permanency of tenure of a full prior, and they therefore retained their own commandery [63]. Many of these varying offices were held, usually at different times, by the same person. At times High Germany and Low Germany each functioned as the equivalent of a separate priory, sometimes governed by a lieutenant of the Prior of Germany, or of the grand preceptor, or of the Master; their officers acted much as any other prior, holding chapters of commanders, using a seal of office and authorizing sales, leases, purchases, pensions, exchanges and other arrangements; probably they also collected *responsiones* [64]. Occasionally Bohemia, Poland and Moravia were also held as separate priories. What was unusual, in comparison with general Hospitaller practice, was that all these priors within the German province were, at least in some ways, subject to what was in effect a superior prior, that is to the Grand Preceptor of *Alamania*, whose office differed, however, from that of grand preceptors in other provinces, especially in so far as it had become permanent or almost permanent.

In Germany there also emerged a figure, not normally found elsewhere, who controlled a group of commanderies but who was not a prior or his equivalent. Such officers can scarcely be distinguished from some earlier local *magistri*, such as the *magister* in Lorraine of 1222 or the *magister* for Alsace and Breisgau of 1252. The latter was Fr. Heinrich de Toggenburg who was later, in 1263, both Commander of Bubikon near Zurich and lieutenant of the Master in High Germany [65]. Probably he was in effect acting as a prior while the Master in Syria was keeping the priory vacant and possibly enjoying its incomes; in that case, the lieutenant retained the commandery and its incomes. Such officers were often involved in local business to which they gave assent, sometimes sealing documents. Local *magistri* who were not acting for the Master may have been chosen by their prior or grand preceptor; they seem not to have held chapters or collected *responsiones*. In 1271, for example, the Commander of Werben was *vicepreceptor* for Saxony and *Slavia* [66]; in 1280 the Commander of Mainz was also *commendator* for the Hospital's houses in Franconia and Wetterau [67], and in 1281 as *commendator Franconie* he assented to and sealed an act of the Commander of Wölchingen [68]. In 1296 the Commander of Boxberg and Hall was *vice magistri* in Franconia and Swabia [69]. In 1297 Fr. Hermann de Mainz was Commander of Trier and *magister tocius balive per partes inferiores Alemanie*; this *baliva* was apparently the Priory of Low Germany, and Fr. Hermann, who retained his commandery, was probably its lieutenant rather than its prior [70].

The Hospital's retreat to Cyprus in 1291 and the conquest of Rhodes between 1306 and 1310 had little immediate effect on its German province; nor did the transfer to Prussia in 1309 of the Teutonic Order's convent or the suppression in 1312 of the Templars who were never strongly established in German lands. After about 1310 Hospitaller grand preceptors were appointed only rarely in the West, but some German control over Bohemia was maintained through the device, used in about 1323, of naming Fr. Albrecht de Schwarzburg, Prior of *Alamania*, as visitor in both Bohemia and *Dacia*[71]. The flow of donations and legacies to the Order continued in Germany[72], as did the entry into the Hospital of a small group of *milites* from the higher nobility who tended to secure the priory's senior positions. In Bohemia the priors had mostly been German but in 1325 the prior, Fr. Berthold de Henneberg, was effectively replaced, technically as his lieutenant, by a native usurper, Fr. Michael de Tinz; thereafter Bohemian nobles, whether Czech- or German-speaking, normally secured the priory[73]. Priors were usually appointed by the Master and Convent at Rhodes. In 1372 they named as Prior of Bohemia a German, Fr. Hesso Schlegelholtz, who was presumably the senior member of the German *langue* on Rhodes; the Bohemian brethren and their king protested to pope and Master that he was a foreigner; and, after various threats and disputes, he was replaced by the Silesian Fr. Zemovits, Duke of Teschen[74]. Two German developments which were unusual in the Hospital were the making of entry payments, known as *elimosina* or in German *Almosen*, and the extensive practice of investing capital in life-rents or *Leibgedinge* in order to produce a pension for an individual Hospitaller. This tended to fill commanderies with numerous *milites* who lived in them on comfortable benefices, usually without going to serve at Rhodes or sending much money there. In the fourteenth century there may have been as many as 700 brethren in the German priory, many of them *milites*, a very considerable number compared with other provinces. The general consequence of these developments was extensive debt and laxity in the German priory[75]. In 1373 there were about one hundred commanderies in the whole German priory including *Dacia*[76], and about 37 in that of Bohemia; in that year twelve commanderies in the Diocese of Prague contained as many as 112 Hospitaller brethren[77].

One particular development, also scarcely paralleled in the Hospital outside Germany[78], was the appearance of local officials who functioned as an intermediate authority between the prior and the commanders but who gradually came to represent not the Hospital's central authority but rather the brethren of their own region. The intermediate authorities of the thirteenth century, the various *magistri* and lieutenants, had derived their position not from their subordinate brethren but from their superiors. In *Alamania* lieutenants were appointed for increasingly small areas, for example in Franconia, in Wetterau and elsewhere, with titles such as *locum tenens, vice prior, preceptor domorum, preceptor generalis* or *commendator*. The newer intermediate administrative circumscription was the *Ballei*, of which there were eventually some eight or more in *Alamania*, with its officer the *Balleier*. In 1319 the commanders of twenty small commanderies in Ostfreisland reached an apparently unique arrangement with their local superior, the Commander or *magister* of Steinfurt, which was in fact outside their own area: they agreed to pay him 44 marks as their annual *responsiones*, while he would visit their houses but would no longer choose their *commendator domorum*, evidently their regional officer and in effect their *Balleier*, who was instead to be elected by the twenty commanders and merely to be confirmed by the *magister* of Steinfurt. The Steinfurt *magister* could intervene to settle election disputes and he was to receive one *solidus* from each commander when making visitations, but the *magister* was no longer to receive either entrance monies, that is the *elimosina* paid to the commanders, or the horses left by deceased commanders. The arrangement was apparently made without any reference to the Master or to the Prior of Germany [79]. The Ostfriesland *Ballei* constituted a special case in that, while it elected its own *commendator domorum*, it continued to depend on a commander whose commandery was outside its own region. In 1412 Fr. Johannes Cruze held a chapter at Groningen as *balivus domorum* for Westfalia, as Commander of Steinfurt and as *magister domorum per Frisiam*; Ostfreisland apparently retained its special status [80].

There were many brethren who scarcely left their local region or *Ballei*, moving from house to house and holding commanderies within what became a restricted circle. Senior local commanders took it in turns to act as *Balleier* in which capacity they held chapters and confirmed the acts of individual commanders but, except in Brandenburg, they seem not to have received an income from the *Ballei* or to have collected or paid *responsiones* for it; they retained their commandery and had no seal as *Balleier*. How they were chosen is not clear. In 1341, at the prior's command, Fr. Albert de Ulenbrok visited the seven commanderies of the *Ballei* of Westfalia, reporting on their debts and obligations and on their personnel which amounted to 144 brethren [81]. In 1362 the representatives of the *Ballei* of Franconia met at Würzburg and, with the prior's approval, they issued extraordinary and detailed reforming statutes dealing with numerous abuses such as debts, pensions, extravagances, personal possessions, lax behaviour and so on [82]. These reforms would, if put into effect, have been most commendable, but what was really happening was that the German Hospitallers were making local arrangements and solving regional problems with little or no reference to their prior or to the central authority of their Order.

In one region this tendency towards local independence had especially significant consequences. By 1319 the area of Brandenburg, which consisted of Saxony, of *Slavia* that is *Sclavonia* or Mecklenburg, of the Mark of Brandenburg and of Thuringia, was already being governed independently under a separate prior or vice-prior, or *preceptor generalis* as he was most usually termed [83], and was paying, apparently to the Convent's receiver in the West, separate *responsiones* amounting to 1462 1/2 marks for twenty houses, according to the local accounts for that region presented to the Hospital's central authorities [84]. Following the suppression of the Templars in 1312 the Hospital faced grave difficulties in this area which was, quite exceptionally, entrusted not to a local man but to the Italian Fr. Paolo de Modena. This caused such resentment that on 12 January 1323 five leading German brethren wrote to the Master suggesting that he be replaced in the *preceptoria* of Thuringia, Saxony and the Mark by the Prior of Germany, Fr. Albrecht de Schwarzburg [85]. In 1330 this region's dues to the Convent were being calculated separately by the chapter-general held at Montpellier [86]; and in 1335, for example, the *preceptor generalis*, Fr. Gebhard de Bortfeld, held a *provincialis capitulum* at Nemerow [87]. However, all that was a matter of regional independence vis-à-vis the priory and not of proto-Protestant feeling.

Following the papal schism of 1378, the Hospital was in an especially difficult divided position in Germany and in 1382, after many disputes, the prior agreed that the *Ballei* of Brandenburg was to elect its own *Balleier*, as in practice it had been doing for some time. The *Balleier* would still owe obedience to the prior, who was to confirm his election and who could still visit the *Ballei*; the *Balleier* was to attend the prioral chapter every year bringing as the *responsiones* of the *Ballei* as much as 324 florins, almost a third of what the whole priory owed to Rhodes; the *Ballei* would not have to pay any special extra taxes imposed on the priory. Among those agreeing to this arrangement were the *Balleier* of Westfalia, High Germany, Wetterau, Cologne and Thuringia; the arrangement was confirmed by the Hospital's chapter-general at Valence in March 1383 [88]. The agreement merely perpetuated the existing situation in which the Brandenburg Hospitallers enjoyed a considerable degree of independence from the prior; it certainly did not make the *Ballei* independent of the Order. Brandenburg continued to provide *responsiones* to Rhodes; in 1490, for example, it had paid 3824 florins for the two previous years [89].

The situation in distant *Dacia* remained ambiguous. Before the fifteenth century almost all its rulers were German brethren. It held prioral chapters which the Norwegian *fratres* attended, but it began to lose its status as a dependent priory and to become a *Ballei*. In 1415 and 1417 there were references to a *prior generalis*, yet in 1417 the Master licensed the *bailliuus Dacie prioratus Alamanie* to create six knight brethren and in 1420 the *bailliuus*, together with the *Balleier* of Westfalia and Brandenburg, was instructed by the Master and Convent to attend the chapter of the German priory with all his commanders. Brandenburg and *Dacia* clearly enjoyed a special status; some thirty years later, in 1454, they both claimed that *certa privilegia* had exempted them from paying any dues except those which they owed directly to Rhodes [90].

Bohemia was a priory which predominantly supported the Roman popes during the papal schism after 1378. At a prioral chapter in 1392 the prior deputed to a subordinate the judgement of a dispute between several Austrian commanders on the grounds that he himself did not understand German: *in lingua theutunica non bene exscitit*. There was a reference at that chapter to the seizure of the privileges of the *Baiulia* of Austria and, while there were no *Balleien* in

Bohemia,the priory was divided into separate groups from Austria, Bohemia, Moravia and *Polonia*, that is Silesia; each of the four had its *locum tenens*. The text arranged the names of the commanders present in groups according to the four areas to which they belonged [91].

After 1310 at least a few brethren from the province reached Rhodes. There were quite numerous interventions by the Master and Convent on matters such as provisions to priories and commanderies, confirmations of appointments made by priors in the West, receptions of new brethren, summonses to the Convent, the collection of monies and so on. For example in 1410 the chapter-general meeting at Aix-en-Provence confirmed the *Balleier* of Westfalia, who had been appointed by an earlier Prior of Germany, in his position for his lifetime; in 1419 this was confirmed by the Master [92]. Financial contributions from *Alamania* were not negligible. For the year 1364/65 the Convent received 1200 florins from Bohemia [93], and for the two years 1373/74 and 1374/75 the whole province provided 6735 florins, constituting 7.6 percent of the total *responsiones* and other dues paid to the Convent from the West which amounted in all to 89,060 florins for those two years; of these Germany paid 2915 florins and Bohemia 3820 florins [94].

Two Germans, Fr. Albrecht de Schwarzburg between 1306 and about 1320 and Fr. Hesso Schlegelholtz who was lieutenant on Rhodes in 1411 and 1412, were extremely influential in the Convent [95]. Otherwise there were so few Germans in the East during the fourteenth century that the *langue* almost disappeared [96], and in 1410 it was confirmed that the commanders of the German priory could elect their own prior as there were too few suitable Germans at Rhodes [97]. In 1422, however, it was established that the Germans should be given full recognition as one of the seven *langues* with rights and duties – *in omnibus honoribus et oneribus* – in the Convent at Rhodes and in the Hospital's castle at Bodrum on the Anatolian mainland, and in the same year the proctors of the German *langue* on Rhodes demanded that the Germans there should be allowed to choose one of their number for the next priory to fall vacant in that province. In 1428 the German *langue* also acquired its own senior official, the *magnus balivus,* and it decided to repair its *auberge* at Rhodes [98]. In 1428 the Germans had demanded an *officium baiuliatus cum stipendio debito in conuentu,* and in 1433 they sought control of the office of Treasurer. The full acceptance of the German seventh *langue* placed the three French-speaking *langues* in a minority in the Convent, and the Germans played a role in the great quarrel of 1446 when the four non-French *langues* made a major challenge to the French predominance [99].

For reasons largely of size and distance, with language and politics also playing a role, the Hospital's German province was of rather marginal value to its central government in Syria and Rhodes. The normal system of priories did not function well in Germany. The central Convent could have divided *Alamania* into more than one province, but that would have given the Germans and others a body of officers and an influence in the Convent which would have been unacceptably large in proportion to their contribution there. Rhodes could name receivers whose task was to collect monies due [100]. It could also send visitors as, for example, when the Prior of Toulouse went to Germany in 1329 [101], but such methods seldom had much effect in a somewhat remote province. The German priory became divided into what were really sub-priories, and these came to acquire a character of their own with the appearance of the *Balleien*, which were partially independent of their own priory. Unlike the Teutonic Order which depended upon men but not upon financial support from Germany, what the Hospital needed at Rhodes, a well-fortified island which could be defended with a comparatively small force, was money rather than manpower. The Convent's contacts with the German province, though threatened after 1420 by the Hussite revolt in Bohemia, never entirely broke down. After 1428 the German *langue* on Rhodes remained active and the German province continued to send to the Convent financial assistance which was limited but by no means negligible. From the Convent's viewpoint, it was in the long term important above all that connections with the brethren of *Alamania* be maintained across the centuries without losing support from the German province.

Notes

[1] For the period before 1310 the majority of documents used are those published or summarized, sometimes misleadingly, in *Cartulaire général de l'Ordre des Hospitaliers de St.-Jean de Jérusalem: 1100–1310*, ed. J. Delaville le Roulx, 4 vols., Paris 1894–1906. The treatment is extremely selective and incomplete, especially for the period after 1310; much thirteenth-century material is scattered throughout the archives and publications, while details on the post-1310 period, drawn in particular from the Hospital's central archives now in Malta, will appear in an introductory work on the Hospital in *Alamania* being prepared by Karl Borchardt, Ekhard Schöffler and Anthony Luttrell.

[2] For essential bibliography, *Der Johanniterorden – Der Malteserorden: Der ritterliche Orden des hl. Johannes vom Spital zu Jerusalem, seine Geschichte, seine Aufgaben*, ed. A. Wienand, 3rd ed., Cologne 1988; W. Rödel, *Das Grosspriorat Deutschland des Johanniter-Ordens im Übergang vom Mittelalter zur Reformation anhand der Generalvisitationsberichte von 1494/95 und 1540/41*, 2nd ed., Cologne 1972; C. Maier, *Forschungsbericht zur Geschichte der geistlichen Ritterorden in der Schweiz (12.–19. Jahrhundert)*, Schweizerische Zeitschrift für Geschichte 43, 1993.

[3] L. Jan, *Pečeti rytířských Duchovních řádů v Čechách a na Moravě 1189–1310 (S přihlédnutím k dalšímu vývoji)*, Zprávy Krajského vlastivědného muzea v Olomouci 246, 1987; his conclusions largely coincide with those here.

[4] The standard work is J. Riley-Smith, *The Knights of St. John in Jerusalem and Cyprus: c. 1050–1310*, London 1967.

[5] Lists in R. Röhricht, *Die Deutschen im Heiligen Lande*, Innsbruck 1894, and idem, *Deutsche Pilgerreisen nach den Heiligen Lande*, Gotha 1889.

[6] Early developments are summarized in Rödel, Wienand and J. Delaville le Roulx, *Les Hospitaliers en Terre Sainte et à Chypre: 1100–1310*, Paris 1904, pp. 428–431.

[7] *Cartulaire*, no. 47; cf. R. Hiestand, *Papsturkunden für Templer und Johanniter: Archivberichte und Texte*, Göttingen 1972, p. 424.

[8] N. von Holst, *Der deutsche Ritterorden und seine Bauten von Jerusalem bis Sevilla von Thorn bis Narwa*, Berlin 1981, pp. 26–29, 218–220, with plans, photos and references; cf. M.-L. Favreau, *Studien zur Frühgeschichte des Deutschen Ordens*, Stuttgart 1974, pp. 12–34; H. Kluger, *Hochmeister Hermann von Salza und Kaiser Friedrich II.*, Marburg 1987, pp. 127–132, citing extensive earlier literature.

[9] *Cartulaire*, nos. 154–155. Both bulls referred to quarrels outside the Jerusalem kingdom, and *per Alamanniam* might have meant „in Germany", in which case there were by 1143 certain otherwise undocumented foundations *ad opus peregrinorum Jerusolimis* in Germany, possibly made to the German hospital in Jerusalem, which should have passed to the Hospital in that year; cf. Favreau, pp. 25–34.

[10] Kluger, p. 127.

[11] *Cartulaire*, nos. 802, 861. In 1163 Fr. Petrus *dictus Alamannus* was prior of the Hospital's *domus* and *ecclesia* in Constantinople and was sent by the Greek emperor on a mission to France: ibid., nos. 321, 323, 326. In October 1188 Fr. Arlabaudus, Prior of *Alamannia*, was with Fr. Armengaud d'Asp who was then acting as Master: ibid., no. 860. The latter was apparently in Syria in and after October 1187, but the relevant documents, or at least their dates, seem puzzling: references in Riley-Smith, pp. 106–107, but the question requires thorough revision.

[12] *Cartulaire*, nos. 81, 246, discussed in K. Lechner, *Die Kommende Mailberg*, in wienand, 1 st ed., Cologne 1970, pp. 414–416, redating *Cartulaire*, no. 81 to 1245/60 rather than circa 1128: amend Delaville (1904), p. 387. The German practice of making donations without a written charter in the first half of the twelfth century means that the earliest donations are known, if at all, only through later confirmations which makes them difficult to date.

[13] *Cartulaire*, nos. 204, 213, 278, 289, 405, 831 et passim; A. Gąsiorowski, *Najstarsze dokumenty poznańskiego domu joanitów*, Studia Źródłoznawcze 8–9, 1963–1964; E. Dąbrowska, A. Tomaszewski, *Recherches sur les Hospitaliers à Zagość en Pologne*, Annales de l'Ordre Souverain Militaire de Malte 24, 1966; M. Skopal, *Založeni komendy Johanitů na Malé Straně*, Pražsky sborník historicki 26, 1933.

[14] Valletta, National Library of Malta, Archives of the Order of Saint John, Cod. 361, f. 314.

[15] Texts in *Cartulaire*, nos. 70, 2653, and G. Lagleder, *Die Ordensregel der Johanniter/Malteser*, St. Otilien 1983, pp. 130–153.

[16] Munich, Bayerische Staatsbibliothek, Ms. Lat. 4620, partly published in *Recueil des Historiens des Croisades: Historiens Occidentaux* 5, Paris 1895, pp. 405–410; fragments of the statutes in German, datable circa 1390, are in Cologne, Historisches Archiv der Stadt Köln, Geistl. Abt. 129 A, f. 1–8.

[17] K. Borchardt, *Spendenaufrufe der Johanniter aus dem 13. Jahrhundert*, Zeitschrift für bayerische Landesgeschichte 56, 1993.

[18] *Cartulaire*, nos. 831, 1180.

[19] There is remarkably little evidence on this point.

[20] *Cartulaire*, nos. 643, 802, 825; cf. Delaville (1904), pp. 387–389. Fr. Martinus was also *preceptor* in 1189: *Cartulaire*, no. 865. He was probably the Martinus *prepositus*, a title he took in other texts (nos. 643, 802, 865) and on his seal (Jan, Fig. 1), who was with the Master and other senior Hospitallers apparently in Syria in October 1188 (*Cartulaire*, no. 860, and supra, n. 11).

[21] Texts in *Cartulaire* summarized in Delaville (1904), pp. 387–390, 428–431. Templar terminology was similarly diverse in this region: M. Schüpferling, *Der Tempelherren–Orden in Deutschland*, Bamberg 1915, pp. 191–203, and M.-L. Bulst-Thiele, *Sacrae Domus Militiae Templi Hierosolymitani Magistri: Untersuchungen zur Geschichte des Templerordens 1118/19–1314*, Göttingen 1974, pp. 211–212, 372–379.

[22] *Codex Diplomaticus et Epistolaris regni Bohemiae*, ed. G. Friedrich, 1, Prague 1904, p. 262.

[23] *Cartulaire*, nos. 643, 861, 959, 1224, 2713. For Fr. Hugo, who was unknown to Delaville, references in Jan, p. 2. Of the priors listed in Wienand, p. 654, Martinus (1189) and Meinardus (1194) were probably grand preceptors; Peter von Straznitz (1245) is not there documented; and Clemens (1249) and many of his alleged successors were Grand Preceptors of *Alamania*.

[24] *Cartulaire*, nos. 1225, 1273, 2329, 3048, 3540.

[25] Ibid., nos. 802, 1302, 1472, 1605, 1832, and Delaville (1904), pp. 390 n. 1, 399, 430; Delaville and Favreau, p. 33, consider that there was a Prior Martinus in 1186.

[26] Delaville (1904), pp. 391, 430; this assumes that Miko and Raimbaud de Voczon were the same person.

[27] *Cartulaire*, nos. 1149, 1971, 2426, 2611, 2713, 3000.

[28] Ibid., nos. 643, 2191, 2193.

[29] Eg. ibid., nos. 1149, 1502, 2180, 2325, 2592, 2778, 3306, 4243.

[30] That Hospitallers fought at Legnica is an unsubstantiated hypothesis; on the Templars, see Bulst-Thiele, pp. 212–213; M. Starnawska, *Notizie sulla Composizione e sulla Struttura dell'Ordine del Tempio in Polonia*, in: *I Templari: Mito e Storia*, ed. G. Minnucci, F. Sarda, Sinalunga–Siena 1989.

[31] *Cartulaire*, nos. 2989, 3000, 3306, 3627, 3816.

[32] Ibid., nos. 3861, 4298, 4834.

[33] Ibid., no. 825; in October 1188 Fr. Arleboldus, *prior Alamannie*, was with the acting Master, apparently in Syria (discussion supra, n. 11).

[34] Ibid., nos. 1265, 1429, 1455, 1622, 1743, 1767, 1804 n. 1, 2146 etc; Delaville (1904), pp. 389–390, 429.

[35] T. Hatt Olsen, *The Priory of Dacia in the Order of Saint John of Jerusalem*, Annales de l'Ordre Souverain Militaire de Malte 18, 1960; T. Nyberg, *Zur Rolle der Johanniter in Skandinavien: Erstes Auftreten und Aufbau der Institutionen*, in: *Die Rolle der Ritterorden in der mittelalterlichen Kultur*, ed. Z. H. Nowak, Toruń 1985.

[36] *Cartulaire*, nos., 1995, 3982, 4133, 4259 para. 1; Delaville (1904), pp. 400–402, 430–431.

[37] B. Eimer, *The Spiritual Orders of Knighthood in Scandinavia under King Erik of Pomerania: Studies in an Exchange Projekt of 1433*, Annales de l'Ordre Souverain Militaire de Malte 30 (1972).

[38] *Cartulaire*, no. 4046.

[39] Despite considerable ambiguities in the texts, this interpretation broadly follows that in Riley-Smith, pp. 366–371; but the decree of 1278 circa did not say that the Grand Preceptor in the West used the Masters's bull, but that he sealed in wax in the same way as the Master: text in J. Delaville le Roulx, *Mélanges sur l'Ordre de S. Jean de Jérusalem*, Paris 1910, III, pp. 3–5 (but p. 6 prints a different text, with omissions, which confuses the point). The 1206 statutes show that the powers of the grand preceptor were decided by the Master and chapter-general: *Cartulaire*, no. 1193.

[40] Ibid., no. 802; however, Delaville (1904), pp. 391, 428, regards Fr. Martinus as a grand preceptor but of *Alamania*.

[41] *Cartulaire*, nos. 2493, 2505, 2547, 2568, 2611, 2713, 2823, 2908; Delaville (1904), p. 392. Ibid., pp. 391, 428, inexplicably regards Fr. Meinardus, *preceptor* (perhaps commander) at Prague alongside a *prior* (probably of Prague) in 1194 (*Cartulaire*, no. 959), as Grand Preceptor of *Alamania*. Fürstenberg's tenure as grand preceptor was apparently interrupted by Fr. Heinrich de Boxburg, *summus preceptor* in March 1260, Fürstenberg apparently then being in Syria: ibid., nos. 2934–2936, 2948, 3045, 3047. The illusion that Fürstenberg was „Grand Prior" of Bohemia helps to invalidate the lists in Wienand, pp. 654–655. Repeated discussions of these titles have failed to understand the nature of a grand preceptor and the resulting lists are therefore unreliable.

[42] Assuming that they did not use the title in the documents because they were Grand Preceptors of Germany; no other prior is known between about 1242 and 1260: Delaville (1904), p. 429.

[43] *Cartulaire*, no. 2526.

⁴⁴ Ibid., nos. 2908, 3219.

⁴⁵ Ibid., nos. 2713, 2823, 2908, 2934–2936, 3045, 3047, 3219, 3386, 3412, 3455, 3470; cf. Delaville (1904), pp. 392–394.

⁴⁶ Ibid., pp. 392–396, 429.

⁴⁷ Cartulaire, no. 4259 para. 1.

⁴⁸ Ibid., I, pp. CXCVII, CCIII–CCVII; Delaville (1904), pp. 142–143, 390, 398–400; E. Reiszig, *A Jerusálem Szent-János-slovag-rend Magyarországon*, 2 vols., Budapest 1923–1928, summarized in H. Thierry, *L'Ordre de Malte en Hongroie*, Rivista del Sovrano Militare Ordine di Malta 2, 1938. For Croatia, see I. Kukuljevic-Sakcinski, *Priorat vranski sa vitezi templari i hospitalci sv. Ivana u Hrvatskoy*, Řad Jugoslavenske Akademije 81–82, 1886–1887; L. Dubronić, *The Military Orders in Croatia*, in: *The Meeting of Two Worlds: Cultural Exchange between East and West during the period of the Crusades*, ed. V. Goss, Kalamazoo 1986.

⁴⁹ *Cismontanis* might have meant in Hungary, and perhaps also in *Alamania* or even beyond; some texts give *Cismarinis* which might have implied the West in general.

⁵⁰ *Cartulaire*, no. 2445. The Hospital was to serve against pagans and Bulgarians; if other schismatics invaded, it was to provide *centum fratres*, while if Christian armies invaded it was to provide 50 (*quiquingenta*: sic) and if Tartar armies invaded, 60 *fratres*. Cf. A. Forey, *The Military Orders and the Holy War against Christians in the Thirteenth Century*, English Historical Review 104 (1989).

⁵¹ Cf. Riley-Smith, pp. 57, 132, 158–163, 325, 334, 359–360, 432, 459 n. 3.

⁵² *Cartulaire*, nos. 2161, 2445, accepting *cismontanis* rather than *cismarinis*. For *frater R. prior provincialis ... in Ungaria* in 1237, see *Vetera Monumenta Historica Hungariam Sacram illustrantia*, ed. A. Theiner, Rome 1859, p. 154. By 1238 *Esclavonia* was part of the Hungarian priory: *Cartulaire*, no. 2205.

⁵³ Ibid., nos. 2526, 2638, 2663.

⁵⁴ Ibid., nos. 3219, 3692.

⁵⁵ Ibid., no. 2932.

⁵⁶ Ibid., nos. 3030, 3572, 4711 (1262–1306).

⁵⁷ Ibid., no. 3729: *AVST ... MOR ... POL ...* are legible on the seal. Between 1278 and 1281 Brunshorn had a variety of titles as grand preceptor, once in 1279 including Hungary: eg. *Cartulaire*, nos. 3678, 3689, 3692, 3718, 3774; he was never Prior of Germany or of Bohemia. In 1278 the Queen of Bohemia entitled Brunshorn as Grand Preceptor of Bohemia, *Dacia*, Austria, Moravia and Poland, omitting *Alamania* but probably through some error: ibid., no. 3678. Wienand, pp. 652, 654, probably requires amendment on these points.

⁵⁸ *Cartulaire*, no. 3252. In 1276 Fay, still Prior of Hungary, was authorized to sail from Barletta for Syria: ibid., no. 3599.

⁵⁹ An Italian, Fr. Filippo de Gragnana, was Prior of Hungary from 1317 to 1329: J. Delaville le Roulx, *Les Hospitaliers à Rhodes jusqu'à la Mort de Philibert de Naillac: 1310–1421*, Paris 1913, pp. 71/72 n. 6, 174–175.

⁶⁰ *Cartulaire*, nos. 4549 para. 13, 4550, 4672 para. 18.

⁶¹ Cf. Riley-Smith, pp. 368–369.

⁶² Delaville (1904), pp. 394–396, 428–431, but without always distinguishing between lieutenants, priors and grand preceptors. For example, it gives as prior of Lower *Alamania* in 1296 Fr. Hermann de Mainz, but the document has him as Commander of Cologne and lieutenant in Lower *Alamania* of the grand preceptor: *Cartulaire*, no. 4305. For the seal of the *prioratus* of High *Alamania* in 1289: ibid., no. 4042.

⁶³ Eg. *Cartulaire*, nos. 3049, 3911, 3950 n. 2, 4250, 4305.

⁶⁴ Cf. Delaville (1904), pp. 394–396.

⁶⁵ *Cartulaire*, nos. 1756, 2599, 3049; it seems anachronistic to employ the term *Ballei* before about 1300.

⁶⁶ *Codex Diplomaticus Brandenburgensis* 6, ed. A. Riedel, Berlin 1846, p. 19.

[67] J. Wibel, *Hohenlohische Kyrchen- und Reformations-Historie* 2, Onolzbach 1753, codex diplomaticus, pp. 92–93.

[68] *Monumenta Boica*, ed. Bayerische Akademie der Wissenschaften 27, Munich 1829, pp. 528–529.

[69] Würzburg, Staatsarchiv, Urk. 4921.

[70] *Cartulaire*, no. 4395 n. 2.

[71] Malta, Cod. 16 no. 15.

[72] Crudes statistics show show that donations in the Province of *Alamania* continued to rise after 1240 while in France and England they fell: W. Rödel, *Erwerbspolitik und Wirtschaftsweise der Kommdenden Mainz und Niederweisel des Johanniterordens: Ein Stat-Land-Vergleich*, in: *Erwerbspolitik und Wirtschaftsweise mittelalterlicher Orden und Kloster*, ed. K. Elm, Berlin 1992; H. Nicholson, *Templars, Hospitallers and Teutonic Knights: Images of the Military Orders, 1128–1291*, Leicester 1993, pp. 58–65.

[73] Delaville (1913), pp. 70–71, 172–173.

[74] *Monumenta Vaticana res gestas Bohemicas illustrantia*, 4 part 1, ed. C. Stloukal, Prague 1949, pp. 230–231, 262–263; cf. Delaville (1913), pp. 172–173, 219.

[75] Brief interim undocumented survey in A. Luttrell, *The Hospitallers in Fourteenth-Century Germany*, St. John Historical Society Proceedings 2, 1988–1990.

[76] Figures based on research in course of publication.

[77] Excellent detail in V. Novotny, *Inquisitio Domorum Hospitalis S. Johannis Hierosolimitani per Pragensem archidioesim facta anno 1373*, Historiky Archiv 19, 1901.

[78] The *ballivatus* of Avalterre, Chantraine or Flanders, comprising a *preceptoria principalis* and 33 *domus*, had something in common with the nearby German *Ballei*: A.-M. Legras, *L'Enquête pontificale de 1373 sur l'Ordre des Hospitaliers de Saint-Jean de Jérusalem* 1, Paris 1987, pp. 148–150.

[79] *Ostfriesisches Urkundenbuch* 1, ed. E. Friedlander, Emden 1878, pp. 44–45.

[80] Ibid., 1, p. 192: cf. G. Noordhuis, *De Johannieters in Stad en Lande: Geschiedenis van de Johannieters in de provincie Groningen (13 de–17 de eeuw)*, Warffum 1990, pp. 22–24; E. Schöningh, *Der Johanniterorden in Ostfriesland*, Aurich 1973, pp. 9–17; idem, *Zur Geschichte der Johanniterballei Westfalen*, Osnabrucker Mitteilungen 81, 1974. On the *Ballei* of Utrecht, see T. van Bueren, *Macht en onderhorigheid binnen de Ridderlijke Orde van Sint Jan: de Commandeursportretten uit het Sint Janskloster te Haarlem*, Haarlem 1991, pp. 13–16; idem, *Tot lof van Haarlem*, Hilversum 1993, pp. 76–78, 87–90.

[81] *Urkundenbuch für die Geschichte des Niederrheins* 3, ed. J. Lacomblet, Düsseldorf 1853, p. 292.

[82] W. Engel, *Die Krise der Ballei Franken des Johanniterordens zur Mitte des 14. Jahrhunderts*, Zeitschrift für bayerische Landesgeschichte 18, 1955; cf. W. Rödel, *Reformbestrebungen im Johanniterorden in der Zeit zwischen dem Fall Akkons und dem Verlust von Rhodos: 1291–1522*, in: *Reformbemühungen und Observanzbestrebungen in spätmittelalterlichen Ordenswesen*, ed. K. Elm, Berlin 1989.

[83] Delaville (1913), pp. 72–75.

[84] Text in J. Miret y Sans, *Les Cases de Templers y Hospitalers en Catalunya*, Barcelona 1910, p. 402.

[85] Malta, Cod.16 no. 15 (possibly 12 January 1324).

[86] Delaville (1913), p. 75, n. 2.

[87] *Codex Diplomaticus Brandenburgensis* 19 (1860), pp. 196–197.

[88] Delaville (1913), pp. 217–218, gives details, but wrongly claims „C'était pour l'Hôpital la perte de la province de Brandebourg".

[89] E. Opgenoorth, *Die Ballei Brandenburg des Johanniterordens im Zeitalter der Reformation und Gegenreformation*, Wurzburg 1963, pp. 34–49; cf. infra, n. 93. Earlier historians misinterpreted events in the light of what happened later in the Protestant Reformation; there was no *Herrenmeister* at the time.

[90] Hatt Olsen (1960), pp. 23–25, 29; idem, *Dacia og Rhodos: en Studie over forholdet mellem Johannitterstormestern pa Rhodos of prioratet Dacia i de 14. og 15. arhundrede*, Copenhagen 1962, pp. 19, 26–27, 77 n. 73, 102–104.

[91] Prague, Státní Ústřední Archiv, Archiv Maltézského velkopřevorstri, no. 951, summarized in L. Jan, *Ivanovice na Hané, Orlovice a johanitský řád*, Časopis Malice moravské 3, 1992, pp. 211–213.

[92] Malta, Cod. 336, f. 142 v; Cod. 342, f. 144.

[93] Malta, Cod. 319, f.187.

[94] A. Luttrell, *The Hospitallers' Western Accounts, 1373/4 and 1374/5*, in: *Camden Miscellany* 30, London 1990, pp. 8–9. In circa 1478 27 houses in High Germany paid *responsiones* of 1578 florins, while 38 houses in Low Germany plus the *Ballei* of Brandenburg (1243 florins) and the Priory of *Dacia* (544 florins) paid 3810 florins, for a total of 5388 florins; no figures were given for Bohemia: Paris, Bibliothèque Nationale, Ms. Lat. 13,824, f. 88v–90 (transcript kindly provided by Anne-Marie Legras). Brandenburg thus provided 23 per cent or the priory's contribution.

[95] Delaville (1913), pp. 7–9, 24, 32–34, 78–79, 185, 187, 209, 214–215, 223, 230–231, 350.

[96] There were a few German brethren in Rhodes between 1330 and 1344: Malta, Cod. 280, f. 1–54. The *ordinationes* agreed in 1373 referred to twelve electors, two from each *langue*, implicitly excluding a seventh *langue* which was presumably that of *Alamania*: Paris, Bibliothèque Nationale, Ms. Franç. 17, 255, f. 71.

[97] Malta, Cod. 336, f. 148v–149.

[98] J. Sarnowsky, *Der Konvent auf Rhodos und die Zungen("lingue") im Johanniterorden: 1421–1476*, infra.

[99] R. Valentini, *Un Capitolo Generale degli Ospitalieri di S. Giovanni tenuto in Vaticano nel 1446*, Archivio Storico di Malta 7, 1936, p. 135.

[100] Eg. Malta, Cod. 316, f. 230; Cod. 319, f. 187v–188.

[101] Delaville (1913), pp. 74–75; see also Hatt Olsen (1960), pp. 28–29.

The Structure of the Aragonese Hospital: 1349-1352

There are excellent studies and publications of texts concerning the early history of the Hospitallers of Aragon who were extensive landholders and formed a leading element in the society of the Aragonese kingdom and its defence,[1] but their functions and organization during the fourteenth century are scarcely known. It seems useful therefore to establish, however approximately, the number and identity of the brethren at a point when the sources make this possible, and also to explore in a preliminary fashion how their corporate life was organized. This information should have been made available in 1373 when Pope Gregory XI instructed his bishops throughout the Latin West to report the names, numbers, status, ages and incomes of the Hospitallers in each diocese, but in Aragon there was resistance to such inquiries so that the inquests were never made and the statistics are lacking for all five of the Hospital's Hispanic priories, that is for Portugal, Castile and Leon, Navarre, Catalunya and Aragon.[2] However, for the Aragonese priory, confusingly known as the *Castellanía de Amposta*, three volumes of the Castellan's registers (cited merely by volume and folio) provide numerous names for the three-year period from 7 April 1349 to 11 April 1352, together with some information on incomes and a little about the brethren's status within the order, but none about their ages.[3] Additional material is contained in the Castellany's six-volume *Cartulario Magno* (CM) compiled between 1349 and 1354;[4] in other documents from the Castellany's archives (Carp. and Caja);[5] in the archives of the Priory of Catalunya;[6] in the registers of the Masters of the Hospital at Rhodes for 1347/8 and 1351/2 (Malta);[7] and in other sources.

---

1. Synthesis and bibliography in Ma. L. Ledesma Rubio, *Templarios y Hospitalarios en el reino de Aragón*, Zaragoza 1982; see also idem, *La encomienda de Zaragoza de la orden de San Juan de Jerusalén en los siglos XII y XIII*, Zaragoza 1967; A. Forey, *The Templars in the "Corona de Aragón"*, London 1973; and R. Sáinz de la Maza, *La orden de Santiago en la Corona de Aragón: la encomienda de Montalbán (1210-1327)*, Zaragoza 1980.

2. A. Luttrell, *Papauté et Hôpital: l'Enquête de 1973*, in A.-M. Legras, *L'Enquête pontificale de 1373 sur l'ordre des Hospitaliers de Saint-Jean de Jérusalem*, I, Paris 1987, pp. 30-31.

3. Madrid, Archivo Histórico Nacional, Órdenes Militares, Códices 599B - 601B; volumes iv-vi (602B - 604B) are also cited: utilized in A. Luttrell, *Las órdenes militares en la sociedad hispánica: los Hospitalarios aragoneses, 1340-1360*, "Anuario de Estudios Medievales", 11 (1981).

4. Madrid, Códices 648B - 653B.

5. Madrid, Órdenes Militares, San Juan de Jerusalén, Llengua de Aragón, Carpetas and Cajas; these documents have not been searched exhaustively.

6. As used in J. Miret y Sans, *Les cases de Templers y Hospitalers en Catalunya*, Barcelona 1910, but without references; this archive has been incorporated into the Arxiu de la Corona d'Aragó at Barcelona and awaits further investigation.

7. Valletta, National Library of Malta, Archives of the Order of St. John, Cods. 317-318; used in J. Delaville le Roulx, *Les Hospitaliers à Rhodes jusqu'à la Mort de Philibert de Naillac: 1310-1421*, Paris 1913, and A. Luttrell, *The Hospitallers in Cyprus, Rhodes, Greece and the West: 1291-1440*, London 1978; see especially idem, *Los Hospitalarios en Aragón y la Peste Negra*, "Anuario de Estudios Medievales", 3 (1966)

* * *

The Hospitallers had no effective overall accounting system and could not themselves have presented neat budgets or clear and complete statistics, but they must have had a shrewd notion of their wealth and weight in the kingdom. They certainly knew about the *monedatge* or *maravedí* returns, since they collected and shared them jointly with the crown. The *monedatge* accounts listed heads of families which had a capital of over 105 *sueldos*, but they omitted all sorts of inhabitants and even whole areas, and as fiscal documents they gave only very crude notions of population statistics. The returns for 1409 and 1414 represented a situation in which the population had fallen considerably since about 1350, but the extent of the Hospital's property had probably remained roughly stationary and its proportion of the kingdom's wealth may not have changed greatly. The 1409/1414 documents contained no information for Zaragoza and other major centres, while there were commanderies in places such as Barbastro and Calatayud which were not of the Hospitaller *señorío* so that their share of the local wealth cannot be deduced; the returns did cover the Castellany's Catalan commanderies but not that in Valencia. The 1409/1414 data included Hospitaller possessions around Caspe, Tortosa, Monzón, Teruel and many other places, indicating in extremely approximate form that the *Castellanía de Amposta* contained 101 out of 420, or 24 percent, of the places listed, and 7,978 *maravedís*, perhaps equal to some 56,000 *sueldos* of Jaca, or 29 percent, of the total incomes; the military orders actually paid a staggering 45.5 percent of the total. With over 7000 *fuegos* listed, and many more omitted, the Aragonese Hospital constituted the greatest lordship in the kingdom. Caspe had 615 *fuegos*, Monzón 530, Castellote 391, Cantavella 322 and so on, down to places with 10, 8, 6, 4 or even one *fuego*[8]. Perhaps a quarter of this population was contained in the Castellany's four Catalan *baylias* which may have contained as many as 2700 *fuegos* or *fochs* before the plague came in 1347, though by 1358 the number had apparently fallen to 1774, with 838 *fochs* in the *baylia* of Miravet; these four *commanduries* covered almost 1400 square kilometres and would in 1358 have had a very low density of just over one *foch* per square kilometre[9]. This Catalan population was partly Muslim, the *aljama* of Azcón being strongly Moorish.[10]

The *Castellanía de Amposta* consisted in about 1350 of 29 *baylias* of which one was at Torrente in Valencia[11] and four, at Orta, Uldecona, Azcón and Miravet, were in Catalunya.[12]

---

8. F. Arroyo Ilera, *División señorial de Aragón en el siglo XV*, "Saitabi", 24 (1974); these figures await further refinement.

9. The dating of the various *fogatges* has been revised: see J. Iglésies Fort, *El Fogaje de 1365-1370: contribución al conocimiento de la población de Cataluña en la segunda mitad del siglo XIV*, "Memorias de la Real Academia de Ciencias y Artes de Barcelona", II ser., 34 (1962), p. 281 *et passim*, and J.M. Pons Guri, *Un fogatjament desconegut de l'any 1358*, "Boletín de la Real Academia de Buenas Letras de Barcelona", 30 (1963/4), pp. 461-463 *et passim*. These were agreed global figures, not the result of a real count. The 1366 *fogatge* gave 2700 *fochs*; a royal letter of 1368, which included some *fochs* from Palau in the *baylia* of Monzón, gave 2754 (v.33-34); and the 1378 *fogatge* gave 1374 *fochs*.

10. Fourteenth/Century materials in J.M. Font Rius, *La carta de seguridad de Ramón Berenguer IV a las morerías de Ascó y Ribera del Ebro: siglo XII*, in *Homenaje a Don José Maria Lacarra en su jubilación del profesorado: estudios medievales*, I, Zaragoza 1977, pp. 274-280.

11. Details on the relatively minor incomes from Valencia are given in Ma. D. Cabanes Pecourt, *Las órdenes militares en el reino de Valencia: notas sobre su economía*, "Hispania", 113 (1969), pp. 515-516, and in a collection of studies in "Torrens," 3 (1984).

12. The demarcation between the Castellany and the Priory of Catalunya was established in 1319. Whether Orta was in the Kingdom of Aragon was disputed at the *cortes* of Perpignan in 1350/1: A. Ubieto Arteta, *Historia de Aragón: la formación territorial*, Zaragoza 1981, pp. 347-354.

A new Castellany was formed in 1319 by amalgamating the Hospitaller and Templar lands in Aragon while creating a separate Priory of Catalunya which included holdings in Roussillon and Mallorca but not the four *baylias* west of the Ebro. Between 1319 and 1324 a list of incomes of the Castellany, *aliquibus expensarum non deductis*, named 30 *baylias*, counting two each for Zaragoza and Huesca, one for Siscar and one for Valencia. The *redditus*, given in *libre jaccenses* did not include the incomes of a number of former Templar churches at Cantavella, Alfambra, Villel, Ricla, Noviellas, Ambel and Monzón which were only subsequently acquired by the Hospital. The *baylias*, whose wealth varied remarkably, were Valencia at 500 *libre*; Amposta, 750; Miravet, 2000; Orta, 800; Azcón, 800; Caspe, 450; Torrente de Cinca, 300; Samper de Calanda, 350; Castellote, 650; Cantavella, 500; Aliaga, 700; Alfambra, 100; Villel, 150; Calatayud, 400; Ricla, 300; Zaragoza, 1300; Zaragoza, the former Templar house, 500; Mallén, 300; Añón, 200; Noviellas, 200; Ambel, 700; Boquiñenich, 50; Castieliscar, 150; Añiés and Pilvet, 50; Huesca, the Hospitaller and Templar *baylias*, 1000; Sant Miguel de Foces, 200; Saliellas, 150; Barbastro, 400; Monzón, 2500; and Siscar and Sosterres, 400. This amounted to 15,600 *libre jaccenses* or 18,850 *libre barchinonenses*; to this were added 1250 *libre barchinonenses* from the *baylias* of Valencia, which were also reported at the beginning of the list as paying 500 *libre jaccenses*, to give a grand total for the Castellany of 20,100 *libre barchinonenses*. The total for the Priory of Catalunya was 19,662 *libre barchinonenses* 10 *soldi*[13]. The four Catalan *baylias*, then given as Amposta, Orta, Azcón and Miravet, provided more than a quarter of the Castellany's total incomes. How much of this total was due as *responsiones* to the Master and Convent at Rhodes is unknown. In 1329 the king wanted the *responsiones* of the Castellany to be fixed during the life of the new Castellan, Sancho de Aragón, at an annual 2500 florins, perhaps about 28,000 *sueldos* of Jaca, while in 1328 he wanted the priory's *responsiones* reduced from 9800 to 8000 florins;[14] however, the sums actually paid remain uncertain. If the Castellany's total annual incomes were about 332,000 *sueldos* of Jaca, it was being expected to pay more than eight percent of them as *responsiones*.

Normally one or more *baylias* in the Castellany were magistral *cambras*; in 1341 Guillem de Guimerà could claim that he held Monzón and the patronage of its churches by grant from the Master at Rhodes, while the Castellan insisted that Guimerà was not its commander but its *arrendador* and that he ruled it as the Castellan's regent (i.20-22). Some *baylias* were prioral *cambras*, technically in the hands — *ad manum* — of the Castellan and governed for him by regents or lieutenants whom he named; from 1349 to 1352 there were apparently three such *baylias*, at Zaragoza, Monzón and Miravet. A number of *baylias*, and not just the prioral *cambras*, had no *comendador* or commander, for the Castellan could appoint a *tenient* or *regidor* who was not always a Hospitaller. In 1350 the Hospitaller Albert de Joya was *tenient* for the Castellan of the places, the *lochs* or *lugares*, of Palau, Cellas and Gavet, which were *membras* of the commandery or *comanadoria*[15] of Monzón (CM vi. 263-266) but, unlike Monzón, were in Catalunya (CM vi. 178-180). Monzón was one of the Castellan's *cambras* and it was being ruled for him by the Commander of Castellote as

13. Text in Miret, pp. 399-400. The female houses at Sigena and Rápita were omitted. Sosterres was also reported under Catalunya as paying 150 *libre*; Siscar and Sosterres were later in the Priory of Catalunya. The sums given actually total 16,850, but 15,600 seems more likely to be correct.

14. Barcelona, Arxiu de la Corona d'Aragó, Reg. 522, f. 76v-78v, 228v-229v.

15. The Latin form for *comendador* was *preceptor*, and for *baylia* it was *baiulia* or *preceptoria*; "encomienda" was not normally used in this period, but *comendadoria* was employed occasionally as was the Latin *comendaria*, while Catalan used *comenador* and *comenadoria*.

rigient por nos la nuestra baylya de Monçon in 1351 when the Castellan sent a letter addressed to him or to his *lugar tenient* which showed that the *baylia* was being administered on the financial side by a lay *bayle* who had rented the *baylya* and its incomes for a year to another layman (iii.74v).

A commander could, with permission, rent his *baylia* to another Hospitaller or to a layman. A *baylia* might include dependent members, *lugares* or *casas*, which could also be rented or be assigned to a separate regent.[16] Two different places, for example Pilvet and Añiés, could jointly constitute a single *baylia*; or a commander might hold two *baylias*, or be *comendador* of one and *regient* of another. At Huesca there were two *baylias*, the *casas nuevas* being the former Templar *baylia* and the *casas antiguas* the original Hospitaller one. Almunia, Cabañas and Alpartil were held by a single commander in 1339 (CM iii.574-575) but were merely *lugares* with a *regient* in 1349 (i. 56). *Baylias, lugares* and *casas* changed their status and component parts from time to time, while there were considerable ambiguities and inconsistencies in the terminology of the scribes, who were often confused themselves.[17] In particular they sometimes gave the title of *comendador* to someone who was more strictly a regent or lieutenant. On 6 April 1352 Simon Pérez de Molina was granted the *regimjento dela baylia nuestra d'Alfambra* to rule it in head and members as its *regidor soberano et mayor* with all its incomes (iii. 137v) yet he was not its *comendador* and seven days later he was addressed as *rigient la baylia nuestra d'Alfambra* (iii. 139).[18] The Hospital had a "palacio" at Almunia[19] which was the seat of a *baylia* in 1338 when the prioral chapter met there (Carp. 611 no. 119), yet it was merely a *lugar* without a commander in 1349. Between 1349 and 1352 there were 29 *baylias*: Alfambra, Aliaga, Ambel, Añón, Azcón, Barbastro, Calatayud, Cantavella, Caspe, Castellote, Castieliscar, Huesca *casas antiguas*, Huesca *casas nuevas*, Mallén, Miravet, Monzón, Noviellas, Orta, Añiés and Pilvet,[20] Ricla, Saliellas, Samper de Calanda, Sant Miguel de Foces, Sigena, Torrente de Ribera de Cinca, Torrente in Valencia, Uldecona, Villel and Zaragoza.

A few brethren held offices such as *mayordomo* to the Castellan or *cambrero* of a large *domus* such as that at Monzón castle, while the Hospitaller priests or chaplains served the chapels of the commanderies and some of the Hospital's many churches where they were variously entitled *abbat, prior* or *vicario*; some Hospitaller priests holding or serving detached churches resided in a Hospitaller *domus* but others lived apart. There were insufficient brethren priests for all the Hospital's churches, many of which were served by secular priests. Knights, sergeants and priests could all be commanders. The Castellan's licences for the reception of new brethren sometimes specified whether they were to be chaplains, knights or sergeants. Between April 1349 and April 1352 the Castellan granted licences for the reception of at least six sergeants and eight priests, but not every licence necessarily resulted in a new Hospitaller. These licences apart, the documents in the registers never, with the exception of a reference of 1352 to Pedro Sánchez de Navas as *sergent* (iii. 102v),

---

16. For the fourteenth century, the best study of an individual *baylia* is Ma. L. Ledesma, *La orden de San Juan en Zaragoza en el siglo* XIV, in *La ciudad de Zaragoza en la Corona de Aragón*, Zaragoza s. d.

17. Thus the lists and maps in A. Ubieto Arteta, *Historia de Aragón: divisiones administrativas*, Zaragoza 1983, pp.65-82, provide numerous names but do not constitute a real description of the Castellany at any one time.

18. Another example *infra*, p...-... n. 50.

19. Illustrated in Ledesma (1982), p. 241.

20. Pilvet, presumably near Añiés in the mountains north of Huesca, must have been deserted in the fourteenth century; it has never been located.

distinguished between *milites* and sergeants, and it is only in some cases clear from the context in the document that a Hospitaller was a priest; the numbers of priests and *milites* given are, therefore, very much minimum figures. There was the case in 1350 of a Hospitaller Juan de Ocón, who may have been very young, being licensed to become a priest (ii.8v). One priest, Bertran de Tarragona, was a doctor in canon law (ii.68).

Brethren without office, whether newly received or retired senior commanders, were assigned an *estaja* at a Hospitaller house where they would be fed and clothed. Also assigned to a *baylia* were the donats, the *donados*, who were members of the Hospital under a vow of obedience but were not professed religious. A payment of 381 *sueldos jacceses* in 1351 for cloth to dress the *donados* in the castle at Monzón (iii.32v-33) suggested that these might be quite numerous. There were still some ex-Templars in the Hospital's houses in 1341 (i. 22-23); there were several at Zaragoza in 1344 (Carp. 694 no. 13); and one, Berenguer dez Coll, was alive in the Priory of Catalunya as late as 1350.[21] The size of a Hospitaller community must have varied, for the lay men and women attached to the *domus* were seldom mentioned in the documents. However, in 1370 the Commander of Orta, Berenguer de Montpahon, was ordered to maintain in the castle there a *miles*, a sergeant, two servants, a Hospitaller priest, a lay chaplain, an altar boy, a woman to clean the house, three stable hands, a baker, a woman to manage the bread oven, three pairs of mules or pack animals and two warhorses, but there was no mention of *donados*:

> ordenamos que uos tengades enel castiello d'Orta, vn freyre cauallero, et otro sargant e dos moços suyos, e dos capellans, vn freyre capellan et otro freyre capellan seglar,[22] vn scalano vna muger para linpiar la casa, tres azembleros et vn fornero, vna fembra por recaudar la pueya del forno, iij pares de azemblas et .ij. caualgaduras vuestras ... (v. 156-157)

At Orta in 1370 there was, therefore, a theoretical total of four Hospitallers in the house. The number of professed brethren in a *domus* at any given time may often have been low. At Zaragoza, almost certainly the largest and most important house in the Castellany, on 2 August 1339 there were present the commander, two chaplains and five *freyres dela casa* (CM iii.297); on 20 March 1340 the commander, the Castellan's lieutenant, the commander of another commandery, a chaplain and five other *freyres* (CM ii. 492-498); on 20 June 1340 the *prior*, the *cambrero*, the *clavero* and three other *conuentuales* (CM iv.340); on 4 October 1340 the commander, the commander of another commandery, one chaplain and four other *freyres* (CM iii.301); and there were at least nine brethren at the house in Zaragoza on 4 February 1350 (Carp. 728 no. 7). At Ricla on 27 December 1345 the commander, a *cauallero* and three *conuentuales* of the *baylia* were present (CM iii.514). Alfambra had only a commander and one other *frater* in 1330 (CM i. 183, 194-195). The registers for the period April 1349 to April 1352 contain no assignations of an *estaja* for 12 of the 29 *baylias*. Of these, Ricla had a community in 1345 and Sigena was a special case, being attached to the female house; the other ten were Aliaga, Barbastro, Cantavella, Huesca *casas nuevas*, Noviellas, Pilvet and Añiés, Saliellas, Sant Miguel de Foces, Torrente de Ribera de Cinca and Uldecona. Possibly some of these *baylias* had no *casa*, no Hospitaller community and no liturgical life. Even if every one of the 29 *baylias* had been occupied by an average of five

---

21. Miret, p. 384.
22. The Ms. mistakenly has the *et* sign instead of a comma after *capellanes*; *capellan* was inserted after *otro* in place of the word *freyre* which should have been crossed out but was not.

brethren, that would only give a total of 145 Hospitallers resident in the houses of the Castellany plus various priest brethren serving Hospitaller churches outside the central houses and some others who were non-resident for various reasons.

A group of professed Hospitaller sisters or *freyras* lived, under the Castellan's jurisdiction, in the prestigious royal foundation at Sigena. They paid *responsiones* and attended chapters, the *prioressa* and four others being at the chapter held at Almunia in 1351. On 14 June 1353 the Castellan licensed the prioress to receive as sisters one of her own relations or *sobrinas* and Affresca de Rexach, who was already some sort of novice or *escolana dela sacrestanja* at Sigena (iii. 156v, 157). On 5 September 1351 the Hospitaller Fortaner de Glera, *vicario* of Sena near Sigena,[23] was permitted to travel in Aragon and Catalunya to manage his own affairs and those of three *freyras* of Sigena:

> Die ut supra el senyor castellan dio carta de licencia a ffray Fortaner vicarjo de Sena que pudies yr por la castellanja et porel priorado de Cataluenya por liurar sus afferes, et por affers delas nobles Religiosas donya Gujsabel d'Alagon, donya Toda Perez d'Alagon, donya Francisca de Castellet, freyras del monasteryo de Xixena, tanto tiempo quanto a el plugujes. corregida:- (iii.22)

The sisters were in difficulties and on 17 September 1351 the Castellan was prepared to lend them money:

> Dia sabbado .xuij dias de setiembre, el senyor castellan dio carta a ffray Johan Martinez d'Alujco comendador de Castellot et regient la baylya de Monço, que con fray Gerau comendador de Xexena en semble, reconociesse las rentas del monsteryr *(sic)*, et si non cumplian fasta el anyo de lij, quelo prestasse, et quelo segurasse la prioressa et las duenyas del conuent, et esto se fazia por que eran numero mas de xxx. corregida: - (iii.70)

This implies that there were over 30 sisters or *duenyas* at this time. Urraca Artal Cornel was already prioress by 7 March 1349 when the subprioress was Isabel Saurnia de Figuarelas.[24] Present at Sigena in an act of 8 August 1362 concerning a male *donado* were the prioress with eight other named sisters and six brethren, who included the *prior* and the *comendador*, and *todo el Conuento de duenyas et de Freires, et de donados del dito monasterio* (Caja 8127[1] i. 285-287). There must also have been a few sisters in the convent at Rápita near Tortosa which had been so abandoned by 1382, on account of the death of its *duenyas*, that instructions were given to recruit new *monjas* and *donadas* and to repair the buildings (vi. 107-107v).[25]

The professed male religious in the *Castellanía de Amposta* between April 1349 and April 1352 amounted at least to 121 *freyres*; in 1353 Martín de Ceylla was *clavero* of Sigena

---

23. The great *retablo* at Sigena (now Barcelona, Museu d'Art de Catalunya n°. 15,916), showing a donor in a black habit with a white Hospitaller cross, was inscribed FRA FORTANER DE GLERA COM [E] NADOR DE SIXENA. Fr. Fortaner became preceptor between 8 August 1362 and 20 September 1365: Caja 8127[1], i. 285-287, and text in J. Arribas Salaberri, *Historia de Sijena*, Lérida 1975, pp. 112-114. The three hitherto unnoticed arms on the painting were those of the prioress Toda Pérez de Alagón who died between 20 September and 5 October 1369: R. del Arco, *El Monasterio de Sigena*, "Linajes de Aragón," iv (1913), p. 234. The painting apparently dates between August 1362 and September 1369.

24. *Infra*, p...; the date is 7 March Era 1387.

25. Miret, pp. 589-590, names a number of *freyras* at Rápita from 1384 onwards.

on 20 May (Carp. 706 no. 36) and four more brethren were mentioned between 14 and 23 June.[26] At least 42 Hospitallers were listed at the chapter of April 1349 (i. 70,72,86),[27] and a minimum of 42 brethren and five sisters attended the chapter of May 1351 (iii.18-18v). Of 17 Hospitallers named at the chapter of June 1346 all but three were alive in 1349,[28] an astonishing survival rate in a period which experienced the great plague of 1347. Three of those named in 1346 and still alive in 1349, Adam Pérez de Nuevalos, Bernat dela Horden and Pere del Bosch, were not mentioned thereafter.

Some Hospitallers appeared in the registers only once in three years, and the number of those never mentioned cannot be estimated. Some brethren died or left the Hospital, while new entrants were received; not all those listed between 1349 and 1352 were in the Hospital simultaneously. These were years of crisis and change; the plague of 1347 seems not to have killed many brethren, but that year saw the revolts of the *uniones* and was followed by protests to Rhodes and rebellion against the new Castellan, Juan Fernández de Heredia, who reorganized the Aragonese Hospital; he persecuted certain Hospitallers and recruited new brethren, some of them his own kinsmen.[29] In addition to the Castellan himself, there were at least eight Hospitallers named Heredia, two of them commanders, between 1349 and 1352, while other kinsmen cannot be identified, except that the Hospitaller Gil Gonçalvez del Espuro was the brother of Juan Gonçalvez del Espuro (iii.67), and the latter was the *cunyado* of the Juan Fernández de Heredia who was regent of Miravet (ii.16v).

Some brethren left the Castellany. Many received licences to travel for a matter of months in neighbouring priories, notably those of Castile and Catalunya, in order to visit their relatives and deal with their personal affairs, while in 1350 a number were permitted to travel to the *perdonança*, the jubilee, in Rome. Hospitaller *baylias* in one priory could be held by brethren from other priories within the same *langue*, and four of the Castellany's *baylias* were in Southern Catalunya. García Gonçalvez Bugia moved from the Castellany to a Castilian commandery and Guillem de Guimerà to a Catalan one. Some brethren listed between 1349 and 1352 were Castilian, Catalan or even Valencian in origin. During 1351 the Castellan complained that commanders and other brethren were moving to other priories.[30] Guillem de Guimerà took complaints against the Castellan made by thirteen other

---

26. Bertran Figuera, assigned *estaja* at Barbastro, 19 June (iii.172v); Eximeno de Borga, *prior* of Campiello, dead by 22 June (iii.205v); Pedro del Orden, *conuentual*, 14 June (iii.157v); Remon dela Raz, chaplain at Calatayud, 22 June (iii,205v).

27. Correct the total of 46 wrongly given in Luttrell (1966), p. 500.

28. Sancho d'Oros and Ramón de Capiella were aged; the Sancho d'Oros of 1358 (iv.81) was not a Hospitaller: Luttrell (1966), p. 500 n. 4. García Gonçalvez Bugia was Commander of Azcón in the Castellany of Amposta and of Población in the Priory of Castile in Jan. 1348 (Malta 317, f.111) and was mentioned in 1357 as a former lieutenant of the latter priory (v.157v). The allusion to a Pedro Fernández de Luna at the chapter of 1346 given in Luttrell (1966), p. 501 n.9, is erroneous; the mention of Pedro Fernández de Luna at the chapter on 8 April 1349 (iii.132v) is a scribal error for Pedro Fernández de Liñan who was at that chapter (iii.187v). Lop or Lop Fernández de Luna, Commander of Mallén in 1341 (i.26,27), is last documented as regent of Ambel, probably some time after July 1348, in a text of 23 June 1349 which showed he had imposed fines on the Moors of Ambel, presumably in connection with their having assisted in the revolt of the *unión* (i.41-42). Lop Fernández de Luna, Archbishop of Zaragoza from 1351, became Bishop of Vich on 3 December 1348 when he was *clericus*: C. Eubel, *Hierarchia Catholica Medii Aevi*, I, Münster 1913, p. 153, 526. He is not previously documented, unless he was the Hospitaller in question. (Francisco de Moxó y Montoliu kindly exchanged information on this subject).

29. Details in Luttrell (1966), pp. 500-502.

30. Malta 318, f. 102v-103: text in Luttrell (1966), p. 512.

Hospitallers to the Master at Rhodes some time before 12 April 1351. The thirteen included four commanders, Bertran Roger de Pallars, Jofre de Inglerola, Marco de Vilagranada and Guillem de Abella; two *priòres*, Guillermo de Villalba and Francisco Bosch; and seven others, Pedro Ruiz de Aranda, Juan de Novalles, Gerau de Pomar *el joven*, Alfonso Fernández Garín, Bernat Çacorvella, Pere Aveniella and Juan López de Fanlo (Malta 318, f. 92-93). Alfonso Fernández Garín and Pedro Martínez de Arcanya had apparently been condemned to death for their part in the *uniones* against the king, though they must have been pardoned as they appeared as simple *freyres* at the chapter of May 1351.[31] Juan de Sant Matheo was also in trouble, for in 1350 his habit was to be restored (ii.9).

There were never more than a very few Hospitallers from the Spanish *langue* at Rhodes or on nearby Kos.[32] The Prior of Catalunya, Pere Arnau Peres Tortes, commanded the galleys at Rhodes in 1347 and in 1348 he founded a hospice there for Catalan Hospitallers;[33] the Aragonese Pedro Martínez de Arcayna also had a *hospitium* at Rhodes at some time before March 1348.[34] In 1350 the senior Hispanic Hospitaller at Rhodes, who traditionally held the office of *Drapier*, was the Castilian Mendario de Valbuena, and Guillem de Rocafulla, probably a Catalan, was *de casa del senyor Maestro* there (ii.lllv). On 20 March 1348 the Master authorized the Castellan to send four Hospitallers to Rhodes when he saw fit (Malta, 317, f.112v) but it is doubtful whether any went. In 1350 the chapter of the Castellany decided to send Sancho López de Casseda to Rhodes (ii.70), and he and Domingo Ximeno were there in 1351 when they handed over certain monies sent by the Castellan to the Master (Malta 318, f.19v). Other Aragonese brethren went to Rhodes not to serve there but to protest against the Castellan, and these included Albert de Joya in 1348, who had been deprived of his habit but was then pardoned and sent back to the Castellany (Malta 317, f.114), and Guillem de Guimerà and Berenguer de Montpahon in 1351 (Malta 318, f. 92-93,94-94v,102).[35]

The Castellan periodically sought licences from the Master of Rhodes to create new brethren. Thus on 2 January 1348 he was empowered to receive four knights, four sergeants and four donats, and on 28 March 1351 to create no less than fifteen knights and five sergeants;[36] presumably there were other such licences. Between 13 June 1349 and 29 August 1350 the Castellan issued at least seven licences for different commanders to receive a total of at least six sergeants and seven chaplains. He may have reserved the reception of *milites* to his own patronage, though in July and August 1353 he did authorize his lieutenant, who was presumably a knight, to receive three *caualleros* (iii.222,228v-229,230). On 17 September 1351 the Castellan authorized the admission of as many Hospitaller priests as were needed at Sigena, and on 20 February 1352 he licensed the reception of another priest (iii.70,87v). The Castellan must have been a knight himself; so were Juan de Mendoza in 1322 (CM iv.345); Gerau de Pomar in 1342 (Carp. 616 no. 15); Pedro Ortiz de Sotes and

---

31. Details in Luttrell (1966), p. 500.

32. Details in Luttrell (1978), XI p. 16; Gómez de Penya Aguda, squire of the Commander of Kos in 1353 (iii. 226v-227), was not a Hospitaller.

33. Details in Luttrell (1978), XI p. 16.

34. At Rhodes in 1337 and had *hospitium* there before 1348: Malta 280, f. 41v; 317, f. 245v.

35. The Hospitaller *Petrus Ortis*, who had killed a slave belonging to the Hospitaller *Johannes de Valensa* on Kos, was in September 1351 to be deprived of his habit and imprisoned: Malta 318, f. 210v, 211, 212v. Pedro Ortiz de Sotes was at Ambel in Aragon in Sep. 1351 (iii.28v), and it was probably Pedro Ortiz de Salzedo of the Priory of Castile (iii.111) who was on Kos.

36. Malta 317, f. 111; 318 f. 95: text of the latter in Luttrell (1966), p. 511.

Pedro Fernández de Heredia in 1346 (CM. i.277); Pere de Albis in 1358 (Caja 8261[1] n°. 283); and Martín de Lihori in 1378 (*infra,* ... n. 51). Fernando de Aragón was of royal descent (Carp. 689 no. 64) and so probably a *cauallero*. Pedro de Aragón was *nobilis* and presumably a *miles* (CM iv.328), while Ramón Dezprats may have been a knight as he was authorized to receive a man who was not a knight as a *freyre cauallero* (iii.222); a Gerau de Pomar was a *cauallero* in 1335 (Carp. 712 no. 57); and Albert de Joya was described in 1362 as a *Cauallero* and as *donrat linatge et persona fort Cauallerosa*.[37] That amounts to only some twelve *milites*, and others must remain unidentified.

After 1346 fewer Hospitallers bore distinguished names. The Counts of Pallars and the Abella family were nobles in Catalunya, and in Aragon the Heredia, Luna, Sessé, Gurrea, Oarriz, Pomar, Bardaxi, Peralta and Vergua were either *ricoshombres* or *caballeros*,[38] though brethren from those families may have come from cadet branches. Licences were granted in July and August 1353 for the reception as *caualleros* of Bernat, son of the *honrado don* Peregrín de Montagudo; of Martín, son of the late Miguel Martínez d'Alet; and of Frances Martínez de Peralta, *cauallero* (iii.222,228v-229,230). The origins of many brethren are obscure. Probably there were rather few *caballeros* and it is doubtful whether the condition that Hospitaller *milites* should be of noble birth was interpreted strictly.[39] The previous generation had seen King Jaume II's daughter Blanca as Prioress of Sigena until 1347, and another daughter Maria as a *freyra* of Sigena; their brother Jaume, entered the Hospital to avoid marriage in 1319, and Jaume II's illegitimate half-brother Sancho was Castellan of Amposta until his death in 1346.[40] Thus at least three children of Jaume II entered the Hospital. Furthermore, Fernando de Aragón, Commander of Uldecona and Monzón in 1346, was of royal descent (Carp. 689 no. 64; *infra,* ... n. 46), and so perhaps was Pedro de Aragón.

In the three years from April 1349 to April 1352 there were at least 123 professed male Hospitaller religious in the Castellany of Amposta; the total may have been 200 or more. Of the 123 brethren whose names are known, only 33 are identifiable as priests though there must have been many more. The number of donats is entirely unknown. The brethren's ages also remain unknown, but 14 out of 23 Hospitallers listed in a document of 1370 (v.152-153) had been Hospitallers at least since 1352. Of 18 commanders and one other *frater* named in a document of 1339 (Carp. 611 n°. 119) no less than eleven were alive in 1349, and of 24 brethren at a chapter in 1328 (CM iv.566) at least seven were alive in 1349. Leaving the identifiable priests aside, at least 47 of the remaining 90 brethren held an administrative post of some sort at some time between 1349 and 1352; how many of the 90 were knights is unknown. These statistics may be compared with those from other priories. In 1338 in 33 Provençal commanderies to the east of the Rhône there were 334 Hospitallers, of whom 72 were knights, 148 sergeants and 114 priests, and 248 donats, of whom 187 were noble. In 1338 there were 34 knights, 48 sergeants and 34 priests resident in the Priory of England. By 1373 plague and warfare had reduced numbers considerably,

---

37. Barcelona, Reg. 1180, f. 39-41v.
38. Pedro Garcés de Cariñena, *Nobiliario de Aragón,* ed. M. Ubieto Artur, Zaragoza 1983; *Actas de las Cortes Generales de la Corona de Aragón de 1362-1363,* ed. J. Ma. Pons Guri, Madrid 1982, pp. 3-4, 10; *Cortes de Caspe y Alcañiz y Zaragoza: 1371-1372,* ed. M. La. Ledesma Rubio, Valencia 1975, pp. 13-14, 26.
39. A. Luttrell, *Latin Greece, the Hospitallers and the Crusades: 1291-1440,* London 1982, I pp. 264-265.
40. J, Martínez Ferrando, *Jaime II de Aragón: su vida familiar,* I, Barcelona 1948, *passim.* Sancho's mother was María Pérez de lo Gronyo: text in *Colección de documentos inéditos del Archivo General de la Corona de Aragón,* ed. P. de Bofarul, XII, Barcelona 1856, p. 354.

and in the Priory of France, which lay north of the Loire, there may have been perhaps 250 or 300 Hospitallers. Of 178 named *fratres* in that priory, 124 were priests, 49 were sergeants and 4 or 5 knights, though other knights may have been at Rhodes; 75 percent of the 124 priests and 81 percent of the 54 military men were over 40 years of age.[41] In Aragon and elsewhere the fighting reserves of a military order could be slender indeed.

* * *

Only fully professed Hospitaller religious appear in the following list. It does not supply every reference to each *frater* or *soror*, some of whom were mentioned repeatedly, but it does record known changes of office or status. A name accompanied solely by a date indicates that nothing more than his existence as a Hospitaller is known about that man's status at that date. The documents in the Castellan's register, almost all in Aragonese, consistently referred to Hospitallers as *fray*, so that there is seldom any doubt whether persons named really belonged to the Hospital. A number of different hands wrote entries in the registers and they were highly inconsistent in spelling proper names, though they did regularly distinguish Pere from Pedro, Guillem from Guillermo and other Catalan from Aragonese forms. The forms given, without modern accents, in the list are those which seem most reasonable, for example "Ruiz" for *Royz* or "Guillem" for *Gujen*; place names are modernized and "commander" is abbreviated to "com".

ADAM PEREZ DE NUEVALOS, prior Remolinos, 26 June 1349 (i.49,52)[42]
ALBERT DE JOYA, *estaja* Orta, 9 Jan. 1350 (ii.9); *arrendador* Pueyo and regent Palau, Celas and Gavet, 5 June 1350 (ii.60v); com. Torrente de Ribera de Cinca, 5 Feb. 1352 (iii.90v)
ALFONSO FERRANDEZ GARIN, 23 June 1349 (i.39); *estaja* Zaragoza, 30 June 1349 (i.66); regent Pleytas and Coglor, 1 Sep. 1351 (iii.13-13v)[43]
ANTONI GARIN, regent Sant Miguel de Foces, 5 Feb. 1352 (iii.90v); replaced as regent Sant Miguel de Foces by 8 Feb. 1352 (iii.84v); prior Sant Miguel de Foces, 11 Feb. 1352 (iii.85v)
ARNALT DE BARDAXI, com. Añón, 26 June 1349 (i.52)
ARNALT VIDANQUE, priest with *estaja* Samper de Calanda, 24 Feb. 1352 (iii.95v); chaplain *casas* of Temple at Zaragoza, 10 Mar. 1352 (iii.113v)
ARNAU DE SALLET, *estaja* Castellote, 13 Sep. 1351 (iii.55)
ARTAL DE LUNA, 2 July 1349 (i.71); *estaja* Miravet, 9 Mar. 1352 (iii.112v)[44]
BARTOLOMEU DELA, 10 Mar. 1350 (ii.31); regent Calatayud, 9 Oct. 1350 (ii.106); replaced at Calatayud by 6 May 1351 (iii.1); lieutenant com. Calatayud, 31 Aug. 1351 (iii.10)
BARTOLOMEU DEZPRATS, com. Sant Miguel de Foces, 8 Apr. 1349 (i.86); replaced at Sant Miguel de Foces by 22 Apr. 1349 (i.57); *regidor* of *lugar* of Ripol, 23 June 1349 (i.40)

---

41. Luttrell (1987), pp. 31, 40-41.

42. Commander of Castielscar, 25 June 1346 (iii.187v); not documented after June 1349.

43. Mistakenly given as *comendador* of Pleytas and Coglor (iii.13-13v); condemned to death before Oct. 1350 for supporting the *uniones* (Carp. 590 no. 200); accused early in 1351 of "vagabonding about the world for two years" (Malta 318, f. 94-94v).

44. Artal the Hospitaller, Pedro and Leonor, *freyra* of Sigena, were children of Pedro Martínez de Luna and Marquesa de Saluzzo: Garcés de Cariñena, p. 89. Elvira, sister of the noble Pedro de Luna, was licensed to become a *freyra* of Sigena on 15 June 1357 (iv.64v). An Elvira Pérez de Luna who married Blas Maça de Vergua, and who was in 1350 a sister of Juan Martínez de Luna, had a daughter Elvira Maça: Barcelona, Reg. 665, f. 11v-12; Reg. 881, f. 81. However, no Juan Martínez de Luna had a brother Pedro; the Elvira of 1357 may have been the same person as Leonor *freyra* of Sigena and sister of Pedro de Luna.

BELENGUER DE PASSANANT, prior Ambel, 13 Apr. 1352 (iii.96)

BELENGUER DE POMAR, prior Chipriana, 4 Mar. 1352 (iii.106v)

BERENGUER DE MIRALLAS, prior castle Monzón, 10 June 1349 (i.29,30)

BERENGUER DE MOLINA, *estaja* Samper de Calanda, 9 Jan. 1350 (ii.9); *estaja* Orta; 14 May 1350 (ii.45); *estaja* Valencia, 9 Oct. 1350 (ii.103v); *estaja* Ambel, 1 Mar. 1352 (iii.102v)

BERENGUER DE MONTPAHON, com. Castellote, 8 Apr. 1349 (i.86); replaced at Castellote by 2 Jan. 1350 (ii.9v); becomes simple *freyre*.[45]

BERNAT ÇACORVELLA, 8 Apr. 1349 (i.86); abbot Alcolea, 12 June 1349 (i.30); *estaja* Caspe, 7 Jan. 1350 (ii.14v); abbot Alcolea, 4 Apr. 1350 (ii.37); *estaja* Calatayud, 6 June 1350 (ii.59v); deprived of Alcolea, 10 May 1351 (Carp. 708 no. 1)

BERNAT DE LA HORDEN, 22 Apr. 1349 (i.58)

BERTRAN DE TARRAGONA, *doctor en decretos*, 8 June 1349 (i.29); abbot Vallobar, 12 June 1350 (ii.68)

BERTRAN DE VERDU, prior Valencia, 22 Apr. 1349 (i.57); also regent Valencia, 20 Feb. 1352 (iii.92)

BERTRAN ROGER DE PALLARS, com. Caspe, 8 Apr. 1349 (i.86)

DOMINGO DE LAVATA, *cambrero* of the castle at Monzón, 12 June 1349 (i.31)

DOMINGO MARTIN alias DOMINGO XIMENEZ MARTIN, prior Alpartil, 22 Apr. 1349 (i.57)

DOMINGO NAVARRO, *clerigo* not yet Hospitaller, 26 June 1349 (i.52); *estaja* Monzón, 14 Sep. 1351 (iii.58v)

DOMINGO SENT, prior Huerto, 8 Feb. 1352 (iii.81v)

DOMINGO XIMENO DE ALBERIT, prior Añón, 26 June 1349 (i.62-64; ii.29v); prior Almunia, 5 Feb. 1352 (iii.80); also *mayordomo* of Castellan of Amposta, 30 Mar. 1352 (iii.131)

ESTEVAN DE SENT GARIELLO, *cambrero* of castle at Miravet, 12 Aug. 1349 (i.114)

EXIMEN DE BOLAS, 8 Apr. 1349 (i.86); com. Saliellas, later in Apr. 1349 (Miret, 409); replaced at Saliellas by 15 June 1349 (i.46)

FERNANDO DE ARAGON, in prison, 1349-1351[46]

FERRANT GONÇALVEZ DE MENA, com Ricla, 8 Apr. 1349 (i.86); replaced at Ricla by 6 May 1351 (iii.1); com. Olmos (Priory of Castile), 13 Sep. 1351 (iii.58v)

FERRANT LOPEZ DE LOARRE, lieutenant prior Alpartil, 2 July 1349 (i.74); *estaja* Zaragoza, 22 Dec. 1349 (ii.10); prior Juncas, 23 May 1350 (ii.54)

FERRANT RUIZ DE VALTIERRA, 8 Apr. 1349 (i.86); *estaja* Caspe, 12 Dec. 1351 (iii.48v-49)

FORTANER DE GLERA, *vicario* Sena, 5 Sep. 1351 (iii.22)[47]

FORTUN GONÇALVEZ DE HEREDIA, com. Ambel, 22 Apr. 1349 (i.57); com. Calatayud, 6 May 1351 (iii.1); replaced at Calatayud by 16 Sep. 1351 (iii.69)

FRANCISCO BOSCH, prior *Villalonga* (Villarluengo?), 12 Apr. 1351 (Malta 318, f. 92v-93)

FRANCISCO DE MIEDES, prior Temple at Zaragoza, 17 Oct. 1349 (Carp. 796 no. 17); lieutenant prior Almunia, 11 Apr. 1352 (iii.136v)

GALCERAN ÇATALLADA, com. Huesca *casas nuevas*, 8 Apr. 1349 (i.86)

GALCERAN DE ULVIA, com. Barbastro, 8 Apr. 1349 (i.86); replaced by 22 Apr. 1349 (i.70); com. Novillas, 6 May 1351 (iii.1)

GARÇI FERRANDEZ DE HEREDIA, 8 Apr. 1349 (i.86); com. Villel, 21 Dec. 1349 (ii.2); apparently replaced at Villel by 19 Apr. 1352 (iii.146v)

GERAU ÇATALLADA, com. Aliaga and Cantavella, 8 Apr. 1349 (i.86); also lieutenant of Castellan of Amposta, 9 June 1349 (i.38)

GERAU DE POMAR, possibly com. Pilvet and Añiés, 8 Apr. 1349 (i.86);[48] if so, replaced at Pilvet and Añiés later in Apr. 1349 (Miret, 409); *arrendador* Remolinos and Boquiñenich, 23/6 June 1349 (i.49); com. Sigena, 6 May 1351 (iii.1)

GERAU DE POMAR *el joven*, possibly com. Pilvet and Añiés, 8 Apr. 1349 (i.86); if so, replaced at Pilvet and Añiés later in Apr. 1349 (Miret, 409); regent Orta, 16 May 1350 (ii.45v); replaced at Orta by 31 Aug. 1351 (iii.10v)

---

45. He was accused late in 1350 of murder and of travelling to Rhodes without licence (Barcelona, Reg. 665, f. 50v-51; Malta 318, f. 94-94v); alive in 1370 (v.156).

46. On 7 July 1351 the pope requested the Master of Rhodes to pardon Fernando de Aragón, a kinsman or *consangineus* of the king, who had been in prison for two years after killing another Hospitaller: Archivio Vaticano, Reg. Vat. 145, f. 26-26v.

47. *Supra*, p...

48. Conceivably it was Gerau de Pomar *el joven* who was Commander of Pilvet and Añiés.

GIL GONÇALVEZ DEL ESPURO, 19 Feb.. 1352 (iii.93v)
GIL SANCHEZ DEL ESPITAL, 5 Feb. 1352 (iii.91)
GONÇALVO DE TORRES, prior Mallén, 25 June 1349 (i.44); replaced by 20 July 1349 (i.90)
GONÇALVO LOPEZ DE HEREDIA, *estaja* Alfambra, 17 June 1350 (ii.68)
GONÇALVO PEREZ DE HEREDIA, 12 Jan. 1350 (ii.9v)
GONÇALVO PEREZ DE MALLORCAS, chaplain San Jaime, Mallén, 24 June 1350 (ii.73); prior Añón, 7 Mar. 1352 (iii.110v)
GONÇALVO RUIZ DE CASTELBLANCH, 18 May 1350 (ii.61)
GUILLEM DE ABELLA, com. Barbastro, 22 Apr. 1349 (i.70); also regent Monzón, 10 June 1349 (i.29); com. Calatayud, 16 Sep. 1351 (iii.69)
GUILLEM DE ESTARANA, abbot San Juan Monzón, Apr. 1349 (Miret, 409)
GUILLEM DE GUIMERA, com. Orta, 8 Apr. 1349 (i.86); replaced at Orta by 16 May 1350 (ii.45v); *estaja* Caspe, 5 Oct. 1350 (ii.101v); com. Tortosa (Priory of Catalunya), 12 Feb. 1352 (ii.86)[49]
GUILLEM DE MONTBALDRON, 16 June 1349 (i.47)
GUILLEM DE PERALTA, 22 Apr. 1349 (i.57); *arrendador* Pinel, 12 Aug. 1349 (i.113)
GUILLEM VEGUER, prior Fortaner, 5 Oct. 1350 (ii.101v)
GUILLERMO DE VILLALBA, prior Cetina, 12 Apr. 1351 (Malta 318, f. 92v-93)
HUGO DE SALIELLAS, *estaja* Ambel, 13 Sep. 1351 (iii.55)
JAYME BALLESTER, *estaja* Villel, 18 Mar. 1350 (ii.31v); regent Villel, 19 Apr. 1352 (iii.146v)
JOFRE DE INGLEROLA, com. Uldecona, 8 Apr. 1349 (i.86)
JUAN DE BONUEL, prior Miravet della Sierra, 16 June 1349 (i.47)
JUAN DE ESTADILLA, regent Ariéstolas and of *la obra del puent de Monçon*, 12 June 1349 (i.30); regent Cofita and Ariéstolas, 2 July 1350 (ii.76v); lieutenant of lieutenant Monzón, 4 May 1351 (CM vi.266)
JUAN DE LA BRAÇA, 25 Mar. 1350 (ii.33)
JUAN DE MARZIELLA, prior Temple, Zaragoza, 1 Nov. 1351 (Carp. 728 no. 7)
JUAN DE NOVALLES, com. Añón, 8 Apr. 1349 (i.86); simple *freyre*, 22 Apr. 1349 (i.57); regent Almunia, Cabañas and Alpartil, 25 June 1349 (i.56); replaced at Almunia, Cabañas and Alpartil by 15 Sep. 1351 (iii.65v)
JUAN DE SANT MATHEO, habit being returned, 6 Jan. 1350 (ii.9)
JUAN DIAZ DE MENDOÇA, 8 Apr. 1349 (i.86); *estaja* Castellote, 27 May 1350 (ii.57)
JUAN FERRANDEZ DE GALVE, 12 June 1349 (i.30-31); *estaja* Azcón, 29 May 1350 (ii.58); regent Alfambra, 16 Sep. 1351 (iii.69); replaced at Alfambra by 6 Apr. 1352 (iii.137v)
JUAN FERRANDEZ DE HEREDIA, Castellan of Amposta, lieutenant of the Master of Rhodes in *Espanya* (*passim*)
JUAN FERRANDEZ DE HEREDIA, 8 July 1349 (i.81); regent Miravet della Sierra, 31 Jan. 1350 (ii.16v); regent Miravet, 6 May 1351 (iii.1v)
JUAN GONÇALVEZ DE ADEMUZ, *estaja* Villel, 12 July 1349 (i.86)
JUAN LOPEZ DE FANLO, 8 Apr. 1349 (i.86); *estaja* Miravet, 24 July 1350 (ii.84v); com. Ricla, 6 May 1351 (iii.1); regent *baylia* of Barbastro and of *casa* of Santafé in *baylia* Monzón, 15 Sep. 1351 (iii.64, 85-85v); also regent *baylias* Sant Miguel de Foces and Saliellas, 8 Feb. 1352 (iii. 84-85, 85v-86)[50]
JUAN LOPEZ DE SESSE, 18 May 1350 (ii.61)
JUAN MARTINEZ DE ALVIÇO, com. Villel, 8 Apr. 1349 (i.86); also regent Miravet, 1 Aug. 1349 (i.105); replaced at Villel by 21 Dec. 1349 (ii.2); com. Castellote and regent Miravet, 2 Jan. 1350 (ii.9v); replaced at Miravet by 6 May 1351 (iii.1v); also regent Monzón, 14 Sep. 1351 (iii.58v)
JUAN MARTINEZ DE OCON, 18 June 1349 (i.48); licensed to become a priest, 6 Jan. 1350 (ii.8v); *estaja* Calatayud, 24 May 1350 (ii.55v); *estaja* Mallén, 20 June 1350 (ii.70)
JUAN ORTIZ DE LAS ERAS, 13 Dec. 1349 (Carp. 724 no. 16)
JUAN TALLADA, abbot Ontiñena, 12 June 1349 (i.30)

---

49. Went to Rhodes with complaints against the Castellan in 1351 (*supra*, p.   ); claimed to belong to the Priory of Catalunya, 5 Oct. 1350 (ii.101v).

50. The texts of 8 Feb. 1352 called him *comendador* and even *comendador sobrano et mayor de las dichas baylias*, of which he was really regent. On 5 Feb. he was, perhaps in error, described as Commander of Ricla (iii.90v); on 12 Feb. 1352 as Commander of Barbastro (iii.87); and on 17 and 18 Apr. as Commander of Barbastro and Saliellas, in a text granting him possession of the *baylias* of Barbastro, Saliellas and San Miguel de Foces (iii.141v, 142v).

JUAN XIMENEZ DE SAYAS, *estaja* Añón, 15 June 1350 (ii.67); *clerigo* regent priory Añón, 7 Mar. 1352 (iii.111)
JUAN YUNYIS DE MONTAGUDO, 29 May 1350 (ii.58)
LOP RUIZ DE ESPEIO, 8 Apr. 1349 (i.86); com. Castieliscar, 22 Apr. 1349 (i.57); replaced at Castieliscar before 29 Feb. 1352 (iii.103v)
MARCO DE VILLAGRANADA, com. Valencia, 8 Apr. 1349 (i.86); com. Ambel, 6 May 1351 (iii.1)
MARCO TALLADA, com. Huesca *casas antiguas*, 8 Apr. 1349 (i.86)
MARTIN DE LIHORI, com. Castieliscar, 8 Apr. 1349 (i.86); com. Mallén and Noviellas, 22 Apr. 1349 (i.57); com. Mallén only, 6 May 1351 (iii.1)[51]
MARTIN DE MONTANYANA, prior Nuevo but recently dead, 30 Mar. 1350 (ii.35v)
MARTIN GONÇALVEZ DE HEREDIA,, *estaja* Mallén, 24 May 1350 (ii.55v)
MATHEO CORVARAN, 16 June 1349 (i.47); prior Nuevo, 30 Mar. 1350 (ii.35v)
MIGUEL DE MORILLAN, *estaja* Caspe, 17 Feb. 1350 (ii.24)
MIGUEL FORTUNYO, 12 Aug. 1349 (i.111)
OCHOVA MIGUEL DE ALDAVA, prior Zaragoza, 4 Feb. 1350 (Carp. 733 no. 40)
PEDRO AYNAR DE ANDUES, *estaja* Zaragoza, 9 Mar. 1352 (iii.112)
PEDRO DE ARAGON, com. Samper de Calanda, 8 Apr. 1349 (i.86)
PEDRO FERRANDEZ DE HEREDIA, 8 Apr. 1349 (i.86)
PEDRO FERRANDEZ DE LINYAN, 8 Apr. 1349 (i.86); com. Pilvet and Añiés, later in Apr. 1349 (Miret, 409); com. Castieliscar, 29 Feb. 1352 (iii.103v)
PEDRO LAYN, *estaja* Monzón, 6 Aug. 1349 (i.108); *arrendador* Grisén, 22 June 1350 (ii.72)
PEDRO LOPEZ DE ANYON, prior Mallén, 20 July 1349 (i.90); prior Ambel, 6 May 1351 (iii.1v); prior Mallén, 7 Mar. 1352 (iii.110v)
PEDRO LOPEZ DE GURREA, 13 Dec. 1349 (Carp. 724 no. 16)
PEDRO LOPEZ DE VERGUA, 8 Apr. 1349 (i.86); com. Sant Miguel de Foces, 22 Apr. 1349 (i.57); also com. Saliellas, 15 June 1349 (i.46); lieutenant of lieutenant Monzón, 19 Oct. 1351 (CM vi.268)
PEDRO MARTINEZ DE ARCAYNA, com. Calatayud, 8 Apr. 1349 (i.86); replaced at Calatayud by 9 Oct. 1350 (ii.106); simple *freyre*, 6 May 1351 (iii.1v);[52] regent Almunia, Cabañas and Alpartil, 15 Sep. 1351 (iii.65v)
PEDRO ORTIZ DE SOTES, apparently at Ambel, 10 Sep. 1351 (iii.28-28v)
PEDRO RUIZ DE SOTES, 18 Jan. 1350 (ii.11)
PEDRO RUIZ DE ARANDA, 12 June 1349 (i.34); *estaja* Calatayud, 1 July 1349 (i.68); *estaja* Monzón, 9 July 1349 (i.81)
PEDRO SANCHEZ DE ALIAGA, 8 Apr. 1349 (i.86)
PEDRO SANCHEZ DE NAVAS, *estaja* Calatayud, 27 July 1349 (i.95); *estaja* Azcón, 29 May 1350 (ii.58); *sergent* with *estaja* Castieliscar, 31 Mar. 1352 (iii.102v)
PEDRO YENEGUEZ NAVARRO, *estaja* Monzón, 4 Aug. 1349 (i.107)
PERE AVENIELLA, 22 Apr. 1349 (i.60)
PERE ÇATALLADA, 8 Apr. 1349 (i.86)
PERE DE ALBIS, com. Torrente de Ribera de Cinca, Apr. 1349 (Miret, 409), also *mayordomo* of Castellan of Amposta, 19 July 1349 (i.89); com. Zaragoza, 22 June 1351 (Carp. 714 no. 52)
PERE DEL BOSCH, 22 Apr. 1349 (i.58)
PERE DE VILARAMON, 10 Sep. 1351 (iii.32)
PERE MALLA, 8 Apr. 1349 (i.86); *estaja* Monzón, 20 May 1350 (ii.52)[53]
PERE PINEDA, 10 June 1349 (i.29); *estaja* Orta, 27 Jan. 1350 (ii.14v); lieutenant of lieutenant of Monzón, 16 Feb. 1352 (CM vi.309)
RAMON DE LIMINYANA, 10 Sep. 1351 (iii.32)
RAMON DE VAL, prior Grisén, 25 June 1349 (i.41)
RAMON DEZPRATS, com. Azcón, 8 Apr. 1349 (i.86)

---

51. In 1378 Lihori had a *deudo de parentesco* with Juan Fernández de Heredia and was a *cauallero*: Barcelona, Reg. 1745, f. 33-33v.
52. Condemned to death for supporting the *unión* and arrested in Barcelona while on his way to Rhodes in Nov. 1350: Carp. 590 no. 200.
53. Probably the Pere Mallada of 5 Feb. 1352 (iii.91).

RODRIGO PEREZ DE HEREDIA, *estaja* Alfambra, 17 Feb. 1350 (ii.25); *estaja* Samper de Calanda, 14 May 1350 (ii.45)
RODRIGO YENIGUEZ DE MOROS, com. Alfambra, 8 Apr. 1349 (i.86); replaced at Alfambra by 16 Sep. 1351 (iii.69); lieutenant of lieutenant Monzón, 20 Jan. 1352 (CM vi.304); simple *freyre*, 5 Feb. 1352 (iii.91)
RUY GONÇALVEZ BUGIA, 8 Apr. 1349 (i.86)
SANCHO DE AGUILLON, *estaja* Huesca *casas antiguas*, 13 Sep. 1351 (iii.55); *estaja* Orta, 8 Feb. 1352 (iii.81)
SANCHO DE OARREZ, 13 Dec. 1349 (Carp. 724 no. 16)
SANCHO DE ODINA, 1 Nov. 1351 (Carp. 728 no. 7)
SANCHO LOPEZ DE CASSEDA, 12 June 1349 (i.30)[54]
SANCHO LOPEZ DE SESSE, com. Zaragoza, 3 June 1349 (Carp. 719 no. 12); com. Orta, 31 Aug. 1351 (iii.10v)
SANCHO MARTINEZ DE BATERNAY,[55] 4 July 1350 (ii.81)
SIMON PEREZ DE MOLINA, *estaja* Villel, 17 Feb. 1350 (ii.25); regent Alfambra, 6 Apr. 1352 (iii.137v)
VITA DE CASTELCLAR, prior Almunia, 22 June 1349 (i.42); replaced at Almunia by 5 Feb. 1352 (iii.80)

FREYRAS OF SIGENA

FRANCISCA DE CASTELLET, 5 Sep. 1351 (iii.22)
GUISABEL DE ALAGON, 5 Sep. 1351 (iii.22)[56]
ISABEL SAURNIA DE FIGARUELAS[57]
MARIA PEREZ DE MONEBA, 6 May 1351 (iii.18)
SANCHA DE SAU, *sacristana*, 6 May 1351 (iii.18)
SANCHA XIMENEZ DE UNCASTIELLO, *clauera*, 6 May 1351 (iii.18)
TODA PEREZ DE ALAGON, 5 Sep. 1351 (iii.22)
URRACA ARTAL CORNELL, *prioressa*, 3 June 1349 (Caja 8127[1] i.174)[58]
VIOLANTE DE RIBELLAS, 6 May 1351 (iii.18)

---

54. Ordered to go to Rhodes on 20 June 1350 (ii.70) but at Sigena on 6 Sep. 1351 (iii.24).
55. Possibly Paternoy near Jaca.
56. Subprioress on 17 Nov. 1347 following the resignation of Blanca de Aragón when the king sent an envoy to overcome a revolt and control the election of Blanca's successor: Barcelona, Reg. 1128, f. 145-145v.
57. Subprioress, 7 Mar. 1349 (*supra*, p...); Miret, p. 537, gives her as prioress in 1380, but M. de Pano, *Las prioras Cornel de la Real Casa de Sigena*, "Linajes de Aragón", 7 (1916), p. 203, shows she was never prioress.
58. Provided by papal bull of 21 Aug. 1347, according to Pano, p. 206; this provision may have provoked the revolt mentioned in Nov. 1347 (*supra*, p... n. 56).

XIV

The Economy of the Fourteenth-Century Aragonese Hospital

The Aragonese members of the Order of Saint John of Jerusalem were fully professed religious who took the standard vows of poverty, chastity and obedience, and who followed the liturgical routine of an order of the Roman Church according to a rule approved by the pope. In the fourteenth century the Hospitallers' fundamental purpose as brethren of a military order was that of armed resistance to the infidel. Their priory in Aragon, an administrative unit known as the *Castellanía de Amposta*, was an important component of Aragonese society, especially after 1317 when the acquisition of the properties of the dissolved Order of the Temple greatly increased the extent of the Hospital's landed holdings. In 1409/14 the Order held over 100, or approximately a quarter, of the *señoríos* or lordships in Aragon, which made it the greatest single landholder in the kingdom, owing at least 56,000 sueldos, amounting to some 29 percent, of the general tax known as the *monedatge*, according to partial statistics which covered less than half the kingdom; it held over 4300 hearths in Aragon and considerable estates with a further 2700 hearths in southern Catalunya. In about 1350 a total of perhaps some 200 Hospitallers lived in 29 preceptories, one of them in Valencia, with probably well over 30,000 dependents subjects. From these houses they recruited brethren and managed their estates so as to produce, in theory, a nucleus of brethren to send to the Eastern Mediterranean and, above all, the monetary surplus owed as *responsiones* to the Convent or headquarters on distant Rhodes which constituted the central point of the Hospital's military confrontation with the Mamluks and Turks[1].

1   A. Luttrell, «Hospitaller Life in Aragon: 1319-1370», in *God and Man in Medieval Spain: Essays in Honour of J. R. L. Highfield*, ed. D. Lomax - D. Mackenzie (Warminster, 1989), provides background, terminology and bibliography; the works there cited of J. Delaville le Roulx, J. Miret y Sans, S. García Larragueta, A. Forey and Ma. L. Ledesma Rubio remain fundamental and contain much supplementary bibliography. Further details and statistics are given in A. Luttrell, «The Structure of the Aragonese Hospital: 1349-1352», in *Primeres Jornades sobre els Ordes Religiosos-Militars als Països Catalans (segles XII-XIX)* (forthcoming), using specially F. Arroyo Ilera, «División señorial de Aragón en el siglo XV», *Saitabi*, xxiv (1974). The Castellany's archives are in Madrid, Archivo Histórico Nacional, Sección de Órdenes Militares, Llengua de Aragón [AHN]; the Castellan's registers are in Madrid, Sección de Códices, 599B-604B [RA i-vi]. Sueldos are normally those of Jaca into which other monies are converted at approximately 10 to 11 sueldos to the florin of Aragon. Part of this research was completed with the assistance of a Vicente Cañada Blanch Fellowship from London University and of support from the Leverhulme Foundation which was provided through the Venerable Order of Saint John of Jerusalem; I am extremely grateful for both.

Technically, the priory or *Castellanía* was governed by the Castellan and by its chapter, but the latter met only irregularly. Castellan and chapter established the main lines of policy and they authorized leasings, modified *responsiones*, granted or confirmed preceptories and supervised much other business; they were also responsible for the monies due to the Treasury at Rhodes[2]. Yet for most brethren and their subjects the Hospital's effective administrative and economic unit was not so much the Castellany as the local preceptories, occasionally known in Aragonese as *comendadorias*, into which the Castellany was divided. Those houses in which one or more Hospitaller brethren were resident were normally governed by a Hospitaller preceptor, or in certain circumstances by a lieutenant known as a *tenient* or *regidor*, who was responsible for the community's religious and disciplinary life as well as for its economic management and for a wide variety of local affairs; preceptors sometimes held more than one house and occasionally they were absentees.

With certain exceptions, each preceptory corresponded to a *baylia*, an economic and financial entity which owed the Castellan a portion of its incomes as *responsiones* and which could, with the requisite licence, be farmed out by its preceptor either to another Hospitaller or to a secular; the farmer was to manage its temporal affairs but did not necessarily exercize jurisdiction as preceptor over the house's Hospitaller brethren. Preceptors or others holding a *baylia* could, with superior permission, lease all or part of it, but could not make permanent alienations or mortgages without special permission. The renting of fields, houses and so forth was often recorded in a contract, the Castellan giving the preceptor or his representative a licence, sometimes rehearsed in the written lease or *treudo*, to fix payments and expenses[3]. The distinction between preceptory and *baylia* became increasingly marked as the administration of the Order at the local level changed into a more exclusively financial operation. The development of the *baylia* into a business investment became especially evident among the more mercantile Catalans. When in 1409 the Master's procurator granted to the lieutenant governing the Priory of Catalunya four magistral *baylias* or *cambras* and all the Master's other incomes in the priory for one year for 2200 *lliures*, the lieutenant simply farmed the whole concession to two merchants of Barcelona for exactly the same sum[4]; the merchants must have expected a profit while the lieutenant was spared the risks and troubles of administering the *baylias* and collecting their incomes.

The collection of local dues was a perpetual concern. A *libro delas responssiones* for the whole Castellany existed by 1370[5]. Preceptors had to present in chapter a series of accounts and receipts to show that they had no debts, that they had paid proper maintenance and dress allowances to those in their houses, and so forth[6]. In 1350 the Preceptor of Valencia was instructed to bring to chapter the accounts for the *baylias* of Miravet and Azcón relating to the years when the late Castellan, Fr. Sancho de Aragón, had held them, as well as some of Fr. Sancho's monies and plate. The personal goods, the *spolia* or in Aragonese *despullya*, of deceased brethren normally went to the Castellan or to the central Treasury, while the revenues of a *baylia* from the day of its incumbent's death until the next chapter, which were known as the *mortuarias*, usually went to the Castellan or to the Treasury, as did the *vagantes* or vacancies which were the profits for the subsequent year. However, those matters depended on the deceased's status while the relevant regulations were continually being changed, especially where they concerned incomes from *camere* or *cameras*, that is of *baylias* which were reserved to the Castellan or the Master or which were within their gift; these incomes were beyond capitular control[8]. Preceptors also paid small sums as their *pitança d'ultramar* which were destined to support the brethren of the Hispanic *langue* or nation serving at Rhodes[9].

---

2   Eg. texts in A. Luttrell, «Los Hospitalarios en Aragón y la Peste Negra», *Anuario de Estudios Medievales*, iii (1966), 509-514.
3   Cf. Luttrell (1989), 106-109.
4   J. Miret y Sans, *Les Cases de Templers y Hospitalers en Catalunya* (Barcelona, 1910), 451.
5   RA v, f. 160.
6   Luttrell (1989), 108-109.
7   RA ii, f. 21 v.-22.
8   A. Luttrell, «The Hospitaller's Western Accounts: 1373/4 and 1374/5», in *Camden Miscellany*, xxx (London, 1990), 4-5 *et passim*. In 1349 the Castellan's three *camere* were Zaragoza, Monzón and Miravet which had in 1320 circa together provided almost a third of the Castellany's incomes: Luttrell (1989), 107.
9   Eg. RA v, f. 187; vi, f. 7 v.

THE ECONOMY OF THE FOURTEENTH-CENTURY ARAGONESE HOSPITAL

The Hospital's rule stated that one third of its incomes was due as *responsiones*, but it gave no clarification as to what expenses were to be taken into account in calculating incomes[10]. Nothing approaching a third of total incomes was actually paid during the fourteenth century, and in reality there were considerable fluctuations in the amounts demanded and much non-payment. Before 1307 the Templar's Aragonese preceptories, which often paid partly in kind, apparently provided about ten percent of their incomes[11]. The amount theoretically due from each Hospitaller *baylia* depended on what had traditionally been owed, and it was in practice determined by the overall sums, periodically varied, which the Convent at Rhodes demanded from the Castellany[12]. There were frequent cases of debt and arrears, though an exception occurred in 1353 when the Preceptor of Huesca Nueva paid 3180 sueldos of *responsiones* in advance for the years 1354, 1355 and 1356, securing a considerable advantage since he would otherwise have owed 4500 sueldos at 1500 sueldos a year[13].

The era of conquest and settlement, with arrangements designed to defend new lands and increase their productive manpower, was largely over by 1300. The Hospitallers' colonization techniques were similar to those of the Templars and their absorption of the Temple's lands after 1317 brought only minimal disruption, but there were variations between one region and another. Though the *domus* itself was often situated in a town, the Castellany's wealth was predominantly agricultural. In Zaragoza and Huesca in particular, there were rents from houses, shops and other properties, but incomes came mainly from rural estates in northern and central Aragon and especially from the irrigated valleys of the Ebro and its tributaries which produced wine, olives, vegetables and, above all, cereals. These lands had been acquired and consolidated through donations, purchases and exchanges, and they were improved and exploited by programmes of irrigation, settlement and planting. Alienations to nobles, to clergy or to others who might claim immunity from the payment of dues were prohibited. The social and legal status of those who lived on the Hospital's domains varied greatly; some were effectively serfs who were tied to the land but were free of the heavier oppressions often inflicted by the nobility and were exempt from much royal interference, while others were reasonably free. The simple peasant with an individual lease was not necessarily an *hombre* or *vasallo* owing military service.

After 1300 the Hospital retained an incalculable, but probably rather small, part of its land under direct management as its demesne or *dominicatura*, together with a number of slaves and oxen available to work it. The brethren preferred to lease properties for rents, which apparently provided the bulk of the Castellany's incomes. Payment was either in cash or kind, as a proportion of produce or in fixed quantities. Individual leases were for short periods, for life or even in perpetuity; there were also improvement contracts *ad plantandum* and share-cropping arrangements *ad medietatem*. Scattered lands were more likely to be rented to individuals, while leasing was especially advantageous where whole communities could be made responsible for a single group payment. The result was a wide range of small peasant exploitations rather than a regime of extensive *latifundias*. *Cartas pueblas* often regulated collective agrarian contracts with farmers, serving to impose contributions and labour services, and to enforce the Hospital's lucrative monopolies on justice and fines, on mills, ovens, smithies, baths and irrigation works in such a way as to extract the maximum proportion of surplus production[14].

---

10 J. Riley-Smith, *The Knights of St. John in Jerusalem and Cyprus: c. 1050-1310* (London, 1967), 344-346; the Hospital was still declaring that it was paying a third in 1291: texts in J. Delaville le Roulx, *Cartulaire général de l'Ordre des Hospitalliers de S. Jean de Jérusalem: 1100-1310*, iii (Paris, 1900), nos. 4147, 4168, 4283.

11 A. Forey, *The Templars in the "Corona de Aragón"* (London, 1973), 323-324; various attempts to use the detailed Templar texts of 1289 and 1307 and the Hospitaller survey of 1320 circa to establish useful overall statistics are frustrated by numerous variables and difficulties in interpreting technical terms and data.

12 Cf. Luttrell (1989), 107-110.

13 RA iii, f. 227 v.-228.

14 Background in Forey, *Templars* (1973), and Ma. L. Ledesma Rubio, *Templarios y Hospitalarios en el Reino de Aragón* (Zaragoza, 1982); see also A. Conte, *La Encomienda del Temple de Huesca* (Huesca, 1986). Ma. L. Ledesma Rubio, *La Encomienda de Zaragoza de la Orden de San Juan de Jerusalén en los siglos XII y XIII* (Zaragoza, 1967), and A. Ubieto Arteta, *El real monasterio de Sigena: 1188-1300* (Valencia, 1966), do not cover the period after 1319. For lists of peasants', vines, trees, animals, poultry, agricultural produce implements, clothing, household goods and their prices in 1273, see A. Forey, «A Thirteenth-Century Dispute between Templars and Hospitallers in Aragon», *Durham University Journal*, lxxx (1988). For a Hospitaller «villa de señorío» studied briefly across seven centuries, G. Carranza Alcalde, *Historia de Mallén* (Zaragoza, 1988).

Parts of southern Aragon had largely been depopulated in the course of the reconquest and were still being settled and defended during the thirteenth century. For example, in 1264 and 1267 the Templars attempted to attract first twenty Christian families and then thirty Muslim families to Villastar between Teruel and Villel. Except at Aliaga which they had not received from the crown, the Hospitallers were not established in the south before acquiring the extensive Templar holdings there after 1317. They inherited the Temple's *carta puebla* at Villastar where a few settlers owed the usual *diezmos* and *primicias*, contributions in produce and wine, taxes on their flocks and some military service. From Villel, with its irrigated gardens surrounding the castle, the Hospital governed some 200 square kilometres of pastoral and hunting country[15]. A broad band of territory, much of it in the possession of the military orders, stretched across the domains of the Order of Montesa in northern Valencia and those of the Hospital, mostly acquired from the Temple, in southern Catalunya and southern Aragon; these were buttressed by the Aragonese possessions of the Order of Santiago centred on Montalbán and those of Calatrava around Alcañiz[16]. This disposition largely lost its original strategic purpose as a security belt, but these extensive land holdings retained that essentially rural character of those great estates which became typical of the lands of the Hispanic military orders once they no longer retained a significant frontier function[17].

The monotonous agrarian world in which many Hospitallers were immersed offered only local excitements and activities. Individual brethren spent much time renewing leases and collecting rents for houses, fields and vineyards, matters recorded in notarial acts often witnessed by several of the Hospitallers present[18]. Some accounts kept by the preceptory at Villel at some point between 1323 and 1339 listed those inhabitants of the town and surrounding areas, including a miller and a shepherd, who paid *censes*, usually a few sueldos, for their *quinchas* or holdings; some had two *quinchas*. There were *huertas* or gardens, vines, a beehive and a shop; the various quarters of Villel contained, in addition to houses, a square, a mill, an oven, some threshing floors, a tower and a tannery. Receipts from Villel, Libros and Villastar totalled 645 sueldos plus some wax and chickens. This was apparently the income for a whole year since the payments were collected partly at Lent, partly at Michaelmas and partly at Christmas. The area paid annual *cena* taxes of 400 sueldos to the king and 133 sueldos 4 dineros to the *gouernador*, presumably the Governor of Aragon. The sums totalled 533 sueldos 4 dineros, of which the town of Villel paid 266 sueldos 8 dineros, the preceptor paid 133 sueldos 4 dineros and the outlying *aldeas* or villages provided the other 133 sueldos 4 dineros *por composicion*; Riodeva gave 66 sueldos 8 dineros, Villastar 44 sueldos 4 dineros and Libros 22 sueldos 2 dineros[19]. An undated account book for the Preceptory of Alfambra north of Teruel showed repeated small cash payments for wine, oil, beef, beans, salt, rice, shoes, nails and an axe, and for work on the mill and its irrigation *açut*. One item concerned 250 eels and another involved four animals which carried goods to Villel for two brethren. The expenditures recorded across nine months amounted to 480 sueldos 8 dineros[20].

15   Ma. L. Ledesma Rubio, «La colonización del Maestrazgo turolense por los Templarios», *Aragón en la Edad Media: Estudios de Economía y Sociedad*, v (Zaragoza, 1983); idem, «La formación de un señorío templario y su organización económica y social: la Encomienda de Villel», *Homenaje a José María Lacarra*, ii (Pamplona, 1986); A. Gargallo Moya, «La carta-puebla concedida por el Temple a los moros de Villastar: 1267», *Actas del III Simposio Internacional de Mudejarismo* (Teruel, 1986).

16   A. Ubieto Arteta, *Historia de Aragón: La formación territorial* (Zaragoza, 1981), 266-275; C. Laliena Corbera, «Les Ordres militaires et le Repeuplement dans le Sud d'Aragon (XIIIe siècle)», in *Les Ordres militaires, la Vie rurale et le Peuplement en Europe Occidentale (XIIe-XVIIIe siècles) = Flaran*, vi (Auch, 1988); see also R. Sáinz de la Maza Lasoli, *La Orden de Santiago en la Corona de Aragón: la Encomienda de Montalbán: 1210-1327* (Zaragoza, 1980); idem, *La Orden de Santiago en la Corona de Aragón: 1327-1357* (Zaragoza, 1988); and, predominantly on Calatrava, C. Laliena Corbera, *Sistema social, estructura agraria y organización del poder en la Edad Media: siglos XII-XV* (Teruel, 1987).

17   On Jaume Vicens Vives' notion of «anti-economic» orders with their «régimen de latifundios», see A. Luttrell, «Las Órdenes Militares en la sociedad hispánica - Los Hospitalarios aragoneses: 1340-1360», *Anuario de Estudios Medievales*, xi (1981).

18   Of the numerous *treudos* in AHN, those for Zaragoza in Carps. 796-843 are sampled in Ma. L. Ledesma Rubio, «La Orden de San Juan de Jerusalén en Zaragoza en el siglo XIV» , in *La Ciudad de Zaragoza en la Corona de Aragón* (Zaragoza, s. d.).

19   AHN, Sección de Códices, 648 B, f. 452-473, datable to the time of Fr. Pedro Sánchez de Fanlo, Prector of Villel between 1323 (*ibid.*, f. 124-126) and 1339 (*ibid.* f. 444).

20   Barcelona, Arxiu de la Corona d'Aragó [ACA], Varia de Cancillería 4 (apparently post-1312); similar Hospitaller text of 1416 for Vallfogona, Catalunya, in Miret 564-568.

THE ECONOMY OF THE FOURTEENTH-CENTURY ARAGONESE HOSPITAL

The Templar preceptory at Villel was already paying 400 sueldos for the *cena* in 1307[21]; in that year it owed a miserable 350 sueldos as *responsiones*[22] while its annual incomes were estimated at 3000 sueldos in 1320 circa[23]. The *censes* at 645 sueldos provided about a fifth of those incomes, and much of the rest must have come from *diezmos* and *primicias*. The crown and Castellany each took a half of the *monedatge*, a tax on property which was collected supposedly every seven years. When the royal collector of that tax came to Villel in 1342 he drew up a list of contributors in collaboration with the *justicia* and sworn *homens buenos*, while the preceptor was quick to insist on the Castellan's rights. The neighbouring communities were levied in roughly the same proportions as for the *cena*. Villel had 253 contributors, Villastar 23, Riodeva 61 and Libros 5, making a total of 342; all the inhabitants of Cabrioncello had moved to Riodeva; Alfambra had 265 contributors, Orrios 43 and Alcalà 142. From all these places the crown and the Hospital seem each to have received 1988 sueldos[24]. The Hospitallers, who continually sought to maintain their lands in cultivation, declared in 1350, soon after the first onset of the great plague, that they would welcome new settlers at Cabrioncello[25].

The wealth which the Castellan and certain individual Hospitallers were able to amass from the Castellany did not derive merely from agrarian activities. Urban rents, profits of justice, fines raised after the great revolts of 1347 and sundry other incomes were significant. There was a minor trade along the Ebro river to the sea; in 1351 the Castellan was granted personal rights to have a *carregador* or small port at Ulldecona whence he was licensed to export wheat, barley, wine and other goods[26], and in 1354 the Hospital contracted to sell wood from Fortaner and Pitarch which was to be delivered in agreed measures at Caspe for 156,000 sueldos of Barcelona, perhaps 143,000 sueldos of Jaca[27]. Quantities of timber from the *baylia* of Aliaga and elsewhere were sold and transported down the Ebro[28]. Waters and mills were also lucrative, if contentious, assets[29]. Basically the Castellany's wealth was agrarian, but the Hospital and its subjects also had their flocks and the disputes which came with them; in 1287, for example, the Hospital's men of Añón were robbed of over 700 sheep[30]. Inventories of the direct possessions of Templar houses made in 1289 showed 28 oxen, probably for agricultural work, at Miravet and 30 at Cantavella; 31 mares and 1380 unspecified others animals, probably sheep and goats, at Miravet; 78 mules, 182 pigs and 1061 other animals at Monzón; 1060 goats at Orta; 539 sheep at Alfambra; and 652 sheep at Cantavella[31]. Declining population did not necessarily result in a switch from agriculture to grazing. In 1412, for example, the chapter of the Castellany granted the grazing land, the *devessa* or *mont*, of Ador to the Moorish *aljama* of Caspe for forty years with obligations to plough and cultivate, to preserve certain trees and to pay rents in cash and kind[32]. Brethren might have their own flocks and herds, and in 1357 Fr. Berenguer de Montpahon, Preceptor of Castellote, was allo-

21   A. Forey, «Cena Assessments in the *Corona de Aragón*: the Templar Evidence», *Gesammelte Aufsätze zur Kulturgeschichte Spaniens*, xxvii (1973), 285.

22   Forey, *Templars* (1973), 415-419, assuming one *mazmodina* was worth 5 sueldos.

23   Text in Miret, 399-400; not all expenses had been deducted from this figure, while it did not include incomes from the Templar churches subsequently acquired by the Hospital. Templar Castellote apparently paid *responsions* of 630 sueldos in 1307: text in Forey, *Templars* (1973), 415-419. Its total incomes were apparently 13,000 sueldos in 1320 circa: text in Miret, 399. They were sold for 8,000 sueldos a year in 1313: texts in Sáinz de la Maza Lasoli (1980), 363-364, 370-371.

24   ACA, Real Patrimonio 2394 (damaged: the figures are uncertain); J. Russell, «The Medieval Monedatge of Aragon and Valencia», *Proceedings of the American Philosophal Society*, cvi (1962), confused the analysis, wrongly supposing that the Hospital's holdings did not pay this tax.

25   ... *Empero si algunos pobladores vienen a poblar et a fazer se vezinos en el dicho lugar nuestro del Cabrioncello, nos los entendamos a fazer mucho mayor gracia:* RA ii, f. 25 v.

26   ACA, Reg. 894, f. 39.

27   Text in Miret, 406-407.

28   Eg. RA. ii, f. 38 v.-39; iv, f. 75 v.; f. 113-114.

29   F. Castillón Cortada, «Política hidráulica de Templarios y Sanjuanistas en el Valle de Cinca (Huesca)», *Cuadernos de Historia Jerónimo Zurita*, xxxv-xxxvi (1979).

30   ACA, Reg. 74, f. 43.

31   Forey, *Templars* (1973), 238-239; Ledesma Rubio (1982), 203-205; statistical analysis, with some confusions, in M.-C. Gerbet, «Les Ordres militaires et l'Élevage dans l'Espagne médiévale (jusqu'à la fin du XVe siècle)», in *Les Ordres militaires, la Vie rurale et le Peuplement en Europe Occidentale (XII-XVIIIe siècles)* = *Flaran*, vi (Auch, 1986), 98-99. There seem to be no fourteenth-century Hospitaller statistics for animals in Aragon.

32   Text in G. Colás Latorre, *La Bailía de Caspe en los siglos XVI y XVII* (Zaragoza, 1978), 173-175.

wed to keep the animals he had when he left the preceptory, since they were his personal *joyas* and did not belong to the *estamiento* of the *baylia*[33]. In 1377 a preceptor in Catalunya left his house deserted in the care of a slave, taking with him the eight oxen which belonged to the *baylia*[34].

Slaves were expensive and the Aragonese Hospitallers apparently possessed few of them after 1300[35], but they did govern Moorish communities which were allowed their religious, legal and fiscal independence. Numerous Moors farmed and irrigated the Order's estates in central Aragon or worked as artisans and builders in their own *mudéjar* style, exploited but protected by the Hospital[36]. At Caspe, for example, the Hospital dealt with two quite separate communities and institutions: a Christian *consejo* and a Moorish *aljama* or *morería*[37]. In 1352 a Moorish «knight» whom the Hospital had purchased and held in captivity at Miravet was granted to a Castilian Hospitaller for him to exchange with a kinsman in Moorish hands[38], and in 1366 the Preceptor of Añón fled to Castile taking with him from Ambel thirty-three Moors of both sexes for whom he demanded ransom as hostages[39]. The *mudéjares* of Azcón in southern Catalunya were badly treated; when in 1323 they protested against increases in their labour services the Hospitallers refused to show the Moors a copy of the royal privilege which they had lost[40], but in 1369 their *alcayt* was confirmed in his right to judge the Moors there and they were to keep their slaughter house[41]. When, in 1394, Fr. Juan Fernández de Heredia was endowing his foundation at Caspe with the Moorish place of Exatiel, its *saraceni* inhabitants did homage on a Koran in the possession of the Hospitaller representative, using Arabic phrases they may not even have understood to swear *Por Uille Ille Alladi, le Ileha, Illehua, e por el Alquiba*[42]. This was the first part of a standard Aragonese version corrupting the Arabic words meaning «By God, except whom there is no God, and by the *qibla*», the *qibla* being the direction towards which Muslims prayed[43].

The Castellany had to share parts of its incomes with the crown, with the secular church and with its own lay chaplains, stewards, lawyers and other employees; it faced expenditures on pensions, interest on loans and the maintenance of its own brethren and houses. Any alienation of rights or incomes in return for annual payments or any change from rents in kind to rents paid in cash was theoretically disadvantageous, since it was difficult subsequently to raise the sums owed in order to keep pace with inflation. Hospitallers could not be certain what might be in the Order's best interests, but they had long been acquainted with the practical side of agrarian business management and local government, with precise accounting, crop yields, prices, and marketing[44]; preceptors must usually have had a realistic understanding of the situation in their own *baylia*, but the Castellany's financial records could scarcely have provided an accurate overall balance sheet of its affairs.

The long-established system of preceptories and *responsiones* suited an institution which needed to create surplus wealth in its Western possessions and to transfer it to the East. The Hospital was unlikely to change its universal Western arrangements, but alternative models were conceivable. In 1320 the new Valencian Order of Montesa surveyed its resources, which in 1325 circa brought in the annual equivalent of 135,000 sueldos of Jaca. The bulk of this income came from *diezmos* and

33   ... *ganados grossos et menudos et otras joyas et cosas en sp[eci]al vnas vacas qu'el tenje d'vna muller de Moriella:* RA iv, f. 61.
34   ACA, Gran Priorato de Catalunya, Armari 24, vol. 20, f. 12 v.-13.
35   However in 1395 the Catalan house at Barberà had a slaves' room, the *cambra hon jaen los esclaus:* text in Miret, 562-564.
36   Ma. L. Ledesma Rubio, «Notas sobre los Mudéjares del Valle del Huerva: Siglos XII al XIV», *Aragón en la Edad Media: Estudios de Economía y Sociedad (siglos XII al XV)*, iii (Zaragoza, 1980).
37   Cf. Colás, 91-107.
38   RA iii, f. 142-142 v.
39   ACA, Reg. 1388, f. 22.
40   J. Ma. Font Rius, «La Carta de Seguridad de Ramón Berenguer IV a las Morerías de Ascó y Ribera del Ebro (siglo XII)», *Homenaje a Don José María Lacarra de Miguel en su Jubilación del Profesorado: Estudios Medievales*, i (Zaragoza, 1977).
41   RA v, f. 126-127.
42   AHN, Carp. 606, no. 21.
43   Cf. R. Burns, *Islam under the Crusaders: Colonial Survival in the Thirteenth-Century Kingdom of Valencia* (Princeton, 1973), 216-218.
44   Cf. T. Bisson, «Credit, Prices and Agrarian Production in Catalonia: a Templar Account, 1180-1188», in *Order and Innovation in the Middle Ages: Essays in Honor of Joseph R. Strayer*, ed. W. Jordan *et al.* (Princeton, 1976).

primicias which functioned in effect as an income tax on the order's subjects; rent payments or *censos*, in cash or kind, were a minor matter. The rearrangement of the former Hospitaller and Templar preceptories in Valencia was carried out by the new order whose first three brethren and first two Masters were former Hospitallers. They were in a position to make sweeping initial changes to a comparatively small and compact institution. The Master of Montesa had to be supported from the Valencian preceptories whereas the Hospitaller Master's incomes came predominantly not from the priories and preceptories but from the Rhodian islands. Other funds, allotted to the *Clavero*, were needed to finance the defence of Montesa castle and of Valencia's, southern Moorish frontier. The preceptory system was drastically revised; the economy was reorganized to maximize incomes from rents since these could more easily be assigned to particular functions, leaving the preceptories largely as financial units rather than as centres of community or liturgical life. The Master received the incomes of one *baylia*, that of Cervera, while Montesa castle was maintained from the revenues of Perpuchent which were paid to the *Clavero*. The preceptories received 38.5 percent of the incomes of the other *baylias* and the remaining 61.5 percent went to a central *fondo comun* which in turn transferred part of those monies to the *Clavero*. Such, crudely, was the situation in 1330, but as the Moorish threat receded the Master acquired control of the *fondo comun* and by 1430 the incomes of the *Clavero* had been much reduced[45].

Following the great revolt of 1347 the Castellan was able to impose on his rebellious subjects many heavy fines and advantageous new collective contracts[46], but the great plague and disastrous weather conditions combined with endless warfare to produce a major depression. The population at Monzón eventually fell from perhaps about 2500 in 1293 to less than half that number in 1397[47]. After 1347 the Hospital faced a death roll of perhaps a quarter or a third of its subjects and the flight of many agricultural labourers who were unable to pay their rents, while in some areas the Castilian invasions caused further casualties, desertions and expenditures after 1356. It became extremely difficult to find new tenants, and the Hospitallers' reaction was direct and explicitly motivated; for several decades it remained essential to try to maintain cultivation and prevent abandonments by keeping men on the land through large-scale reductions and postponements of rents[48]. Only a fraction of the Castellany's revenues, the total of which was virtually incalculable, was exported to Rhodes, especially as the *responsions* and other dues were seldom, if ever, paid in full. Very large sums went to the crown as war subsidies or were corruptly diverted to the Castellan and other Hospitallers, or to their kinsmen and clients, but these monies may well have come from extraordinary impositions, alienations or loans rather than from regular incomes. The annual *responsiones* theoretically due to Rhodes stood at well over 27,000 sueldos in 1329˙and at about 40,000 sueldos in 1364/5[49]. For the two years 1393/4 and 1394/5 the *responsiones* and other dues actually paid to the Receiver-General amounted to no more than 40,000 sueldos, that is 20,000 sueldos a year[50].

The institutions of preceptory and *responsiones* continued to create and transfer wealth for the Hospital. The growing practice of renting and sub-renting *baylias* probably brought some financial advantage at the cost of an erosion of community life in many preceptories. The Aragonese brethren were certainly capable of progress and innovation, but after 1317 they merely absorbed the Templar's preceptories into the Hospital's existing administrative framework, which was broadly similar to that of

---

45   L. García-Guijarro Ramos, *Datos para el Estudio de la Renta feudal maestral de la Orden de Montesa en el siglo XV* (Valencia, 1978); see also E. Guinot Rodríguez, *Feudalismo en Expansión en el Norte valenciano: Antecedentes y desarrollo del Señorío de la Orden de Montesa - Siglos XIII y XIV* (Castellón, 1986), and E. Díaz Monteca, «Notes documentals per l'Estudi de la Unió al Maestrat de Montesa: s. XIV», *Boletín de la Sociedad Castellonense de Cultura*, lxi (1985). The Montesa statistics are crude and Guinot's terminology ambiguous, but the outlines seem clear; they offer only a rough and hypothetical guide to the Hospital's situation.

46   Luttrell (1989), 102; *idem*, «The Aragonese Crown and the Knights Hospitallers of Rhodes; 1291-1350», *English Historical Review*, lxxvi (1961), 17-18.

47   A. Sesma Muñoz, «Demografía y Sociedad: la Población de Monzón en los siglos XIII-XV», *Homenaje a José María Laccara*, ii (Pamplona, 1986).

48   Text and details in Luttrell (1966).

49   Luttrell (1989), 113-115.

50   Valletta, National Library of Malta, Archives of the Order of St. John, Cod. 329, f. 65-69 v./73-73 v.

the Temple. Soon after 1319 the Castellany's incomes were estimated at 332,000 sueldos a year[51]. If the *responsiones* due from it were well over 27,000 sueldos in 1329, the *responsiones* expected amounted perhaps to about ten percent of incomes, as apparently had also been the case with the Aragonese Templars[52]. After 1347 the number of brethren to support probably dwindled, while wool production and stock raising may well have increased. Incomes seem to have come above all from taxes on produce rather than from fixed rents. Rigorous, sometimes brutal, management and the rewriting of contracts after 1347 served to reinforce monopolies and increase the Order's share of production. The Hospitallers were well aware of the need to expand agrarian output by continuing to encourage settlers and to irrigate new land, and they were wisely prepared to reduce rents in order to avoid leaving fields uncultivated during hard times. The Hospital may have been an essentially agrarian and reactionary organization but it succeeded quite competently in countering and surviving the economic crises of the fourteenth century.

---

51 Hospitaller text in Miret, 379-402; the interpretation of the figures given is debatable.
52 Profits of presumably more than 8000 sueldos apparently paid *responsions* of 630 sueldos at Templar Castellote (*supra* 729, note 23), suggesting, with many reservations, a rate of less than 8 percent.

XV

The Hospitaller Priory of Catalunya in the Fourteenth Century*

The brethren of the military–religious Order of the Hospital of St John of Jerusalem had been established in Catalunya since the early twelfth century. By 1319, however, they were confronted with many changes.[1] The city of Acre and the surviving remnants of the Latin kingdom of Jerusalem had been lost in 1291, but by 1310 the Hospitallers had completed the conquest of Rhodes and had moved their Convent, or headquarters, to that island. The French king's assault on the Templar order in 1307 and its dissolution by the pope in 1312 gave all the military orders a profound shock and raised searching questions about their proper role. The transfer of the Templars' lands greatly increased the Hospital's territories but involved administrative difficulties which led in Catalunya to the foundation of a new Hospitaller priory in 1319. These events did not alter the fundamental organization of the military orders or the canonical status of their individual members. Hospitallers continued to be religious who belonged to a regular order. Whether priests, *milites*, sergeants or sisters, they all took vows of poverty, chastity and obedience which bound them to a common liturgical life of

---

*This is an English version of 'El Priorat de Catalunya: el Segle XIV', *L'Avenç* [Barcelona], 179 (March 1994), pp. 28–33.

[1]The principal documentary source is the Archivo del Gran Priorato de Catalunya (AGP) now in Barcelona, Arxiu de la Corona d'Aragó (ACA); it was used extensively in J. Miret y Sans, *Les Cases de Templars y Hospitalers en Catalunya* (Barcelona, 1910), and partially in J.-M. Sans i Travé, 'Guillem de Guimerà', *Arrels: Miscel.lania d'Aportacions històriques i documentals de l'Espluga de Francoli*, III (Espluga de Francoli, 1989). Additional studies, using the fragments of the Hospital's central archives now in Malta, are: J. Delaville le Roulx, *Les Hospitaliers à Rhodes jusqu'à la mort de Philibert de Naillac: 1310–1421* (Paris, 1913); A. Luttrell, *The Hospitallers in Cyprus, Rhodes, Greece and the West: 1291–1440* (London, 1978); idem, *Latin Greece, the Hospitallers and the Crusades: 1291–1440* (London, 1982); idem, *The Hospitallers of Rhodes and their Mediterranean World* (Aldershot, 1992). See also P. Bertran, 'L'Orde de l'Hospital a Catalunya: els Inicis', *L'Avenç* [Barcelona], 179 (March 1994). There are studies concerning individual commanderies: eg. L. Ma. Figueras Fontanls, *El Senyoriu de Celma: una aproximació històrica* (Valls, 1985). The activities of the priory conceived as a whole rather than as a series of studies of individual commanderies require more attention; especially important are the prioral registers for 1377–1379 and 1399–1400 in AGP 537–538.

2

prayer according to a rule and statutes which had papal approval. All were dedicated to a holy war against infidels and pagans, but it was more important than ever that they were forbidden to become crusaders. Technically the crusade depended on occasional papal proclamations which by the fourteenth century frequently directed crusades against Latin and other Christians; on the other hand, the holy war waged against the infidel by the military orders was theoretically continuous, perpetual and independent of papal proclamation, while they were forbidden to fight fellow Christians. Many Hospitallers, including the priests and sisters, never actually bore arms against an infidel, but all helped to sustain their order through their membership and prayers and by raising the monies sent as *responsiones* to sustain the Convent. After 1291, however, Latin Syria was lost and in the Hispanic peninsula the reconquista had become slow and, especially for the Catalan brethren, distant.

From about 1310 onwards the overall government of the Hospital and its major military activities were centred at Rhodes, but the Order held lands, privileges, exemptions, houses, churches, hospices, cemeteries and other rights and possessions throughout the Latin West. These properties were organized in provinces, such as that of Spain, which were divided into priories; the priories were subdivided into commanderies.[2] Each commandery or *domus* was supposedly a centre of religious life and liturgy in which new members were recruited and to which elderly ones could retire. It was a unit of economic exploitation, known in Catalan as a *battlia,* which was destined to support its own resident community and to produce *responsiones* in surplus cash. The commandery was also a point of contact between the brethren and the general public on whose support they ultimately depended. The commander or *preceptor,* who could be a *miles,* a sergeant or a priest, governed the *domus* and its members, held weekly chapters and was responsible for paying the *responsiones.* The *battlia* or *baylia* involved no element of obedience or jurisdiction over brethren but constituted the purely secular and economic part of the commandery. A commander could, with superior licence, rent his *battlia* to another Hospitaller or to a secular, but he could not normally alienate, sell or pawn it.

*

* *

The internal life of the commanderies scattered across Catalunya naturally depended on their relationship with the rest of a society in which ideas were changing, and in particular on the policies of the government. By 1300 the crown, which had been extremely generous to the military orders in the earlier expansive phase of the reconquista, was seeking to recover territories, incomes

---

[2]Those who talk of the military orders as having an 'estructura feudal' are using the term in an extremely wide sense which has nothing whatsoever to do with the fief.

and rights which it had alienated, and it feared and resented powerful exempt corporations under foreign control. When in 1308 and 1309 the Templars in Aragon defended their castles against royal attacks, King Jaume II claimed that the Templars' lands within his domains should be used to create a new national order devoted to the war against the infidel within the Hispanic peninsula. When the pope granted the Templars' lands to the Hospital in 1312 the Hispanic kingdoms were excluded from that arrangement, and only in 1317 was it finally agreed that the Hospital would have the Templars' lands in Aragon and Catalunya, but that both the Hospitaller and the Templar properties in Valencia would pass to the new order of Montesa which should defend the Granada frontier. Included in this agreement was the provision that the rulers of the Hospital in Aragon and Catalunya could not enter into the administration of their offices until they had in person done *juramentum* and *homagium* to the king, a concession which was effectively to allow the crown a veto on appointments to the government of the Order within its kingdoms.[3]

Despite the loss of its Valencian territories, the Aragonese priory, known as the *Castellanía de Amposta*, became so large that in 1319 it was divided into two. The new Priory of Catalunya included Majorca and three commanderies in Roussillon, which formed part of the Kingdom of Majorca until the Aragonese king reconquered it in 1344. In order that the *Castellanía* and the priory be approximately equal in size, the four commanderies in Southern Catalunya south of the Ebro, including the great Templar castle at Miravet, remained in the *Castellanía*. In 1320 the Priory of Catalunya consisted of 29 *domus*, including that of Majorca, and the female house at Alguayre. At that time total incomes, apparently calculated before the deduction of expenses, were 19,662 *lliures* of Barcelona; of this sum the Commandery of Mas Déu, which seems to have included all the incomes from Roussillon, was valued at 3000 *lliures*. The Templar properties at Barcelona and Perpignan were sold before 1319, but the rest of the Templars' Catalan houses, excluding Orta, Ascó and Miravet which remained in the *Castellanía*, apparently produced over half the total of 19,662 *lliures*. The incomes of the *Castellanía* were 20,100 *lliures* of Barcelona.[4] In about 1410 approximately 24 per cent of the lordships in Aragon belonged to the Hospital which possessed more than 4300 *focs* or hearths in that kingdom with a further 2700 in Southern Catalunya; in 1366 the Priory of Catalunya possessed at least 2281 *focs*.[5]

---

[3]Luttrell (1978), XI, pp. 6–7; map in *Gran Enciclopèdia Catalana*, VIII (Barcelona, 1975), p. 503.

[4]Text in Miret, pp. 399–400; the totals seem acceptable, though the original is lost and the figures as given do not add up correctly.

[5]A. Luttrell, 'The Structure of the Aragonese Hospital: 1349–1352', in *Actes de les Primeres*

Nominations to the Priory of Catalunya made by the Master and chapter-general at Rhodes were repeatedly contested by successive kings. The first prior, Fr Ramon de Ampurias, a noble of licentious habits who had once been excommunicated, was frequently involved in debts, violences and property disputes.[6] The Master of the Hospital attempted to circumvent royal resistance by naming lieutenants who would not owe homage, by having incomes from the Kingdom of Majorca paid directly to Rhodes, by invoking papal intervention, and by reserving the priory and its incomes to himself. In response, the crown could impose embargos on men and money leaving for Rhodes. The royal candidate was excommunicated in 1331. In 1347 Fr Pere Arnau Perestorts, then serving at Rhodes as General of the Hospital's galleys, was elected prior; King Pere III attempted unsuccessfully to oppose him, since he had previously fortified the castles of the Hospital in Roussillon in defence of the King of Majorca. There were further scandals in 1364 when the prior, Fr Vidal Alquer, was suspended after incurring huge debts and illegally selling and mortgaging Hospitaller properties. In 1372 the priory was given to the *Castellán de Amposta*, Fr Juan Fernández de Heredia, and in 1379, soon after he had become Master of Rhodes, he appointed Fr Guillem de Guimerà as Prior of Catalunya.[7]

The nomination of the prior was not simply a matter of patronage but involved issues vital to the crown. Hospitaller brethren sat in the parliament or *corts*, served in royal armies and played a significant part in the administration of the many areas they controlled. Their privileges, jurisdictions and exemptions were extensive. The main matters of dispute concerned taxation, military service and jurisdictions. The priory could not avoid all obligation to provide troops, who were mostly not Hospitaller brethren, for royal campaigns and especially for service against the infidels of Granada. For example, in 1320 the priory commuted its obligations on the Granada frontier for 30,000 *sols*, and in 1342 the king summoned 40 *equites* from the priory for service on the Granada frontier. The king was especially annoyed when brethren from the priory fought against him in Roussillon during his war with Majorca in 1344. There were repeated demands for subsidies and aids for campaigns in Sardinia, Castile and elsewhere, and for coronations, royal marriages and so on. The king also attempted, in 1329 and 1331 for example,

---

Jornades sobre els Ordes Religioso-Militars als Països catalans: segles XII–XIX (Tarragona, 1994); J. Iglesies Fort, 'El Fogaje de 1365–1370: Contribución al Conocimiento de la Población de Catalunya en la segunda midad del siglo XIV', *Memorias de la Real Academia de Ciencias y Artes de Barcelona*, ser. II, XXIV (1962), pp. 281–285.

[6]Miret, p. 404; Delaville, pp. 64–66; Luttrell (1978), XI, pp. 8–11; idem (1992), III, p. 74; G. Meloni, 'L'Attività in Sardegna di Raimondo d'Ampurias, dell'Ordine dell'Ospedale di Gerusalemme', *Anuario de Estudios Medievales*, XI (1981).

[7]Delaville (1913), pp. 66–67, 122, 171–172, 181-183; Luttrell (1978), XI, pp. 7–16.

to reduce the amount of money leaving Catalunya for Rhodes in the form of *responsiones*.[8]

*

* *

In 1377 there were 25 commanderies and one female convent in the priory, plus 10 other places where there was a church ruled by a Hospitaller priest as its *prior*.[9] In 1373 the three Roussillonais houses of Mas Déu, Bayoles and Orla contained 9 priests, 3 sergeants and 3 *milites*, an average of 5 *fratres* per house.[10] In about 1350 the *Castellanía de Amposta* had possibly some 200 brethren in 29 commanderies, maybe 5 or 6 per house. The number of *milites* varied greatly from one priory to another; the Priory of Catalunya perhaps had 200 or 250 brethren and maybe some 40 *milites*, a few of them at Rhodes, plus perhaps 10 to 20 *sorores* at Alguayre.[11] The prior administered his brethren and houses through letters, by travelling around the priory and at an annual chapter. The prior had no fixed seat and no central archive, though documents were deposited in a number of major houses. Chapters were held at varying seats, and especially at Espluga de Francoli. By 1377, at the latest, the prior had a register for his outgoing letters, and in particular it recorded admissions and expulsions of brethren, litigations, leases of property, licences to travel, mandates for brethren to take up residence in a particular house, liturgical matters, the renting of *battlias*, copies of inventories of certain commanderies and, above all, business concerning *responsiones* and money. In 1377 the priory's commanders were summoned to a chapter to choose the unrealistically large number of 16 knights and 16 squires for the Hospital's coming expedition against the Turks, and to bring the monies they owed. They were instructed to take to the chapter 'the inventories of the state of your houses which should be sealed with the seals of the brethren of the houses, and that the brethren should be paid their clothing allowance and the companions should be paid their wages'.[12]

---

[8]Luttrell (1978), XI, pp. 8–16; P. Ortega, 'Aragonesisme i Conflicte Ordes/Vassalls a les Comandes templeres i hospitaleres d'Ascó, Horta i Miravet : 1250–1350', *Anuario de Estudios Medievales*, XXV (1995).

[9]AGP 537 *passim*.

[10]Archivio Vaticano, Collectorie 438, f. 1–24.

[11]Figures, extremely hypothetical, in Luttrell (1992), XV, p. 103; cf. P. Bertran i Roigè, 'Les Ordinacions del Convent d'Alguaire', *Cuadernos de Historia Económica de Catalunya*, XVII (1977).

[12]Examples in AGP 537, f. 1–1v *et passim* used in Miret, where some texts from it are published; on Hospitaller life in Aragon, Luttrell (1992), XV, *passim*; on the prior's residence and itinerary, P. Bertrán i Roigé, 'Les Despeses del Gran Prior de Catalunya de l'Orde de Sant Joan de Jerusalem: 1419', *Miscel.lania de Textos Medievals*, VI (Barcelona, 1992).

Of the 25 commanderies of the priory in 1377, at least 11 had originally belonged to the Templars and six or more other places which had once been Templar houses were in Hospitaller hands but were not then being administered as commanderies. The Hospital had town houses in Barcelona, Lleyda, Tortosa and Vilafranca de Panedès, but most of its commanderies were rural in character, some of them fortified. They had chapels and cemeteries, stables and living quarters for the brethren and for other dependents, and these were sometimes arranged around a courtyard with outer walls and towers. In a few places the Hospital also controlled a lay parish.[13] The largest and richest house was at Mas Déu. This was in ruins by about 1495 when it was reported 'that the said place of Mas Déu is a strong castle, walled and moated and furnished with a thick wall and with many towers, a ditch and a drawbridge and other dispositions necessary to a strong place.'[14] In 1373 the commander at Gardeny had his own room, and in 1377 the commander and the senior priest at Bayoles both had a room and a bed; in 1395 Barberà had 'the room where the slaves sleep'.[15] The commanders administered discipline. They faced much local violence and repeated disputes over jurisdictions. They leased out urban houses and agricultural lands, and were responsible for economic and financial matters. In theory the commander presided over a religious community but by the late-fourteenth century some houses had been leased to seculars or had only one or two brethren in residence. Thus in 1373 at Orla in Roussillon there was a commander who was a priest and one sergeant, four *boverii*, two *famuli* and an *ancilla* or female servant.[16] A series of accounts and inventories showed that the commanderies and their chapels were reasonably, though not luxuriously, furnished; on the other hand, they mentioned few arms or objects indicative of any military preparedness.[17]

The military orders had long acquired and grouped estates through donations, purchases and exchanges, and they showed considerable expertise in their management and financial accountability.[18] Though there were some

[13]Summaries and plans in J. Fuguet Sans, *Templers i Hospitalers*, I: *Guia del Camp de Tarragona, la Conca de Barbarà, la Segarra i el Solsonès* (Barcelona, 1997).

[14]Cited in J. Brutails *et al.*, *Inventaire sommaire des Archives Départementales: Pyrénées – Orientales: Archives Ecclésiastiques Série G* (Perpignan, 1904), p. 40.

[15]Texts in Miret, pp. 555–559, 560–561, 562–564.

[16]Archivio Vaticano, Collectorie 438, f. 10v–12v.

[17]For example, texts in Miret, pp. 555–564.

[18]T. Bisson, 'Credit, Prices and Agrarian Production in Catalonia: A Templar Account, 1180–1188', in W. Jordan *et al* (ed.), *Order and Innovation in the Middle Ages: Essays in Honor of Joseph R. Strayer* (Princeton, 1976); A. Conte, 'Trets precapitalistes en l'Economia templera a la Corona d'Aragó: l'Exemple d'Osca', *L'Avenç*, 161 (1992). The agricultural management of the priory awaits study.

rents from town houses, the main revenues came from agriculture with seigneurial rights over justice, ovens and mills also providing incomes. Some estates were farmed directly, for example by the four *boverii* of 1373 at Orla, where in 1377 the commander had taken away the house's eight oxen and had left it uncultivated in the charge of a slave.[19] Like other large landed corporations, the priory certainly suffered the economic decline and demographical disasters which resulted from poor climate, warfare and above all the great plague which arrived in 1347. Many lands were leased for rents, and after 1347 the only way to retain their cultivators and avoid the abandonment of the land was to lower rents and incomes. Thus in 1359 the prioral chapter reduced tributes at Artesa in the Commandery of Gardeny since the place was almost completely depopulated as a result of the plague and its lands were uncultivated. In 1377 the same was true near Lleyda where 'in the place of Escaravat there lives no one.'[20] Unlike many religious orders, the Hospitallers could not merely live off their incomes in kind or cash but had also to produce a surplus in money to send to Rhodes. This may have encouraged a preoccupation with finance as opposed to production which increasingly showed itself in the leasing of *battlias*, in whole or in part, to laymen. Thus in 1409 when the proctor of the Master of Rhodes rented to the prior's lieutenant four Catalan commanderies and other incomes belonging to the Master for one year at 2200 *lliures*, the lieutenant simply subrented the whole concession to two merchants of Barcelona at the same price. That was a purely financial operation through which the lieutenant renounced all profit but avoided trouble and risk; the *battlias* involved had become merely financial units.[21] Towards the end of the fourteenth century the leading Catalan Hospitallers were engaging in numerous transactions in which they bought, sold, rented, exchanged and mortgaged the priory's properties, jurisdictions and incomes under a variety of contracts and investments.[22]

These money-oriented activities of the leading brethren partly reflected their origins in a society in which the provincial nobility mingled with the urban patriciate, above all that of Barcelona. Many Catalan Hospitallers were priests or sergeants, and the *milites* must have been a minority. The *milites* included men of noble families such as Fonollet, Guimerà, Maissen, Erill, Sarrera and Pomer. But despite the regulations of the Order, there were other Hospitaller *milites* who would not have been knights in secular life. There were no formal proofs of nobility in the fourteenth century, though evidence of a noble self-awareness was evident in the many items

---

[19]AGP 537, f. 12v–13.
[20]Text in Miret, pp. 410–411; Luttrell (1978), XIV, pp. 505, 507.
[21]Texts in Miret, pp. 449–453.
[22]Texts and references in Sans i Travé, pp. 19–20, 54–69 *et passim*.

mentioned in the inventories as bearing the *senyals* or arms of noble brethren. Pressures grew to exclude the bourgeoisie, perhaps because economic conditions reduced the total wealth of the priory. This was reflected in the growing tendency for commanders to hold two or more houses and for small houses to be united into a single commandery. In 1437 attempts were made to exclude the non-military burgesses of Barcelona who protested their nobility, and when in 1438 the son of a 'notable merchant of Barcelona' attempted to become a Hospitaller *miles* and alleged the noble connections of his mother, a commission was formed to take evidence so that 'his lineage, customs and life should be seen and known'.[23] Fr Guillem de Guimerà, prior from 1379 until his death in 1396, had quite exceptionally a personal tomb, but he was a notoriously corrupt Hospitaller who served frequently in the *corts* and had held the highest office as deputy of the Governor General of Catalunya. His administrative and military talents coupled with royal favour brought him success and eventually the priory, but he died leaving enormous debts. As the second son of the lord of Ciutadilla, Guimerà belonged to the petty nobility. He could afford considerable expenses, especially on buildings adorned with his arms in his commandery at Barberà and on the marrying of his two illegitimate daughters. Since his borrowings and mortgagings had been made without superior authorization they were technically illegal, for a religious could neither own nor alienate property, and so after his death the Order refused to repay his creditors.[24]

The number of Catalan Hospitallers at Rhodes was not large, but the island served as a base for Catalan merchants and pirates in the East and there was a small Catalan community there.[25] Service at Rhodes was a path to promotion for Catalan brethren, who might also secure the office of *drapperius* or Drappier reserved to the *langue* of Spain at Rhodes. The most important Catalan to reside there was the Roussillonais Fr Pere Arnau Perestorts who became Prior of Catalunya while at Rhodes. In 1348 he donated a house at Rhodes for Catalan Hospitallers so that in future they should not have to beg for lodgings as he himself had had to.[26] There were always a few others at Rhodes; for example, Fr Pere Tholoni, Commander of Barcelona, in 1365; Fr Rigaut de Nicosia, Commander of Gardeny, in 1366; Fr Francesc Zammar, licensed to sell houses and lands at Rhodes, in 1381; Fr Ramon de Majorca, lieutenant of the Drappier and Commander of the Duchy of Athens, in 1382; and Fr Garsia de Maissen, lieutenant of the Drappier, in 1403. In 1393 the Drappier, the Catalan Fr Pere de Vilafranca,

---

[23]Texts in Miret, pp. 430–431, 555–564; cf. Luttrell (1982), I, pp. 264–265; idem (1992), XV, p. 105 n. 60; Figueras, pp. 136–137.

[24]To Sans i Travé, add especially AGP, Armari 24, Legs. 1 and 5A.

[25]Luttrell (1978), XIII, *passim*.

[26]Luttrell (1978), XI, p.16.

was repairing the 'hospice of the *langue* of Spain' at Rhodes, and in 1403 eight Hispanic brethren, four of them from the Priory of Catalunya, constituted the *langue* of Spain and received a new *frater* , a Catalan.[27] At times the Catalan financial contribution was as meagre as that of its manpower, and the crown must certainly have profited more from the priory than did the Convent at Rhodes. In 1329 the king proposed that the *responsiones* be limited to 2000 florins, a figure he changed in 1331 to 3000 florins; in 1347 the amount theoretically owed was 5000 florins; in 1364 the Hospitallers' treasurer at Avignon accounted for only 700 florins received from Catalunya.[28] The two years 1370/71 and 1371/72 produced at least 4520 florins.[29] In 1373/74 the treasurer at Avignon received 2742 florins of *responsiones*, 1711 florins of a special impost and 950 of arrears, a total of 5403 florins; in 1374/75 he received 2900 florins of *responsiones* and 1769 of impost, totalling 4669 florins. The grand totals received at Avignon in those years were 42,230 and 46,830 florins, of which the Catalan priory contributed approximately 11 per cent.[30] During the papal schism which began in 1378 many priories refused to pay *responsiones* to Rhodes, yet considerable sums continued to be sent from Catalunya to the treasurer at Avignon: 2183 florins in 1380, 2000 florins of arrears for 1382/84, increasing to 20,327 florins paid jointly with the *Castellania de Amposta* in 1385/86 and 7738 florins from Catalunya alone in 1386/87.[31] The chapter of the Priory of Catalunya complained in 1398 that only nine of 21 priories were contributing; the Catalans had to pay 3600 florins a year plus heavy and sometimes ruinous special imposts or *taylles,* sometimes amounting to one third of all incomes, which included 2000 florins demanded from the prior, 1000 florins from Mallorca, 600 from Mas Déu and 500 from Granyena.[32]

The first hundred years of the Priory of Catalunya was a period of unequal achievements in which quarrels and the corruption were accompanied by limited but real contributions to the maintenance of the Hospitallers at Rhodes. The crown was only partly successful in its aim of controlling appointments and attaining the quasi-nationalization of the priory. The Catalan Hospital retained most of its landed property and was to use it to some effect in the future when two Catalans became Masters of Rhodes, Fr Antoni

---

[27]Valletta, National Library of Malta, Archives of the Order of St John, Cod. 319, f. 123v, 131v; 321, f. 108, 217v–218; 326, f. 149; 333, f. 56.

[28]Luttrell (1978), XI, p.10 *et passim.*

[29]Malta, Cod. 16 no. 35.

[30]Text in A. Luttrell, 'The Hospitallers' Western Accounts, 1373/4 and 1374/5', in *Camden Miscellany,* XXX (London, 1990), pp. 8, 11, 18.

[31]Malta, Cod. 48, f. 7, 58, 88, 118, 143v–145v, 146; these are partial figures.

[32]Text in Miret, pp. 456–458; cf. Figueras, pp. 134–137.

Fluvià from 1421 to 1437 and Fr. Ramon Zacosta from 1461 to 1467, and the Catalan priory was to make considerable contributions to the defence of Rhodes during the dangerous period after the Mamluk conquest of Cyprus in 1426 and during the sieges of Rhodes between 1440 and 1444 and again in 1480.[33]

---

[33]Miret, pp. 434–440; Luttrell (1978), XIII pp. 389–390.

XVI

GLI OSPEDALIERI E UN PROGETTO PER LA SARDEGNA: 1370-1374

Pietro IV d'Aragona durante il suo lunghissimo regno, iniziato nel 1336 e conclusosi nel 1387, cercò costantemente una soluzione al problema della Sardegna dove ai difficili rapporti con i « giudici » o re d'Arborea si aggiungevano altri problemi riguardanti, in particolare, la politica di Genova nel Tirreno ed i rapporti con il papato che, da quel lontano 1297 – anno dell'infeudazione da Bonifazio VIII a Giacomo II d'Aragona – considerava il « regno di Sardegna e Corsica » un possedimento della Chiesa di Roma [1]. Per la soluzione di questi problemi Pietro IV tentò una molteplicità di iniziative di tipo militare e diplomatico e, nel 1370, preoccupato per le conseguenze che avrebbe potuto avere sull'isola regnicola e sulla stessa corona d'Aragona la guerra scoppiata qualche anno prima con Mariano IV d'Arborea, propose un curioso ed improbabile progetto di scambio di terre.

Dopo la distruzione dell'ordine dei Templari, avvenuta tra il 1307 e il 1312, numerose furono le iniziative tendenti alla fondazione di nuovi ordini militari o alla trasformazione di quelli esistenti [2]. Nel 1317 le terre già possedute dai Templari e quelle appartenenti agli Ospedalieri nel regno di Valenza andarono a costituire il patri-

---

[1] Sulle vicende della Sardegna negli anni 1297-1420 vedi F. CASULA, *Profilo storico della Sardegna catalano-aragonese*, Cagliari 1982; IDEM, *La Storia della Sardegna da Mieszko I di Polonia a Ferdinando II d'Aragona*, Sassari 1985; vedi anche L. BROOK, F. CASULA, M. COSTA, A. OLIVA, R. PAVONI, M. TANGHERONI, *Genealogie Medioevali di Sardegna*, Cagliari 1984.

[2] H. FINKE, *Papsttum und Untergang des Templerordens*, 2 voll., Münster 1907; A. LUTTRELL, *Gli Ospitalieri e l'Eredità dei Templari: 1305-1378*, in *I Templari: Mito e Storia*, a cura di G. MINUCCI e F. SARDI, Sinalunga-Siena 1989, pp. 67-86.

504

monio del nuovo ordine di Montesa e, intorno a quell'anno, Roberto d'Angiò re di Napoli propose che tutti i beni dei Templari siti nei regni di Giacomo II d'Aragona venissero incamerati nei possedimenti regi in cambio della rinuncia del monarca aragonese alle sue pretese alla Sardegna, che sarebbe stato dato a Federico d'Aragona in cambio della Sicilia [3].

Qualche anno più tardi, nel 1322/23, Roberto d'Angiò intervenne ancora una volta sulla questione, proponendo che, sempre in cambio della rinuncia di Giacomo II alle sue pretese al regno di Sardegna, uno dei figli del re aragonese incamerasse nella sua *senyoria* tutti i beni degli Ospedalieri i quali, nel 1317, erano entrati in possesso dei beni che i Templari avevano in Aragona e in Catalogna. Se questa soluzione non fosse apparsa idonea il sovrano angioino proponeva di utilizzare i beni dell'ordine di Montesa siti nel regno di Valenza [4]. Uno scambio di questo genere era stato attuato proprio nel 1317 per iniziativa del papa Giovanni XXII che aveva trasferito ad un suo nipote tutti i possessi dei Templari e degli Ospedalieri nella contea Venaissin, compensando l'Ospedale con terre nell'Italia del sud [5].

Nel 1345 incirca cominciò una serie interminabile di trattative, portate avanti soprattutto da fra' Juan Fernández de Heredia, il Castellán de Amposta priore degli Ospedalieri in Aragona, tendenti ad ottenere il passaggio a quest'ordine delle terre possedute in Aragona dagli ordini castigliani di Santiago e di Calatrava in cambio dei beni che erano appartenuti ai Templari in Castiglia e che teoricamente erano stati assegnati all'Ospedale [6].

Intorno all'agosto del 1370 Pietro IV riprendeva questo progetto e, per mezzo dei suoi ambasciatori Ramón de Peguera e Francesch Roma, che si trovavano ad Avignone per trattare della questione sarda con il papa Urbano V, al quale spettava approvare ogni mutazione dei possessi degli ordini [7], il re Pietro propose che le terre

---

[3] Documento pubblicato da H. FINKE, *Acta Aragonensia*, II, Berlino-Leipzig 1908, p. 718.

[4] Documento pubblicato da A. ARRIBAS PALAU, *La conquista de Cerdeña por Jaime II de Aragón*, Barcellona 1952, pp. 372-374.

[5] Documento pubblicato da C. FAURE, *Étude sur l'Administration et l'Histoire du Comtat Venaissin du XIII au XV siècle: 1229-1417*, Parigi 1909, pp. 204-207.

[6] Alcuni dettagli in A. LUTTRELL, *La Corona de Aragón y las Ordenes Militares durante el siglo XIV*, in *VIII Congreso de Historia de la Corona de Aragón*, II parte 2, Valencia 1970, pp. 67-77.

[7] Non è il caso di studiare qui tutti i dettagli di queste lunghe trattative, con i re-

aragonesi degli ordini castigliani di Calatrava e di Santiago venissero annesse ai possedimenti dell'ordine di Montesa oppure che, considerate lo stato di guerra tra Aragona e Castiglia, venissero rese di fatto indipendenti dai loro maestri castigliani e che i loro precettori dovessero essere *naturals* del re d'Aragona [8].

Il sovrano avanzava, inoltre, un'ardita proposta che nelle sue intenzioni avrebbe potuto risolvere la difficile ed annosa questione sarda: i « giudici » d'Arborea avrebbero dovuto lasciare la Sardegna rinunciando a tutti i loro possessi in quest'isola in cambio di varie terre possedute dagli Ospedalieri in Italia [9]. La proposta venne rinnovata nel novembre dello stesso anno e sostenuta con la tesi che tale scambio sarebbe stato vantaggioso anche per l'Ospedale dal momento che la Sardegna era molto fertile e in grado di fornire vettovaglie e altri prodotti a Rodi: *per ço car la terra de Serdenya es molt fertil e porien sen acorrer de viandes en Rodes e en altres parts.* I precettori italiani allora reggenti le terre che sarebbero passate in possesso del « giudice » sarebbero stati trasferiti in precettorie ma sostituiti successivamente da *naturals* del re provenienti dalla Catalogna o dall'Aragona, oppure inviati *en la terra ferma deça mar,* ossia nella penisola iberica, mentre in Sardegna sarebbero stati nominati subito dei precettori catalani o aragonesi. Tutto questo sarebbe stato preceduto, naturalmente, da una stima accurata del valore delle terre italiane e sarde. Se il papa, il maestro dell'ordine e gli stessi Ospedalieri non fossero stati d'accordo, il re si dichiarava disposto ad offrire loro alcune città reali della Sardegna [10].

Questo singolare progetto non ottenne alcun consenso e nel

---

lativi problemi della datazione di carte e capitoli, alcuni dei quali copiati nei registri reali soltanto verso il 1373/74, quindi qualche anno dopo la loro utilizzazione ad Avignone. Il documento dell'[agosto?] 1370 si trova nell'Archivio della Corona d'Aragona di Barcellona (in seguito: A.C.A.), Reg. 1240, ff. 101-104, ed è stato pubblicato da J. VIVES, *Galeres catalanes enviades al papa Urbà V*, in « Analecta Sacra Tarraconensia », VIII (1932), pp. 82-85; documento del 29 settembre 1380 in A.C.A., Cartas Reales Pedro IV n. 6403; del 18 ottobre [1370] in E. PUTZULU, *Tre note sul Conflitto tra Mariano IV d'Arborea e Pietro IV d'Aragona,* in « Archivio Storico Sardo », XXVIII (1962), pp. 131-158: 143-144 (al documento è attribuita questa data da L. D'ARIENZO, *Carte Reali Diplomatiche di Pietro IV il Cerimonioso, re d'Aragona, riguardanti l'Italia,* Padova 1970, p. 379, n. 754); del 10 novembre 1370 in A.C.A., Reg. 1227, f. 133; e del 1370 (?) in Reg. 1240, ff. 99-100v.

[8] A.C.A., Reg. 1240, f. 103 (brano omesso in VIVES, *Galeres catalanes,* cit., p. 84).
[9] A.C.A., Reg. 1240, f. 104 (pubblicato da J. VIVES, *Galeres catalanes.* cit., p. 85).
[10] A.C.A., Reg. 1227, ff. 119-120 (senza data).

1371 Pietro IV d'Aragona pensava ad una spedizione armata che, però, non raggiungeva la Sardegna [11].

Nel 1373, quando Juan Fernández de Heredia lasciò l'Aragona per stabilirsi alla corte del papa Gregorio XI ad Avignone, Pietro IV pensò di riproporre il vecchio progetto che mirava essenzialmente a estromettere dai territori della corona d'Aragona gli ordini militari castigliani [12]. Già il 14 novembre 1372, dietro espressa richiesta del re d'Aragona, il pontefice aveva incaricato il suo legato in Castiglia di svolgere delle inchieste e di calcolare il valore dei beni che erano appartenuti in quel regno ai Templari e di quelli posseduti dagli ordini di Santiago e di Calatrava in Aragona e in Catalogna per poter far uno scambio equo [13].

Il 31 agosto 1373 Pietro IV diede istruzioni a Fernández de Heredia perché presentasse al papa alcune proposte riguardanti, tra l'altro, la nomina di un cardinale aragonese e la soluzione della questione sarda [14]. Si trattava probabilmente di varii capitoli senza data relativi all'istituzione di un nuovo ordine militare, intitolato a San Giorgio, con i beni aragonesi degli ordini castigliani di Calatrava e di Santiago; l'ordine avrebbe dovuto essere indipendente dalla Castiglia ed avere come primo maestro un Ospedaliere, fra' Berenguer de Montpahon. Questo capitolo venne però sostituito da un altro che proponeva la creazione di un nuovo ordine con i soli beni dell'ordine di Calatrava, mentre i beni dell'ordine di Santiago sarebbero stati aggiunti solo quando si sarebbe resa vacante la precettoria; quest'ultima soluzione aveva probabilmente lo scopo di evitare l'opposizione del potente precettore di quell'ordine, fra' Ferrán Gómez de Albornoz. L'abate di Poblet avrebbe dovuto svolgere le mansioni di visitatore del nuovo ordine [15].

Tra le proposte del 1373 non figurava il vecchio progetto relativo ad una possibile soluzione della questione sarda attraverso uno scambio tra le terre sarde del « giudice » d'Arborea Mariano IV e

---

[11] G. Todde, *Pietro IV d'Aragona e la Sardegna dopo la Sconfitta d'Oristano (1368-1371)*, in « Archivio Storico Sardo », XXVIII (1962), pp. 225-242.

[12] A. Luttrell, *Gregory XI and the Turks: 1370-1378*, in « Orientalia Christiana Periodica », XLVI (1980), pp. 401-403.

[13] Documento pubblicato da J. Vincke, *Documenta selecta mutuas Civitatis arago-cathalaunicae et Ecclesiae Relationes illustrantia*, Barcellona 1936, pp. 493-494.

[14] A.C.A., Reg. 1240, f. 110.

[15] A.C.A., Reg. 1240, ff. 105-106v (senza data); la stessa proposta anche ai ff. 112-113 (senza data).

quelle possedute in Italia dall'ordine degli Ospedalieri. Ma probabilmente nella primavera del 1374 il progetto veniva ripreso: Pietro IV
inviava ad Avignone Ramón de Vilanova perché sottoponesse al
pontefice questo suo piano che l'inviato considerava ormai l'unica
via possibile per una soluzione del problema sardo: ... *no veu sino
vna via, que lo senyor papa faes que lo jutge lexas al senyor Rey tot
quant ha en Cerdenya et que li(n) fos feta esmena deça en terra ferma
dels bens del orde del espital de Sant Johan ha en Italia, et que al
espital de ço que daria deça fos feta esmena coujnent et bona en la dita illa de Cerdenya co es tot lo jutjat d'Arborea et que altre manera lo
dit mossen en R(amon) noy veu* [16].
Nel dicembre del 1375 Pietro IV inviava al pontefice diversi mes-
saggi riguardanti i problemi degli ordini di Calatrava e di Santiago [17] e nel novembre del 1376 chiedeva a Juan Fernández de Heredia di esercitare la sua influenza sul pontefice per risolvere sia la
questione degli ordini militari castigliani che il problema sardo [18].
Dopo la morte di Pietro IV nel 1387 il figlio ed erede al trono,
Giovanni I, dovette affrontare i problemi lasciati in sospeso dal pa-
dre, e nel febbraio del 1393 scriveva ad Avignone allo stesso Juan
Fernández de Heredia, divenuto Maestro dell'Ospedale nel 1377,
parlandogli della questione sarda e proponendo di nuovo i vecchi
progetti relativi agli ordini militari castigliani [19].
Per la soluzione di quest'ultimo problema Martino I, succeduto
al trono d'Aragona nel 1396 alla morte del fratello Giovanni, presentò al papa una nuova proposta: nel 1402 chiedeva infatti che tutti i beni degli ordini di Santiago, di Calatrava e degli Ospedalieri
nei suoi regni diventassero *Maestrats*, ossia ordini « nazionali », e
che i maestri di tutti e tre, e anche di quello di Montesa, venissero
nominati dal re; i tre nuovi *Maestrats* avrebbero avuto i compito di
lottare sul mare contro gli infedeli dell'Africa [20].

---

[16] A.C.A., Reg. 1240, ff. 114-117 (senza data, ma il 26 aprile 1374 il re scriveva al
papa comunicandogli l'arrivo di Ramón de Vilanova, cfr. D'ARIENZO, *Carte Reali*, cit.,
p. 387).
[17] A.C.A., Reg. 1240, ff. 188v-190v.
[18] Documento pubblicato da J. VIVES, *Les galeres catalanes pel Retorn a Roma de
Gregori XI en 1376*, in « Analecta Sacra Tarraconensia », VI (1930), pp. 184-185.
[19] Cfr. il documento pubblicato da E. PUTZULU, *La mancata spedizione in Sardegna
di Giovanni I d'Aragona*, in *Atti del VI Congresso internazionale di Studi Sardi*, I, Cagliari 1962, pp. 65-66.
[20] Documento pubblicato in MARTIN DE ALPARTILS, *Chronica actitatorum temporibus
domini Benedicti XIII*, a cura di F. EHRLE, I, Paderborn 1906, pp. 330-331.

508

Giovanni I e Martino I, figli ed eredi di Pietro IV, pur occupandosi durante i loro regni della questione sarda ancora aperta e praticamente irrisolta, non riproposero l'improbabile ed anacronistico progetto di scambio tra i beni italiani degli Ospedalieri e le terre del « giudice » d'Arborea.

XVII

THE HOSPITALLERS OF RHODES
BETWEEN TUSCANY AND JERUSALEM : 1310-1431 *

Tuscan interest in Jerusalem did not end with the final collapse of the Latin kingdom in 1291. Men and women continued to leave bequests for the holy land, to participate in occasional crusades and to visit Syria as pilgrims. Increasingly too, they interiorized or domesticated such enthusiasms by taking part in holy wars against the Visconti and other enemies of the papacy in Italy, while the Jerusalem journey was replaced by substitute pilgrimages to Rome or to shrines in Tuscany or even by spiritual paths of prayer [1]. One permanent reminder of an enduring Syrian connection was the Hospital of Saint John of Jerusalem which held some forty or more preceptories or *commende* spread across Tuscany and Northern Lazio [2]. This order had evolved in Jerusalem early in the twelfth century to provide care and shelter for the poor and sick, and especially for Western pilgrims, and it had only gradually acquired a predominantly military character [3]. The Hospital became a rich and powerful institution ; in 1291 it was compelled to retreat to Cyprus, and in 1306 it launched the conquest of Rhodes. Its subsequent operations were directed mainly against the Turks, but it was not entirely deflected from Jerusalem. Occasional military action against the Mamluks in Egypt and Syria continued, while Rhodes became a station for many pilgrims travelling to or from Syria ; in 1403 the Hospitallers even attempted to revive their hospice in Jerusalem itself [4]. Meanwhile a small population of Tuscans,

* The Leverhulme Foundation and the Venerable Order of Saint John of Jerusalem at Clerkenwell most generously supported much of the present research.

1. Various contributions in *Toscana e Terrasanta nel Medioevo*, ed. F. CARDINI, Florence, 1982.
2. The Tuscan Hospital has scarcely been studied. Fragments of the principal sources for the period, the central and prioral archives, survive in Valletta, National Library of Malta, Archives of the Order of Saint John of Jerusalem, and in Florence, Archivio di Stato, Corporazioni Religiose Soppresse, n°ˢ 132-133 (Inventario 137) : details of both in *Cartulaire général de l'Ordre des Hospitaliers de S. Jean de Jérusalem : 1100-1310*, ed. J. DELAVILLE LE ROULX, 4 vol., Paris, 1894-1906, I, p. XIV-XXVII, CXXV-CXXX, CCXXV-CCXXVII. The present preliminary study makes partial use of the Malta archive but none of that in Florence.
3. J. RILEY-SMITH, *The Knights of St. John in Jerusalem and Cyprus : c. 1050-1310*, London, 1967.
4. A. LUTTRELL, "Rhodes and Jerusalem : 1291-1411", in *Byzantinische Forschungen*, 12, 1987, p. 189-207.

Hospitallers, merchants and others, developed on Rhodes [5]. The Hospital at Rhodes thus constituted a spiritual and physical axis, suspended between Tuscany and Jerusalem, which linked together the overlapping, but essentially distinct, institutions of the pilgrimage, the crusade and the holy war against the infidel.

*
* *

The Hospital, established in Tuscany during the twelfth century, was an order of religious whose military activities never entirely replaced their original medical and charitable functions. By 1206 the Order included two separate classes of military brethren, the *milites* and the sergeants, whose fundamental task was to wage a perpetual holy struggle against the infidel, normally in the East ; this war was not technically a crusade, and indeed Hospitallers were expressly forbidden to fight against fellow Christians or to take the cross as crusaders. Their rich endowments in the West were greatly increased when they received the lands of the Temple, another military order suppressed in 1312. These European properties were divided into preceptories which were grouped in priories. The preceptory formed the centre of the brethren's communal and liturgical life and of their economic activity, and normally it produced a monetary surplus to be sent to the Convent or headquarters in the East as *responsiones* [6]. The location of each preceptory depended in part on the vagaries of individual donations. Some *commende* possessed a hospital or hospice for the sick, the poor or the aged. Such houses were sometimes situated on major routes, some of them leading to the East, to Rome or to Santiago de Compostela, so that they gave shelter to pilgrims and others [7] ; one example was the *mansio* by the bridge at Poggibonsi said in 1323 to receive Hospitaller brethren travelling along the Via Francigena to Rome [8]. Some preceptories were located inside or just outside major cities, such as Pisa, Florence or Siena, in which they enjoyed considerable urban

5. A. Luttrell, "Interessi fiorentini nell'economia e nella politica dei Cavalieri Ospedalieri di Rodi nel Trecento", in *Annali della Scuola Normale Superiore di Pisa : Lettere, storia e filosofia*, 2 ser., 28, 1959, p. 317-326.

6. Cf. A. Luttrell, "Templari e Ospitalieri in Italia", in *Templari e Ospitalieri in Italia : la Chiesa di San Bevignate a Perugia*, ed. M. Roncetti et al., Perugia, 1987, p. 19-26.

7. See in general A. Luttrell, "The Hospitallers' Hospice of Santa Caterina at Venice : 1358-1451", in *Studi Veneziani*, 12, 1970, p. 369-383 ; for Tuscany, see T. Szabò, "Templari e viabilità", and other contributions in *I Templari : mito e storia. Atti del Convegno internazionale di Studi alla Magione templare di Poggibonsi — Siena (29-31 maggio 1987)*, ed. G. Minnucci and F. Sardi, Sinalunga-Siena, 1989, p. 297-307 et passim. The fourteenth-century evidence for charitable expenditures in the West is scanty. The number of Templar houses on the Santiago route has been exaggerated : A. Forey, *The Templars in the "Corona de Aragón"*, London, 1973, p. 306, note 249.

8. P. Guicciardini, "Due Magioni del S. M. O. di Malta presso Poggibonsi", in *La Diana*, 3, 1928, p. 245-246, note 3. L. de Filla et al., *La Chiesa di San Giovanni in Jerusalem alla Magione di Poggibonsi*, Siena, 1986, contains the best architectural study of Tuscan *commenda* buildings. On the Hospital's brick-built tower-*domus* of Turri near Poggibonsi alienated in 1323, see R. Stopani, "Gli itinerari della Via Francigena nel Senese : fonti scritte e testimonianze storico-territoriali", in *La Via Francigena nel Senese : storia e territorio*, ed. R. Stopani, Florence, 1985, p. 40-41 and fig. 54.

rents [9], while others, such as the fortified house at Alberese above the Via Aurelia south-west of Grosseto, were in isolated areas. The former Benedictine monastery at Alberese was a special case on account of its strategic situation close to the port at Talamone, but it provided an example of the dangers of repeated violent occupation by secular forces, while in about 1377 quarrels over its control led the Sienese to sequester goods of the Hospital in the city and *contado* of Siena reputedly to the value of 25,000 florins [10].

Many preceptories were quite small and poor. The house of San Giovanni Malanotte at Lucca had the extraordinarily large income of 2,300 *libre* a year in 1260 [11], but an inquiry of 1373 into eight houses in the Diocese of Arezzo showed that one, at *Capraria* in the *contado* of Arezzo, was abandoned and overgrown. Only one, Sant'Appollinare at Montebello, had a preceptor who was a *miles*, Fr. Giovanni de Pacis of Florence aged about 33, and he was an absentee who governed the house through a lay factor. The other six preceptories were held by three sergeants who did not wear the *habitum militis*. Fr. Alberto Mei of Siena, aged about 60, held San Jacopo al Prato where there were two other Hospitallers, one of them a chaplain, and two other *clerici* ; he also held San Giovanni at Monte San Savino. The other houses had to pay salaries to secular priests. Fr. Luto Pagni dei Guasconi of Arezzo, aged about 45, held the former Templar house of San Giorgio at Arezzo and the hospital of Sant'Egidio at Quercia Frassenaria in the *contado* of Arezzo. Fr. Roberto Alberti Franchischi of Siena, aged about 45, was Preceptor of San Giovanni at Asciano and also of San Giovanni at *Bottachino de Valleclavium*. Except for the absentee *miles*, these men were rather elderly. Any communal and liturgical life must have collapsed in houses where there was only one Hospitaller or none at all ; no mention was made of expenses on alms or hospices. The lands at *Bottachino* had been ruined by floods and brought no income. Elsewhere the sums for which it was estimated the house could be rented out, once all expenses and the *responsiones* had been paid to the prior, were : San Jacopo al Prato for 30 florins after 29 florins had been paid to the prior ; Arezzo for 25 florins after the prior had been paid 25 ; Asciano for 30 or 35 florins after 30 had been paid ; Montebello for 36 or 40 florins after paying 33 ; Quercia Frassenaria for 6 florins after 4 had been paid ; Monte San Savino for nil after 12 florins had been paid to the prior [12]. In

9. For a group of urban preceptories, A. Luttrell, "The Hospitallers of Rhodes at Treviso : 1373", in *Mediterraneo medievale. Scritti in onore di Francesco Giunta*, II, Soveria Mannelli, 1989, p. 755-775.

10. E. Fedi, *L'Abbazia di S. Maria dell'Alberese presso Grosseto*, Naples, 1942, with much detail.

11. *Rationes Decimarum Italiae nei secoli XIII e XIV*, 2 vol., ed. M. Giusti and P. Guidi, Vatican, 1932, I, p. 247.

12. Arch. Vat., Instrumenta Miscellanea 2979 ; the estimates varied with the witnesses. An inquest made into the whole Priory of Pisa in 1333 is lost, but its existence is known from an extract in Siena, Archivio di Stato, Capitoli 171, n° 31. On the 1373 inquests, A. Luttrell, "Papauté et Hôpital : l'Enquête de 1373", in *L'Enquête pontificale de 1373 sur l'Ordre des Hospitaliers de Saint-Jean de Jérusalem*, I, ed. A.-M. Legras, Paris, 1987, p. 3-42. There was a *hospitalis* at Quercia Frassenaria in 1275-1279 : *Rationes Decimarum*, *op. cit.* note 11, I, p. 79, 99.

1308 certain Templar houses were estimated to have overall incomes expressed without any deductions : Santa Sofia at Pisa 240 florins, Santa Margherita at Arezzo 40 florins, San Jacopo at Florence 80 florins and the unidentified hospital at *Caporsi*, which was *in districtu Florentie* and in the Diocese of Fiesole, possibly at the modern Montorsoli near Florence, 60 florins [13]. Following the arrival of the great plague in 1348, the year 1373 marked a low point in economic and demographic decline. In fact, in 1351 the house at Alberese was already so dilapidated by warfare and plague that it had almost no income and required repairs [14].

A group of houses in Tuscia Romana or Northern Lazio also belonged to the Priory of Pisa. Some of these had been Templar preceptories such as two small castles just north of Tuscania at Castell'Araldo, secured for the Hospital by Fr. Battista Orsini Prior of Rome only in about 1420, and San Savino, which the Hospital never acquired. Hospitaller houses included those of San Giovanni at Ponte di Rigo on the Via Cassia north of Aquapendente, San Manno on Lake Bolsena, San Giovanni at Sugarella west of Tuscania and an *oratorium* at Canino, all granted with the Preceptories of Corneto and Tuscania to Fr. Achile Mattei Pecorosco of Siena also in 1420, at which time they were in secular hands [15]. Another inquest of 1373 concerned the Dioceses of Viterbo, Tuscania, Orte and Narni. This showed that two preceptories at Viterbo and Orte in the Priory of Rome were held by Fr. Niccolò de Sachetti of Florence, a *miles* aged over 50. The Preceptor of San Giovanni e Vittore at Commenda north-west of Viterbo held both the hospital of Santa Lucia just outside Viterbo, which was managed by a married couple both of whom were *oblati* or donats of the Order, and the church of Santa Lucia, the properties of which were leased to a layman. At Corneto, the modern Tarquinia, the hospital of San Giovanni was a rare exception in having twenty beds and a doctor for the poor and infirm ; it was held by a Hospitaller priest aged about 25 who paid 12 florins a year to a cleric, 22 florins to a married pair who managed it, and 5 florins 48 *soldi* as *responsiones*. The Preceptor of Corneto, aged about 60, held three churches, one the parish church of San Clemente and the other two dedicated to San Matteo and to San Salvatore ; he paid 40 florins *responsiones* and spent 8 florins going with a *socius* to the annual chapter at Siena. The Preceptor of San Leonardo at Montalto, aged about 36, paid 7 florins *responsiones* and, as an absentee, he held the Preceptory of Benedetto at Burlegio near Viterbo where the house and

---

13. Arch. Vat., Instrumenta Miscellanea 440. The Preceptory of *Caporsoli* was in the Diocese of Fiesole : T. BINI, "Dei Tempieri e del loro processo in Toscana", in *Atti della Reale Accademia Lucchese*, 13, 1845, p. 478. Montorsoli is suggested in B. CAPONE, *Quando in Italia c'erano i Templari*, Turin, 1981, p. 122.

14. Malta, Cod. 318, fol. 161v.

15. A. LUTTRELL, "Two Templar-Hospitaller Preceptories North of Tuscania", in *Papers of the British School at Rome*, 39, 1971, p. 90-124, with further detail in A. KINGSLEY PORTER, "S. Giovanni Gerosolimitano di Corneto-Tarquinia", in *Arte e storia*, 32, 1913, p. 325-330, and G. SILVESTRELLI, "Le chiese e i feudi dell'Ordine dei Templari e dell'Ordine di San Giovanni di Gerusalemme nella regione romana", in *Rendiconti della Reale Accademia dei Lincei : Classe di scienze morali, storiche e filologiche*, 26, 1917, p. 491-539 ; 27, 1918, p. 174-176 ; see also A. GILMOUR-BRYSON, *The Trial of the Templars in the Papal State and the Abruzzi*, Vatican, 1982, p. 90, 93-94.

church were ruined but where there was an income of 50 florins, 10 of which were paid as *responsiones*. San Leonardo at Tuscania, with two ruined churches, was held by Fr. Jacopo Chelis of Poggibonsi, aged about 40, and it paid 10 florins *responsiones* [16]. There was also a house of Santa Maria in Capità near Bagnoregio [17] and, in 1320, a *hospitalis pauperum* with a rector and brethren at Montepulciano [18].

In 1337, from the Preceptory at Commenda between Viterbo and Montefiascone, Fr. Giovanni de Rivara, who was Prior of Pisa and of Rome and also *gubernator* of the Preceptory or *fortalicium* at Alberese where he had a room, summoned 29 preceptors holding 37 named preceptories to a prioral chapter at Siena where they were to pay their dues. The chapter met in the cloister of San Leonardo at Siena, the 24 brethren named as present being the prior ; 18 preceptors, who included the Preceptor of Péccioli who was also the *camerarius et gubernator* of the *domus* of the Hospitaller sisters of San Sepolcro at Pisa ; the two *gubernatores* of the Preceptories of San Giovanni at San Gimignano and of San Leonardo at Pisa, the latter being Fr. Guglielmo, son of Giordano della Rocca of the Diocese of Turin ; the *gubernator* of the hospital of San Leonardo at Siena ; and two other named brethren. The list of those present also gave the name of another preceptory, that of Santa Maria in Capità. The document actually named a total of 39 preceptories, eight of them in Tuscia Romana [19]. There was no indication of the total number of brethren in the priory [20]. In 1373 the eight houses around Arezzo supported only six brethren, one of them an absentee *miles*, one a priest and four sergeants, but those were small houses. The number of *milites* was low. A few brethren, such as the Strozzi, Albizzi and Gambacorti, came from leading families. Fr. Gerardo de Gragnana, who was at Anagni as Prior of Pisa and a papal *cubicularius* in 1299, was at Limassol in Cyprus, both as Hospitaller of the Order and later as Marshal, in 1303 [21] ; his family seem to have been lords of Gragnana in the Garfagnana [22]. Fr. Giovanni Melegario, prior in 1307 and 1309, came from Parma and had in 1296 been Preceptor of Padua [23]. Fr. Giovanni de Rivara, Prior of Pisa at least from 1323 to 1348, Prior of Rome from 1330 onwards and papal Rector of the Marche from 1339 at least until 1347 [24], was surely a *miles* since his family

16. Paris, Bibl. Nat., ms lat. 5155, fol. 46-52, partially published in A. LUTTRELL, "The Hospitallers around Narni and Terni : 1333-1373", in *Bollettino della Deputazione di Storia Patria per l'Umbria*, 82, 1985, p. 5-22.
17. M. CAGIANO DI AZEVEDO, "Da un luogo fortificato etrusco a una *Maison* dei Templari", in *Studi castellani in onore di Pietro Gazzola*, I, Rome, 1979, p. 45-48.
18. Malta, Cod. 1126, fol. 309.
19. Siena, Archivio di Stato, Caleffo Nero, Capitoli 3, fol. 9-23 (especially fol. 19-19v) : the preceptories are listed *infra*, p. 135-137.
20. The text stated that those listed *sunt due partes et ultra fratrum dicti prioratus*, but must have intended preceptors rather than *fratres*.
21. *Cartulaire, op. cit.* note 2, nᵒˢ 4471, 4586, 4620-4621.
22. D. PACCHI, *Richerche istoriche sulla provincia della Garfagnana*, Modena, 1785, p. 89.
23. Padua, Archivio di Stato, Commenda di Malta, Filza 1.
24. *Infra*, p. 134 ; J. DELAVILLE LE ROULX, *Les Hospitaliers à Rhodes jusqu'à la mort de Philibert de Naillac : 1310-1421*, Paris, 1913, p. 77-78.

were Marchesi of Saluzzo in Piedmont [25]. Later Fr. Jacopo degli Obizzi, the Hospital's proctor at the Council of Pisa in 1409, was *miles* [26], as was Fr. Leonardo de Buonafede who died in 1412 [27]. Some of these brethren came from important business and landholding families, possibly from a minor branch of their family, while others bore obscure names [28]. The Hospitallers must have had a general sense of who was socially acceptable as a *miles*, but it doubtful whether their criteria corresponded to any secular definition of knighthood, itself a debatable matter, or whether they distinguished clearly between the shifting and indefinable groupings of *grandi, magnati, gente nuova* and others. Licences for Piero son of Francesco Baroncielli of Florence and for Berto Corsini of Florence to be received as *milites* were issued in 1347 and 1365 respectively [29], while the prior was ordered to receive Francesco Benedetti as *miles* in 1351 [30]. Fr. Nerio de Malavolti of Siena, lieutenant of the prior in 1358 [31], was presumably a *miles* ; Giuliano de Benini of Florence was licensed to be received as a *miles* in 1409 [32] ; and there were, of course, others.

There were normally few Tuscan Hospitallers serving on Rhodes, where Italian brethren were not numerous. A Fr. Giovanni de Pisa was at Rhodes in 1337 and 1340, and in 1337 the Pisan priory was called upon to send one Hospitaller there ; Fr. Giovanni de Pisa was still on Rhodes when the Hospital granted him an old-age pension in 1366 [33]. A special case was the Florentine Bartolomeo di Lapo Benini who was in Rhodes as an agent of the Bardi bank and in 1339 became a Hospitaller there. In 1341 the Bardi paid him 1,450 *libbre* for advancing their dealings with the Hospital, and he maintained the family business there through his brother Bindo Benini in Venice ; he held houses and a garden in the country outside Rhodes

25. L. D'ARIENZO, *Carte reali diplomatiche di Pietro IV il Cerimonioso, re d'Aragona, riguardanti l'Italia*, Padua, 1970, p. 131.

26. D. MANSI, *Sacrorum conciliorum nova et amplissima collectio*, XXVII, Venice, 1784, p. 337.

27. G. RICHA, *Notizie istoriche delle chiese fiorentine*, III, part 1, Florence, 1755, p. 305.

28. According to G. B. UCCELLI, *Il convento di S. Giusto alle Mura e i Gesuati*, Florence, 1865, p. 84, Niccolò de Ciupo Squarcialupi of Poggibonsi and his wife Bice made their will in 1362 and separated, both to take the Hospitaller habit. Niccolò's epitaph described him as *frater* and *miles*, but the date 1313 remains obscure : S. DÜLL, "Die Inschriftendenkmäler von Santa Reparata", in *Römische historische Mitteilungen*, 27, 1985, p. 170-171, 200, and fig. 10-12. Possibly the couple really became *donati*, which would explain their will and the puzzling presence of the tombslab in a non-Hospitaller church. Hospitaller burial monuments were rare. That of Fr. Pietro de Imola in Florence was that of a Prior of Rome who died there in 1329 circa : ID., "Das Grabmal des Johanniters Pietro da Imola in S. Jacopo in Campo Corbolini in Florenz : zur Renaissance-Kapitalis in erneuerten Inschriften des Trecento", in *Mitteilungen des Kunsthistorischen Institutes in Florenz*, 34, 1990, p. 101-122. Other Tuscan Hospitaller funerary inscriptions are later in date. That at Lucca on the *sepulcrum* of *Frater Paulus quondam Mei Figlani de Senis*, Preceptor of Lucca, was dated 1396 : text in P. M. PACIAUDI, *De cultu S. Johannis Baptistae antiquitates christianae*, Rome, 1755, p. 297, note 1. Those at Florence of Fr. Giovanni de Rossi dalla Pogna (1398) and Fr. Leonardo Buonafede (1412) are in RICHA, *op. cit.* note 27, III, part 1, p. 304-305.

29. Malta, Cod. 317, fol. 170 ; Cod. 319, fol. 228.

30. Malta, Cod. 318, fol. 161.

31. Malta, Cod. 316, fol. 252v-253.

32. Malta, Cod. 335, fol. 136.

33. Malta, Cod. 280, fol. 41, 42, 45v ; Cod. 319, fol. 207v.

town. By 1348 he was Prior of Messina; by 1351 he held the Priories of Pisa and Rome; in 1364 he was also Prior of Venice; in 1373 and 1374 he was Admiral of the Order [34]; but on 10 September 1374 at Rhodes he was judged too aged and decrepid to act as Admiral, and so he was again appointed prior [35]. In 1359 another Florentine, Fr. Niccolò Benedetti, was named papal captain at Smyrna with the stipulation that his brothers, who included Fr. Francesco Benedetti who was received as *miles* in 1351, had the right to succeed him as captain; they were licensed to send galleys to trade at Alexandria, ostensibly as a way of financing the defence of Smyrna, and to retain for themselves any territory they might conquer from the Turks [36]. However Fr. Niccolò Benedetti made some false move, for in 1364 the Master had kept him in prison for almost five years [37]. There were occasional examples of Tuscan Hospitallers at the Convent in Rhodes. In 1374 the Master, while in port at Corneto, issued a licence for Fr. Giovanni Barti of the Priory of Pisa to go to Rhodes. Fr. Leonardo degli Strozzi was on Rhodes in 1402, when he was granted the Preceptory of Prato, and in 1409 the Master, then at Pisa, instructed his lieutenant at Rhodes to receive as *miles* a certain *Loctus Laurencij de Lestufa* of Florence who was going to Rhodes with horses and arms. Fr. Nani de *Centenay* of the Priory of Pisa was being sent from Rhodes to Italy in 1413, while in 1421 Fr. Achile Mattei Pecorosco of Siena was licensed to leave the island [38].

The contribution in money was apparently more regular. The eight evidently rather poor preceptories around Arezzo were estimated in 1373 to owe the prior about 133 florins a year of *responsiones*, giving a low average of some 16 ½ florins a house. The priory's *responsiones* owed to the Convent at Rhodes were fixed at 1,000 florins in 1317 [39] and at about

34. LUTTRELL, art. cit. note 5, p. 320; ID., *The Hospitallers in Cyprus, Rhodes, Greece and the West : 1291-1440*, London, 1978, VI, p. 169; ID., "A Hospitaller in a Florentine Fresco : 1366-68", in *Burlington Magazine*, 114, 1972, p. 366; for the Rhodian properties, Malta, Cod. 321, fol. 225. Benini, Prior of Pisa and Rome, was at Rhodes on 30 May 1366 : Malta, Cod. 319, fol. 303-304. He was still prior on 13 September 1371 when the pope wanted him to return to his priory to assist in governing the papal possessions in Italy; in February 1373 he was not prior but Admiral and was summoned to give advice at Avignon; on 16 July 1373 the pope requested the Master and Convent to permit Benini, then Admiral, and Fr. Palamedo di Giovanni, Prior of Pisa, to exchange offices, but Benini was still Admiral in September 1373 and, as far as was known at Avignon, in December 1374 : *Lettres secrètes et curiales du pape Grégoire XI (1370-1378) intéressant les pays autres que la France*, 3 fasc., ed. G. MOLLAT, Paris, 1962-1965, n⁰ˢ 294-295, 1479, 1995, 2200, 3028.

35. Arch. Vat., Reg. Vat. 286, fol. 166v-167v.

36. K. SETTON, *The Papacy and the Levant : 1204-1571*, I, Philadelphia, 1976, p. 234-236. In 1353 the pope instructed that if the Archbishop of Smyrna were to die, the Master at Rhodes was to appoint Niccolò Bellincioni of Florence, *civis* of Rhodes, as Captain of Smyrna : *Innocent VI (1352-1362). Lettres secrètes et curiales*, ed. P. GASNAULT et al., I, Paris, 1959, n⁰ˢ 619, 689. Bellincioni, a former employee of the Bardi company, did business for the Hospital in the Levant : LUTTRELL, art. cit. note 5, p. 321.

37. Arch. Vat., Reg. Vat. 246, fol. 174v-175.

38. Malta, Cod. 320, fol. 55; Cod. 332, fol. 140-140v; Cod. 335, fol. 131v; Cod. 339, fol. 180; Cod. 346, fol. 132.

39. Arch. Vat., Reg. Vat. 66, fol. 337.

800 florins in 1330 [40]. In both 1373/1374 and 1374/1375 the priory paid 1,210 florins, that is 17 percent of the 6,784 florins paid by all the Italian priories and 2.8 percent of the total Western contribution of 42,230 florins in the year 1373/1374. In both those financial years the figure consisted of 922 florins of *responsiones* plus a special taille of 288 florins [41]. This total for a priory with some 40 preceptories would give an average of 23 florins per house.

The Hospitallers continued to play a minor role in sustaining Tuscan awareness of the holy land. Apart from its brethren and its churches and houses, parishes and hospices, the Hospital was present in paintings and frescoes. Two panels done in 1329 by Pietro Lorenzetti at Siena each portrayed a Hospitaller ; one stood next to a pope, possibly Honorius III, approving the Carmelite rule, while the other stood beside Honorius IV as he confirmed a change in the Carmelite habit [42]. Bindo di Lapo Benini, who had before 1374 restored or enlarged the Hospitallers' Florentine hospital of San Giovanni, made a donation in 1374 to that hospital on behalf of his brother, then Prior of Pisa [43] ; Bindo may have commissioned the altarpiece from this church which shows John the Baptist and was probably painted by Nardo di Cione in about 1365 [44]. Bindo was also the donor of a painting done by Giovanni del Biondo in 1364 of John the Baptist dressed as a Hospitaller and wearing the Order's cross [45]. The Hospitallers' church at Cascina was covered with frescoes painted by Martino di Bartolomeo in 1398 for Fr. Bartolomeo de Palmieri of Cascina, then Preceptor of San Pietro at Siena [46]. The most grandiose Tuscan representation of the crusade was contained in the fresco painted between about 1366 and 1368 by Andrea da Firenze in the Dominican chapter house at Santa Maria Novella in Florence, one part of which showed the pope flanked by numerous distinguished personages. This scene, which

40. The joint figure for the two Priories of Rome and Pisa was 1,600 florins : Malta, Cod. 280, fol. 7.

41. Text in A. LUTTRELL, "The Hospitallers' Western Accounts : 1373/4 and 1374/5", in *Camden Miscellany*, XXX, London, 1990, p. 10-21 ; in 1374/1375 the Priories of Rome and Pisa were shown as paying identical sums of 922 plus 288 florins, which suggests that the two priories paid jointly.

42. H. VAN Os, *Sienese Altarpieces : 1215-1400*, I, Groningen, 1984, p. 90-99, and fig. 112-113, and J. CANNON, "Pietro Lorenzetti and the History of the Carmelite Order", in *Journal of the Warburg and Courtauld Institutes*, 50, 1987, p. 23, and plates 4a-b ; neither author notices the Hospitaller figures. On artistic interchanges, A. DERBES, "Siena and the Levant in the Later Dugento", in *Gesta*, 28, 1989, p. 190-204.

43. UCCELLI, *op. cit.* note 28, p. 84-85 ; W. and E. PAATZ, *Die Kirchen von Florenz*, II, Frankfurt, 1941, p. 273, 279, 284. The date was 1374 not 1373.

44. M. DAVIES, *National Gallery Catalogues : The Early Italian Schools before 1400*, ed. D. GORDON, London, 1988, p. 84-86, and plate 58.

45. R. OFFNER and K. STEINWEG, *A Critical and Historical Corpus of Florentine Painting*, IV, 4, part 1, New York, 1967, p. 70-72, and plate XVII (4) ; the picture may have been a portrait, conceivably of Fr. Bartolomeo Benini. A figure in a Santa Caterina of about 1378 by Giovanni del Biondo wore a Hospitaller cross but apparently represented a son of the original donor, Noferi di Giovanni di Bartolomeo Bischeri, added possibly in about 1407 : *ibid.*, p. 107-111, and plate XXIV.

46. P. STEFANINI, "La chiesa e i beni dei Cavalieri di Malta in Cascina", in *Archivio Storico di Malta*, 9, 1938-1939, p. 1-41, with photographs ; the donor, with a red tunic and no cross, seems not to be dressed as a Hospitaller as Stefanini claims.

must have been familiar to many Florentines and others, apparently had a crusading iconography with genuine portraits of King Pierre of Cyprus, captor of Alexandria, of Count Amedeo of Savoy, who had retaken Gallipoli from the Turks, of Cardinal Gil de Albornoz, reconqueror of Algeçiras and leader of the crusade in the papal states, and of the Hospitaller Fr. Juan Fernández de Heredia, papal captain general and defender of Avignon. This last, soon to become Master of Rhodes, wore a white eight-pointed Hospitaller cross, and so, probably, did another unidentified figure in the crowd [47].

Such visual crusading propaganda received practical application on a minor scale when the pope launched a Hospitaller *passagium* which invaded North-West Greece in 1378. The Florentine Fr. Niccolò degli Strozzi, who had been sent on a papal mission to Rhodes in 1374 and who subsequently became Prior of Pisa, received personal exhortations to participate from Caterina of Siena, who urged him to follow the path of martyrdom ; in April 1377 he was in Venice seeking shipping, and in April he was at Vonitsa in Epirus where apparently he died soon after, possibly in the defeat of the Hospitaller force by the Albanian Ghin Boua Spata. This *passagium* was in part a Florentine expedition since various kinsmen of Maddalena Buondelmonti, widow of Leonardo Tocco lord of Cephalonia, received papal licences, at a time when Florence was under interdict, to supply and accompany the expedition ; one of them, Esau Bondelmonti, eventually became Despot of Epirus [48].

After 1378 the Pisan priory was alienated from Rhodes and to some extent divided against itself by the repercussions within the Hospital of the schism in the papacy. The Master Fr. Juan Fernández de Heredia, who resided at Avignon from 1382 until his death in 1396, maintained an allegiance to the Avignon popes, as did the Convent at Rhodes and certain Italian Hospitallers. Some brethren were uncertain how to react ; they sought confirmation of their offices from both parties, they paid *responsiones* to neither, or they switched from one allegiance to another. Probably on 16 February 1381 the prior, Fr. Giovanni Siffi, had to replace the rebellious Preceptor of San Gimignano, Fr. Angelo Giovannini, with Fr. Luigi di San Gimignano [49]. The Roman pope, Urban VI, appointed the Neapolitan Fr. Riccardo Caracciolo as "anti-Master" in April 1383 and many Italian brethren supported him [50]. A number of Tuscan brethren attended the Urbanist "chapter general" which opened at Naples on 28 March 1384. They included four procurators of the Priory of Pisa who

47. LUTTRELL, "A Hospitaller", art. cit. note 34. While that article requires considerable revision, the suggested iconography seems valid ; ID., *Latin Greece, the Hospitallers and the Crusades : 1291-1440*, London, 1982, I, p. 256, note 50. Note that eleven Dominicans from Santa Maria Novella departed on the Smyrna crusade of 1345 : M. PAPI, "Santa Maria Novella di Firenze e *l'Outremer* domenicano", in *Toscana e Terrasanta, op. cit.* note 1, p. 99-100.

48. LUTTRELL, art. cit. note 5, p. 322-324 ; ID., *The Hospitallers and the Crusades, op. cit.* note 47, XII, p. 279-280 and XV, p. 412-417.

49. According to L. PECORI, *Storia di San Gimignano*, Florence, 1853, p. 438-439, with the evidently erroneous date of 6 February 1480.

50. LUTTRELL, *The Hospitallers in Cyprus, Rhodes, op. cit.* note 34, XIII ; DELAVILLE LE ROULX, *op. cit.* note 24, p. 248-264.

played a leading part in the proceedings and were all appointed to the ruling council and to other offices : Fr. Bartolomeo Castellani of Florence, Preceptor of Alberese and Prato, Fr. Leonardo degli Strozzi, Preceptor of Arezzo, Fr. Giovanni Cecchi, Preceptor of San Jacopo *inter vineas* or in Campo Corbolini at Florence, and Fr. Bartolomeo de Cascina, Preceptor of San Pietro at Siena. The Urbanist prior, Fr. Francesco degli Strozzi, refused to attend and was subsequently deposed. The procurators accused Fr. Lorenzo and Fr. Angelo Giovannini of attacking and robbing Fr. Bartolomeo de Cascina's preceptory ; they also indulged in much other litigation to their own personal advantage [51].

One result of this split was apparently that the Tuscan *responsiones* no longer reached Rhodes [52]. The priory was represented by at least four and probably six or more brethren at an Urbanist chapter held at the Preceptory of San Sepolcro at Pisa in November 1385 [53], and by 2 December following Caracciolo had appointed Fr. Francesco degli Strozzi as prior, in accordance with a request from the comune of Florence [54]. Strozzi was replaced on 17 May 1386 when Caracciolo named Fr. Priamo Gerardi de Gambacorti as the Master's lieutenant in the priory [55], and a little later, by 1392, Gambacorti was the Romanist prior, a post he still held in 1410 [56]. Caracciolo was himself in Florence in February 1392 following his intervention as a papal envoy negotiating a peace between Milan and the Florentines [57]. While there, in March 1392 Caracciolo acted, in consultation with the new prior, to establish a community of Hospitaller sisters with a hospice for the poor in the Hospitaller house near the modern Porta Romana which had been the hospital of San Giovanni, restored and enlarged some time before 1374 by Bindo di Lapo Benini ; Fr. Leonardo de Buonafede, *miles* and "anti-Treasurer" of the Hospital, drew up a constitution for the sisters [58]. On 7 April 1395 the Florentine comune protested to Caracciolo against his deposition of Gambacorti from his office as prior [59]. The "anti-Master"

51. Malta, Cod. 281, fol. 1-9 ; *infra*, p. 135. Cod. 281, Caracciolo's register for 1384 to 1386, contains much detail on the Priory of Pisa.

52. Italian payments progressively disappeared from the Western accounts kept in Southern France : Malta, Cod. 48, *passim* ; Cod. 322, fol. 52-53v ; Cod. 326, fol. 68v-70. In March 1383 just 45 ½ florins were received from the Priory of Lombardy : Cod. 48, fol. 58.

53. Malta, Cod. 281, fol. 75v-76v.

54. Text in G. MÜLLER, *Documenti sulle relazioni delle città toscane coll'Oriente cristiano e coi Turchi fino all'anno MDXXXI*, Florence, 1879, p. 143.

55. Malta, Cod. 281, fol. 91-91v.

56. DELAVILLE LE ROULX, *op. cit.* note 24, p. 351.

57. *Ibid.*, p. 257-259 ; LUTTRELL, *op. cit.* note 34, XXI, p. 242.

58. UCCELLI, *op. cit.* note 28, p. 84-85, with further detail in G. BOSIO, *Dell'istoria della sacra religione et ill^{ma} militia di San Giovanni Gierosolimitano*, II, 2nd ed., Rome, 1629, p. 144-145 ; E. VIVIANI DELLA ROBBIA, *Nei monasteri fiorentini*, Florence, 1946, p. 105-110, with details on Buonafede's career and on the original organization of the house and its first five sisters, the "gentildonne" Pietra d'Andrea Viviani Gennai, the first prioress, Margherita Lapi Cambi, Francesca d'Agostino of Panzano, Giovanna di Filippo (family unknown) and Francesca di Masio Ricci.

59. Text in MÜLLER, *op. cit.* note 54, p. 146, assuming that its address to *Magistro Rhodiensi* did refer, as it had in 1385 (*ibid.*, p. 143), to Caracciolo : LUTTRELL, *op. cit.* note 34, XXI, p. 242.

died on 18 May 1395 and ten days later an assembly was held at Rome at which various officers were confirmed or appointed. It was attended from Tuscany by Fr. Leonardo de Buonafede, Preceptor of Arezzo and still "anti-Treasurer", Fr. Lodovico de Pontremoli, Preceptor of Val di Nievole, Fr. Lodovico de Nasina, Preceptor of Tuscania, and Fr. Pietro de Pistoia [60]. On 28 October 1399 the Prior of Pisa was among those due to be summoned to a "chapter general" to elect a new "anti-Master" [61].

The Avignon connection survived, and to some extent the Master continued to confirm and appoint in the Tuscan priory. The Avignonese prior Fr. Giovanni Siffi attended the chapter general at Valence in 1383 and, while others evidently controlled the priory in Tuscany, Siffi was at Rhodes, still technically as prior, in 1387 and 1393 [62]. The Hospitallers at Avignon continued to use the Florentine bankers of the Alberti group and Florentines continued to trade at Rhodes [63]. After Fr. Riccardo Caracciolo's death in 1395 no new "anti-Master" was appointed and the schism within the Hospital moved towards an end. On 1 November 1400 the Rhodian Master Fr. Philibert de Naillac, accepting that Fr. Leonardo de Buonafede was Preceptor of San Jacopo at Florence, licensed him to go to Rhodes [64], and after 1409 Buonafede became a leading agent in the reconciliation of the various "Roman" priories with the main body of the Order [65]. Yet Buonafede had not abandoned the Roman pope Boniface IX who on 5 September 1401, and at Buonafede's request, granted indulgences to finance the repair of the hospital of San Giovanni *inter arcus extra muros* at Florence [66]. In 1409 Naillac travelled from Rhodes to the General Council at Pisa where he was guardian of the papal conclave. There the schism in the Hospital was more or less ended and from Pisa the Master issued many acts giving effect to the ensuing reorganization [67]. While there he regulated the affairs of the Hospitaller sisters of San Giovannino in Pisa [68]. On 10 may 1410 Naillac recognized Fr. Priamo Gambacorti as Prior of Pisa [69], a post he held until 1448 [70].

A special place in this axis linking Avignon, Florence and Rhodes was that of Giovanni Corsini, brother of Cardinal Pietro, Archbishop of Florence. Giovanni Corsini was actively involved at Avignon, on Cyprus and elsewhere in the crusade schemes of Gregory XI, who in 1374 sent him

60. Text in S. PAULI, *Codice diplomatico del sacro militare ordine gerosolimitano, oggi di Malta*, II, Lucca, 1737, p. 104-107.
61. Arch. Vat., Reg. Lat. 70, fol. 36-36v.
62. Malta, Cod. 48, fol. 214v-216v ; Cod. 322, fol. 55, 282-282v ; Cod. 327, fol. 46.
63. Details in LUTTRELL, art. cit. note 5, p. 322-326.
64. Malta, Cod. 330, fol. 95.
65. DELAVILLE LE ROULX, *op. cit.* note 24, p. 261, note 1.
66. Malta, Cod. 1126, fol. 384-385.
67. DELAVILLE LE ROULX, *op. cit.* note 24, p. 304-309.
68. Malta, Cod. 336, fol. 168-169 ; the text named eight sisters from various parts of Italy. On San Giovannino, next to San Sepolcro, at Pisa, see E. TOLAINI, *Forma Pisarum : problemi e ricerche per una storia urbanistica della città di Pisa*, Pisa, 1967, p. 78, 198.
69. Malta, Cod. 336, fol. 163v-164v.
70. DELAVILLE LE ROULX, *op. cit.* note 24, p. 351 and note 1 ; *infra*, p. 134.

to Genoa, Naples and Rhodes [71] ; by 1383 he was titular Seneschal to the King of Armenia [72]. He made loans to King Pierre I of Cyprus [73] and to the Hospital at Rhodes [74], where he acquired much property at Phanes, at Diaschoro where he held the *casale* in fief, and in the town where in 1374 he had a lease on buildings once belonging to the Florentine Peruzzi [75]. He apparently accompanied the Hospitallers to Constantinople when they assisted the Emperor Manuel II recover his throne in 1390 [76] ; there during or just before May 1391 he acquired the "tunic of Christ", which came from the empress, and a "thumb" of John the Baptist, from a noble lady, the thumb passing eventually to the cathedral in Florence [77]. Giovanni Corsini was buried in the chapel of Saint Catherine which by 1388 he had founded in the Augustinian church at Rhodes [78]. His brother Pietro was a cardinal-protector of the Hospital by 1373 [79] and in 1392 he was residing in the Hospitaller preceptory of Saint-Jean at Avignon [80], staying in that town until his death in 1405 [81].

Certain unscrupulous Hospitallers operated in Tuscany by selling indulgences there. Thus on 18 January 1320 the pope instructed the Bishop of Gubbio to capture, to investigate and to punish or absolve the Hospitaller Fr. Giovanni de Rossi of Lucca and his accomplice who were preaching with false papal letters ; presumably they were selling indulgences or at least collecting money [82]. Over a century later, in 1431, the Florentine chancellor complained to the pope that a Hospitaller *miles*, accompanied by a loquacious Franciscan and other followers and scribes, was appearing on a high platform, demonstrating various letters and seals to the populace and making exaggerated claims concerning the powers conceded by the pope to the Hospitallers which they claimed allowed them to grant indulgences and absolutions for personal redemption. People came running with money, clothes, silver and gold, so that the place was

71. A. BENVENUTI PAPI, "Corsini, Giovanni", in *Dizionario biografico degli Italiani*, XXIX, Rome, 1983, p. 638-640 ; see also LUTTRELL, *op. cit.* note 47, XV, p. 400, 407. There is much unpublished material on Giovanni Corsini.

72. Malta, Cod. 322, fol. 282v.

73. *Grégoire XI*, *op. cit.* note 34, n⁰ˢ 13, 20.

74. Malta, Cod. 48, fol. 40v-41, 193-194 ; Cod. 321, fol. 232v.

75. Arch. Vat., Reg. Aven. 296, fol. 156v-158 ; Malta, Cod. 320, fol. 37v-39 ; Cod. 339, fol. 207-208.

76. A. LUTTRELL, "The Hospitallers of Rhodes confront the Turks : 1306-1421", in *Christians, Jews and Other Worlds : Patterns of Conflict and Accommodation*, ed. P. GALLAGHER, Lanham, 1988, p. 98.

77. Latin text in E. GAMURRINI, *Istoria genealogica delle famiglie nobili toscane et umbre*, III, Florence, 1673, p. 152-154 ; Gamurrini states that Corsini had the "thumb" from the emperor while in his service, but that is not what the text says.

78. *Ibid.*, p. 154. A treaty was concluded in this chapel in 1388 : text in L. BELGRANO, "Seconda serie di documenti riguardanti la colonia di Pera", in *Atti della Società Ligure di Storia Patria*, 13, 1877-1884, p. 953-965.

79. Text in LUTTRELL, art. cit. note 41, p. 13.

80. M. DYKMANS, "Les palais cardinalices d'Avignon", in *Mélanges de l'École française de Rome : Moyen Age — Temps modernes*, 83, 1971, p. 415.

81. J. CHIFFOLEAU, "Corsini, Pietro", in *Dizionario biografico degli Italiani*, XXIX, Rome, 1983, p. 671-673.

82. *Jean XXII (1316-1334) : Lettres communes*, ed. G. MOLLAT, III, Paris, 1906, n° 12057.

like a market with the scribes writing out and sealing documents, while the Hospitaller ate great dinners and enjoyed other luxuries [83]. Pope Eugenius IV agreed on 28 July 1431 that they should be punished [84].

*
* *

The Tuscans, who had no effective fleet and no Levantine colony, quickly grasped the possibilities of establishing a presence on Rhodes. Fulco de Peruzzi witnessed the contract made at Limassol in 1306 which preceded the invasion of the island, on which the Bardi and Peruzzi almost immediately set up branches, lending the Hospital vast sums of money, importing and exporting goods, and doing business of all kinds. The Florentine merchant Francesco Balducci Pegolotti knew the island and its commercial conditions well, and when in about 1345 the great Florentine houses went bankrupt a number of their Tuscan employees remained on Rhodes, trading on their own account, lending money, entering the Order's bureaucracy and becoming citizens of Rhodes. By about 1370 the Alberti of Florence had become the Hospital's principal bankers, while Florentines continued to trade on the island and the first galley fleet to leave Pisa, in 1422, called at Rhodes [85]. A different type of Tuscan visitor was the Florentine humanist Cristoforo Buondelmonti, a priest who went to Rhodes in about 1423 to learn Greek and who spent a number of years there, leaving descriptions and maps of the Rhodian islands in his widely circulated Liber Insularum Archipelagi [86].

The Hospitallers never forgot their origins in Jerusalem or their obligations to the poor, to the sick and to pilgrims. In addition to their Western hospices, there was always a hospital at their Convent or headquarters, at Jerusalem, Acre, Limassol and Rhodes [87]. After the Muslim conquest of Jerusalem in 1187, Christian pilgrims lodged outside the walls in the former Hospitaller stables, and from about 1336 they were accommodated in the ruins of the Hospital's original hospital run by the Franciscans within the walls; the Hospitaller origin of this building was known to pilgrims [88]. A good number of travellers visited Rhodes on their

83. Text in N. Iorga, Notes et extraits pour servir à l'histoire des croisades au XIV* siècle, II, Paris, 1899, p. 299-301.

84. Arch. Vat., Reg. Vat. 370, fol. 25-25v.

85. Details in Luttrell, art. cit. note 5; relations between the Hospital and the Florentine banks are not studied here. Four members of the Peruzzi company are documented on Rhodes between 1336 and 1340, and six members of the Bardi between 1314 and 1339 : A. Sapori, Studi di storia economica : secoli XIII-XIV-XV, II, 3rd ed., Florence, 1955, p. 724, 727-729, 733-734, 740, 745, 752.

86. H.L. Turner, "Cristoforo Buondelmonti and the Isolario", in Terrae Incognitae, 19, 1987, p. 11-28; manuscripts listed in A. Luttrell, The Later History of the Maussolleion and its Utilization in the Hospitaller Castle at Bodrum = The Maussolleion at Halikarnassos, II, part 2, Aarhus, 1986, p. 193-194.

87. Riley-Smith, op. cit. note 3, p. 247-249, 331-332, 405-408; detail in I. Pappalardo, Storia sanitaria dell'Ordine Gerosolimitano di Malta dalle origini al presente, Rome, 1958; general introduction in L. Smugge, "Die Anfänge des organisierten Pilgerverkehrs in Mittelalter", in Quellen und Forschungen aus italienischen Archiven und Bibliotheken, 64, 1984, p. 1-83.

88. S. Schein, "Latin Hospices in Jerusalem in the Late Middle Ages", in Zeitschrift des Deutschen Palästina-Vereins, 101, 1985, p. 82-92.

way to or from Jerusalem. As early as 1314 an Englishman who arrived in Rhodes on his way to Jerusalem with papal letters of recommendation to the Master was provided on Rhodes with a companion, who subsequently robbed him of 152 florins [89]. Papal recommendations to the Master on behalf of individual pilgrims continued [90], but problems remained ; an envoy travelling to Cyprus had to wait at Rhodes for a ship from 29 November 1398 until 29 January 1399 [91]. Pilgrims in Cyprus could also use Hospitaller houses ; in 1418 Nompar de Caumont travelling from Famagusta to Nicosia stayed en route with the Hospitallers at a place called *Mores*, and at Nicosia he lodged in a "great hostel" at the Hospitaller preceptory where in the chapel he saw an arm of Saint George and part of his lance, a head of Saint Anne, the body of Saint Euphemia and other relics [92]. In 1403 the Hospital challenged the Venetian and Franciscan quasi-monopoly of the profitable pilgrim traffic on sea and land by negotiating a treaty with the Sultan Faraj by which the Order would have rights and facilities to control travel to Jerusalem and to maintain six Hospitallers or others in it, and to establish consuls at Jerusalem and Ramla. The treaty was never ratified or implemented [93]. The Hospital did, however, have a consul at Alexandria at least from 1381 onwards [94].

Many pilgrims travelled on ships which did not call at Rhodes or were diverted by pirates or bad weather. The Earl of Derby and his extensive retinue spent much money at Rhodes on provisions, services, repairs and luxuries in 1393 ; Fr. John de Raddington, Prior of England, apparently accompanied him to Jerusalem [95]. Pilgrims arrived from distant parts such as England and Germany, and some died on Rhodes [96] ; in about 1400 the Russian archimandrite Grethenios was at Rhodes, as in 1416 was another Russian, the monk Epiphanius [97]. Some pilgrims arranged credit facilities at Rhodes ; thus in 1409 the Master, then at Pisa, gave instructions for money to be advanced on Rhodes to the Archbishop of Lisbon and to the King of Portugal's confessor. In the same year Pierre de Nony, *intimus et affinis* of the Master, was to visit Rhodes on his way to Jerusalem. In 1413

89. *Calendar of the Patent Rolls : Edward II, AD. 1313-1317*, London, 1898, p. 277.

90. E.g. in 1354 and 1373 : *Innocent VI (1352-1362) : Lettres secrètes et curiales*, ed. P. GASNAULT, II, Paris, 1962, n° 1244, and *Lettres secrètes et curiales du Pape Grégoire XI (1370-1378) relatives à la France*, 5 fasc., ed. L. MIROT and H. JASSEMIN, Paris, 1935-1957, n° 1454.

91. L. DE MAS LATRIE, *Histoire de l'île de Chypre sous le règne des princes de la maison de Lusignan*, II, Paris, 1852, p. 450.

92. *Le voyage d'Oultremer en Jherusalem de Nompar, seigneur de Caumont*, ed. P. NOBLE, Oxford, 1975, p. 49.

93. Full detail in LUTTRELL, art. cit. note 4 ; background in D. JACOBY, "Pèlerinage médiéval et sanctuaires de Terre Sainte : la perspective vénitienne", in *Ateneo Veneto*, 173, 1986, p. 27-58.

94. Malta, Cod. 321, fol. 213 ; Cod. 339, fol. 120, 151v ; E. ASHTOR, *Levant Trade in the Middle Ages*, Princeton, 1983, p. 365, note 566.

95. *Expeditions to Prussia and the Holy Land made by Henry Earl of Derby*, ed. L. TOULMIN SMITH, London, 1894, p. 225-229.

96. E.g. R. RÖHRICHT, *Deutsche Pilgerreisen nach dem Heiligen Lande*, revised ed., Innsbruck, 1900, p. 93, 96 ; C. TYERMAN, *England and the Crusades : 1095-1588*, Chicago, 1988, p. 282-284, 286.

97. B. DE KHITROWO, *Itinéraires russes en Orient*, Geneva, 1889, p. 168, 196.

magister Florent Bouquaut, donat of the Hospital and a former judge at Rhodes, was also leaving that island on a Jerusalem pilgrimage [98].

Some pilgrims left written descriptions of Rhodes, where they could find rest and lodgings, seek a new ship, meet fellow-countrymen among the Hospital's brethren, visit the town and list the holy relics they saw [99]. Some stayed in the Order's hospital there [100], which was said in 1357 to shelter pilgrims, the poor, the sick and others : *Quod in hospitali Rodi tam peregrinis quam pauperibus infirmis, et aliis provideatur ut pertinet, et est fieri antiquitus* [101]. In 1391 the Neapolitan Hospitaller, Fr. Domenico de Alamania, founded a hospice dedicated to Santa Caterina in the *borgo* of the city [102]. The pilgrim Niccolò da Martoni described it in 1394/1395 with its several fine chambers, its many beds and its relics, but he noted that it was reserved for nobles and that other pilgrims had difficulty in finding accommodation in Rhodes [103]. Pero Tafur, visiting Rhodes in about 1437, described Santa Caterina in which pilgrims received all necessities, except their food, and where they found a church and chaplains to serve them [104]. In 1410 or 1411 Fr. Domenico de Alamania, by then lieutenant of the Master at Rhodes, sought to transfer his foundation to the Franciscans, but on his death in 1411 the Hospitallers refused to carry out that project [105]. The noble pilgrim Niccolò da Este was greeted at Rhodes in 1413 by a group of Italian Hospitallers and friends who entertained him handsomely while his companions stayed in the Santa Caterina hospice ; on his return journey he too saw and listed a collection of relics [106]. In fact, there were numerous

98. Malta, Cod. 337, fol. 129 (pencil fol. 77) ; Cod. 339, fol. 157. Bouquaut became a donat in the Priory of France in 1389, and in 1397 he was Master in Arts and Bachelor in Law, and was received as a donat for life on condition that he became a professed *frater* within two years : Paris, Arch. Nat., MM 31, fol. 85, 97v, 246v (information kindly provided by Anne-Marie Legras). He actually became not a *frater* but a judge at Rhodes.

99. No complete list of visitors' accounts exists ; some are used in G. SOMMI PICENARDI, *Itinéraire d'un chevalier de Saint-Jean de Jérusalem dans l'île de Rhodes*, Lille, 1900, and in E. NASALLI ROCCA DI CORNELIANO, "Rodi nel quattrocento : come la videro i pellegrini in Terra Santa", in *Annales de l'Ordre Souverain Militaire de Malte*, 26, 1968, p. 5-13.

100. This was not the grander hospital built after 1440 but the fourteenth-century hospital which has yet to be located with certainty but is possibly the building which now houses the archaeological institute.

101. Malta, Cod. 69, fol. 21v.

102. Inscription and plans in A. GABRIEL, *La cité de Rhodes : MCCCX-MDXXII*, II, Paris, 1923, p. 102-106 ; curiously, its foundation text (Malta, Cod. 326, fol. 129-131 : extracts *ibid.*, II, p. 227-228) made no mention of its purpose. The building is in course of excavation to which Anna Maria Kasdagli kindly provided a visit in 1990. G. PINTO, "I costi del pellegrinaggio in Terrasanta nei secoli XIV e XV (dai resoconti dei viaggiatori italiani)", in *Toscana e Terrasanta, op. cit.* note 1, p. 282, wrongly gives Alamania as German.

103. "Relation du pèlerinage à Jérusalem de Nicolas de Martoni, notaire italien : 1394-1395", ed. E. LEGRAND, in *Revue de l'Orient Latin*, III, 1895, p. 642.

104. *Andanças é viajes de Pero Tafur por diversas partes del mundo avidos : 1435-1439*, ed. M. JIMENEZ DE LA ESPADA, Madrid, 1874, p. 48-49.

105. LUTTRELL, art. cit. note 4, p. 199-200.

106. *Viaggio a Gerusalemme di Nicolò da Este descritto da Luchino dal Campo*, ed. G. GHINASSI = *Miscellanea di opusculi inediti o rari dei secoli XIV e XV*, I, Turin, 1861, p. 115, 142-143.

132

relics on Rhodes [107] and in 1419 the Lord of Caumont, who visited the chapel on Mount Phileremos and saw other churches, listed the indulgences which these relics afforded the visitor and which made them a spiritual part of the pilgrim itinerary ; visitors to the hospital also secured indulgences [108]. The earliest surviving account of Rhodes by a Tuscan pilgrim is that of the cleric Mariano da Siena who reached the island in 1431 together with fourteen Hospitallers who disembarked there. On his return visit he described not only the relics but also the plague which, he reported, had killed some 8000 Christians in less than six months [109].

Occasionally pilgrims were acting as spies on reconnaissance. Thus on 13 August 1347 the Master at Rhodes issued a safe-conduct for the Florentine Carthusian Amico di Buonamico and six companions who were with him at Rhodes on their way to Jerusalem *pro explorationibus faciendis* [110]. On 15 May 1348 papal letters described this Carthusian as a military expert from the convent of Galluzzo near Florence who was about to return from Avignon to Rhodes where he would serve against the Turks ; the pope had transferred him to the Hospitaller Order [111]. Hospitaller brethren sometimes became pilgrims themselves. On 11 June 1331 the pope licensed Fr. Hélion de Villeneuve, the Master of Rhodes himself, to visit the holy land [112]. Other pilgrims apparently went to Santiago in Galicia. Fr. Raymond Cays, Preceptor of Arles, was licensed to go there on 23 January 1347, and on the following 1 September Fr. Étienne de Lobaresio was given a licence to leave Rhodes for Santiago da Compostela and *alia oratoria*. On 25 January 1348 the Prior of Catalunya, Fr. Perearnau Perestortes, then at Rhodes, was licensed to travel to Jerusalem and other places in the East and to Santiago or elsewhere in the West accompanied by a Hospitaller chaplain and one other Hospitaller *socius* ; he was to secure any licence, papal or otherwise, which might be needed [113]. A few Aragonese brethren received licences to attend the papal jubilee at Rome in 1350 [114]. A steady stream of licences for Hospitaller pilgrims was issued. On 7 October 1374 the Prior of Auvergne, Fr. Robert de Châteauneuf, was permitted to make any *peregrinatio seu viagium* he wished [115] ; Fr. Petrus Bole was licensed to go

107. A. LUTTRELL, "The Rhodian Background of the Order of Saint John on Malta", in *The Order's Early Legacy in Malta*, ed. J. AZZOPARDI, Malta, 1989, p. 10-14, with important complementary materials in F. TOMMASI, "I Templari e il culto delle reliquie", in *I Templari : mito e storia, op. cit.* note 7, p. 191-210.

108. NOMPAR DE CAUMONT, *op. cit.* note 92, p. 51-52.

109. *Del viaggio in Terra Santa fatto e descritto da ser Mariano da Siena nel secolo XV*, ed. D. MORENI, Florence, 1822, p. 9, 120-121 ; cf. F. CARDINI, "Nota su Mariano di Nanni rettore di San Pietro a Ovile in Siena", in *Toscana e Terrasanta, op. cit.* note 1, p. 177-187.

110. Malta, Cod. 317, fol. 224.

111. *Clément VI (1342-1352). Lettres closes, patentes et curiales intéressant les pays autres que la France*, 3 fasc., ed. E. DÉPREZ and G. MOLLAT, Paris, 1960-1961, I, n°s 1646-1649.

112. DELAVILLE LE ROULX, *op. cit.* note 24, p. 85, note 7.

113. Malta, Cod. 316, fol. 14 ; Cod. 317, fol. 31, 86.

114. Madrid, Archivo Histórico Nacional, Sección de Códices, 600 B, fol. 65, 100.

115. Malta, Cod. 320, fol. 38v ; the prior's name is given in DELAVILLE LE ROULX, *op. cit.* note 24, p. 207, note 7.

from Rhodes to the holy sepulchre *et alia sanctuaria* on 4 July 1381 [116]. This must have been not uncommon since in 1382, when Fr. Lodovico Vaignon travelled from Rhodes to Cyprus to plot the overthrow of the Avignonist "schismatics" at Rhodes, he did so successfully using the pretence that he was on pilgrimage [117]. On 12 February 1390 Fr. Johan Merklin, Preceptor of Würzburg, was licensed to go to Rhodes and to Jerusalem, and on 17 March 1392 Fr. Bernabono de Pozzo was permitted to leave the Priory of Lombardy for Rhodes and for Jerusalem and other holy places [118], and licences for brethren to leave Rhodes for Jerusalem continued to be issued [119].

A special feature of the Jerusalem pilgrimage was the ceremony by which certain nobles were dubbed knights in the holy sepulchre. In 1419 the Gascon noble Nompar de Caumont found a young Navarrese knight at Rhodes and took him to Jerusalem where he dubbed and knighted Nompar in the holy sepulchre where he took a series of special vows [120]. At least one Hospitaller may have been knighted in the same way. Possibly in about April 1413 the Master's Lieutenant at Rhodes ordered Fr. Nicolaus *de Boehemia* to receive as a brother of the Hospital in the Priory of *Alamania* a certain Johan de Zemtruvel, with the special condition that he had previously been knighted by another knight in the church of the holy sepulchre at Jerusalem [121]. On 27 June 1413 Fr. Johan Zemtruvel was licensed to leave Rhodes [122], presumably providing a rare example of a man who had been knighted in Jerusalem and been received as a Hospitaller *miles* on Rhodes. That was one way in which the island formed a link between Jerusalem and the West. In Tuscany, as elsewhere, the Hospital's brethren and preceptories contributed to the maintenance among the populace of sentiment for the holy war against the infidel and for pilgrimage to the holy places in Jerusalem.

116. Malta, Cod. 321, fol. 213.

117. Luttrell, *The Hospitallers in Cyprus, Rhodes, op. cit.* note 34, XXIII, p. 42.

118. Malta, Cod. 324, fol. 101 ; Cod. 325, fol. 145.

119. E.g. Fr. Louis de Gletens, 31 March 1412 (Malta, Cod. 339, fol. 173v) ; Fr. Gracian, 18 April 1412 (fol. 173v) ; Fr. Guillaume de Chalon, 26 July 1413 (fol. 181v) ; Fr. Marot Hugonelli, Preceptor of Marseilles, [7] September 1415 (fol. 126v) ; Fr. Hugues *Goy* (?), 8 January 1416 (fol. 128). All but Hugonelli and Chalon came from the Priory of Auvergne. Chalon was of the Priory of France : Cod. 338, fol. 27-27v. A son of the Count of Tonnerre, Chalon went several times to Rhodes : Luttrell, art. cit. note 4, p. 42. No evidence seems to survive for any Tuscan Hospitaller pilgrim within the period studied.

120. Nompar de Caumont, *op. cit.* note 92, p. 32 ; J. Sumption, *Pilgrimage : an Image of Mediaeval Religion*, London, 1975, p. 266, mistakenly regards the Navarrese knight as a Hospitaller and states that he was to dub Nompar as a Hospitaller knight ; he thus wrongly presents dubbings conducted at the holy sepulchre under the auspices of the Hospitallers and others as a general practice.

121. Malta, Cod. 339, fol. 179v (undated) : *fuit preceptum fratri cuidem* (sic) *Nicolao de Boehemia ut faciat fratrem religionis Johannem de Zemtruvel prioratus Alamanj prius per alium militem milicie cingulo decoratum etc. in ecclesia sanctj sepulcrj Jh(erusale)m etc.*

122. Malta, Cod. 339, fol. 181.

HOSPITALLER PRIORS OF PISA : A PRELIMINARY NOTE

Gerardo de Gragnana	... 26 June 1299... (*Cartulaire*, n° 4471)
Giovanni Melegario	... 30 January 1307-25 February 1309... (FEDI, *op. cit.* note 10, p. 109-111 : *Cartulaire*, n° 4850)
Gregorio de Parma	... 21 July 1317-August 1321... (Arch. Vat., Reg. Vat. 66, fol. 337 : J. RAYBAUD, *Histoire des Grands Prieurs et du Prieuré de Saint-Gilles*, I, Nîmes, 1904, p. 270)
Giovanni de Rivara	... 30 October 1323-17 July 1348... (Florence, Archivio di Stato, Corporazioni Religiose Soppresse, n° 132, sezione 191 : *Clément VI (1342-1352). Lettres closes, patentes et curiales*, 3 vols., ed. E. DÉPREZ, J. GLÉNISSON and G. MOLLAT, Paris, 1925-1959, II, n°ˢ 3919-3920 ; *Clément VI*, ed. DÉPREZ-MOLLAT, *op. cit.* note 111, n° 2157)
Bartolomeo di Lapo Benini	... 12 May 1351-before February 1373 (Malta, Cod. 318, fol. 159 : *supra*, p. 123)
Palamedo di Giovanni	... 16 July 1373-10 September 1374 (*supra*, p. 123 note 34 : Arch. Vat., Reg. Vat. 286, fol. 166v-167v)
Bartolomeo di Lapo Benini	10 September 1374-28 September 1375... (*supra*, p. 123 : Arch. Vat., Reg. Vat. 286, fol. 166v-167v)
Niccolò degli Strozzi	... *ca* April 1377-*ca* April 1378... (LUTTRELL, *op. cit.* note 47, XV, p. 415-417)
Bartolomeo Castellani Lieutenant of the Master in the priory	... 1 May 1380... (*ibid.*, p. 417)
Giovanni Siffi	... 16 February 1381-26 July 1393... (*supra*, p. 125, 127)
Vacant ?	
Priamo Gambacorti	10 May 1410-*ca* January 1448 (*supra*, p. 127)[123]

---

123. Gambacorti was suspended in 1419 and restored in 1420 : DELAVILLE LE ROULX, *op. cit.* note 24, p. 351, note 1.

PRIORS OF PISA OF THE ROMAN OBEDIENCE : ca 1384-1410

The complex affairs of the Roman obedience of the Priory of Pisa are partly illustrated in the surviving register of the "anti-Master", Fr. Riccardo Caracciolo (Malta, Cod. 281). Caracciolo's "chapter general" met at Naples from 28 March to 6 April 1384 and a number of Tuscan brethren attended (fol. 1-9v) ; the prior, Fr. Francesco degli Strozzi, did not appear, though he was apparently a Roman appointment since the Avignon prior, Fr. Giovanni Siffi, continued to be recognized by the Master Fr. Juan Fernández de Heredia and by the Convent at Rhodes (supra, p. 125, 127). Strozzi was therefore condemned to lose his position if he failed to appear before Caracciolo, and an unidentified lieutenant of the Master, possibly Fr. Bartolomeo Castellani, was appointed (fol. 5, 6-6v). Following his failure to respond in person, Strozzi was declared to be deposed on 12 May 1385 (fol. 58v-59) and Castellani was named in his place on 16 July (fol. 61-62) ; but Castellani died some time before 25 September 1385 when four magistral procurators, Fr. Leonardi degli Strozzi, Fr. Alberto Franceschi of Siena, Fr. Lorenzo Giovannini and Fr. Jacopo degli Obizzi, were named for the priory (fol. 72-73). On 25 November Caracciolo, then at Pisa, appointed Fr. Bartolomeo de Cascina and Fr. Alberto Franceschi of Siena to act as his lieutenants in the priory (fol. 75v). By 2 December, following pressure from Florence, he had named Fr. Leonardo degli Strozzi as prior (supra, p. 126) ; on 17 May 1388 he appointed Fr. Priamo Gerardi de Gambacorti as his lieutenant in the priory (fol. 91-91v), and from some point before 1392 until 1410 Gambacorti was the Romanist Prior of Pisa (supra, p. 126).

PRECEPTORIES OF THE PRIORY OF PISA IN 1337

Alberese [124]
Asciano, San Giovanni [125]
Borgo d'Arbia
Borgo Fabrice, San Giovanni (possibly Fabbrica near Montepulciano)
Cerbaiola [126]
Corneto, San Clemente
Corneto, San Matteo
Corneto, San Salvatore
Florence, San Jacopo [127]
Foresto, San Giovanni (Diocese of Arezzo)
Frigido, San Leonardo (near Massa di Carrara) [128]

124. San Benedetto, 1307 : text in FEDI, op. cit. note 10, p. 110-111.
125. An inscription of 1323 mentioned repairs to the church of Santa Maria and San Giovanni Battista, Asciano, done by the preceptor, Fr. Federigo Spadafuori : text in E. REPETTI, Dizionario geografico fisico storico della Toscana, I, Florence, 1833, p. 151-152.
126. Cerbaiola was in the comitatus of Florence in 1440 : Malta, Cod. 355, fol. 117v-118. Its patron was San Leonardo in 1389 : Cod. 324, fol. 115.
127. Cf. PAATZ, op. cit. note 43, II, p. 400-410 ; V, p. 95-97.
128. The Hospitaller hospice with parts of a Romanesque church and its carved doorway survive at San Leonardo al Frigido : R. STOPANI, La Via Francigena in Toscana : storia di una strada medievale, 2nd ed., Florence, 1984, p. 47.

136

Gradoli, San Manno
Grosseto (first house)
Grosseto (second house) [129]
Lucca, Malanotte [130]
Lucca, San Pietro
Massa Marittima, San Giovanni [131]
Montalto di Castro [132]
Montebello (Diocese of Arezzo) [133]
Montecatino, San Giovanni
Montechiello [134]
Orvieto (first house)
Orvieto (second house) [135]
Péccioli (north-west of Volterra) [136]
Pescia, Sant'Aluccio
Pisa, Santa Maria Maddelena
Pisa, San Sepolcro [137]
Pistoia [138]
Poggibonsi, San Giovanni
Ponte di Rigo [139]
Pontremoli [140]
Prato [141]
San Gimignano, San Jacopo
San Gimignano, San Giovanni [142]
San Giovanni e Vittore (Commenda south of Montefiascone)

129. A single house dedicated to San Leonardo and San Benedetto, 1385 : Malta, Cod. 281, fol. 84.
130. San Giovanni, 1307, and San Giovanni *de Malanotte*, 1358 : Fedi, *op. cit.* note 10, p. 109-110, and Malta, Cod. 316, fol. 252v.
131. *Caperolla* or *Capriolani* de Massa, 1420 : Malta, Cod. 344, fol. 171v ; Cod. 345, fol. 158.
132. San Leonardo, 1373 : *supra*, p. 120.
133. Sant'Appolinare, 1373 : *supra*, p. 119.
134. Montechiello de *Chioli*, 1347 : Malta, Cod. 317, fol. 170-170v.
135. San Giovanni, 1358 : Malta, Cod. 316, fol. 252v.
136. The former Templar house of Montelopio near Fabbrica at Péccioli : Bini, art. cit. note 13, p. 458. A text of 1384 mentioned apparently separate houses of San Giovanni di Montelopio and of Péccioli : Malta, Cod. 281, fol. 14v-15v.
137. Tolaini, *op. cit.* note 68, p. 78, 93-94, and note 199.
138. San Giovanni, *Pisterio*, 1386 : Malta, Cod. 281, fol. 91-91v.
139. San Giovanni, Ponte di Rigo, 1420 : *supra*, p. 120. A mid-eighteenth century map shows the preceptory's properties around the bridge of the Via Cassia : R. Stopani, "L'evoluzione del tracciato della Via Francigena tra Val d'Orcia e Val di Paglia", in *L'abbazia di San Salvatore al Monte Amiata : documenti storici — architettura — proprietà*, ed. W. Kurze and C. Prezzolini, Florence, 1988, p. 35.
140. N. Zucchi Castellini, "La commenda di San Leonardo e l'Ospedale di S. Giovanni in Pontremoli", in *Studi storici : miscellanea in onore di Manfredo Giuliani*, Parma, 1965, p. 226, 234-237 ; but correct the notion that it became a preceptory only in 1420.
141. San Giovanni, 1384 : Malta, Cod. 281, fol. 17v-18v.
142. San Jacopo belonged to the Temple, and San Giovanni and San Bartolo to the Hospital : C. Talei-Franzesi, "Cenni su l'Ordine Gerosolimitano in San Gimignano", in *Miscellanea storica della Valdelsa*, 51, 1943, with details of frescoes in San Jacopo ; I. Moretti and R. Stopani, *Chiese romaniche in Valdelsa*, Florence, 1968, p. 182-184, 188-191.

Santa Maria in Capità (Bagnoregio)
Scerpenna
Siena, San Leonardo
Siena, San Pietro in Camollia
Silvitella, San Pietro (possibly near Monterone)
Sugarella (west of Tuscania) [143]
Tuscania, San Leonardo

These *domus* or preceptories are those mentioned with the name of their preceptor, who sometimes held two or more houses, in documents of the prioral chapter at Siena in 1337 (*supra*, p. 121). Alberese was described as a *domus seu fortalicium* of which the prior was *gubernator*. The list is probably incomplete, and some houses remain to be located. Certain Hospitaller houses, such as that called Turri near Poggibonsi, sold in 1323, were alienated or otherwise lost before 1337. A preceptory might be divided ; or several houses might be regrouped in one ; or estates might be reshuffled ; or the house, and name, of a preceptory might be moved from one place to another within a preceptory ; or the dedication might be altered. It is, therefore, difficult to establish the precise number of houses at any given time while the changing of dedications causes much confusion. The text of 1337 did not include, or did not name, six of the eight preceptories in the Diocese of Arezzo in 1373 : San Giorgio, Arezzo [144] ; San Giovanni, *Bottachino ; Capraria*, possibly Capraia in Casentino [145] ; Sant'Egidio, Quercia Frassenaria ; San Giovanni, Monte San Savino [146] ; and San Jacopo al Prato, presumably in the Pratomagno. The 1337 texts also omitted San Sepolcro at Florence, usurped in 1327 and 1331 by various Florentines to whom it had been leased by the former prior, Fr. Gregorio de Parma [147] ; Sant'Angelo at *Subterra* near Pescia documented in 1333 [148] ; the former Temple *mansio* at Colle di Buggiano in Valdinievole near Lucca mentioned in 1326 and 1395 [149] ; the *hospitalis pauperum* at Montepulciano in 1320 [150], Montepulciano itself being a preceptory in 1347 [151] ; and other houses as well. Hospitaller texts of 1384 mentioned houses of San Giovanni Montelopio, of Péccioli, of Laiatico, of Valdera, of Santa Croce at Ponsacco just south of Pontedera, of Certalla near Montelopio, and of Sant'*Auzini* at Civitavecchia. Other documents referred to Santa Caterina at Serravalle in 1385 and San Giovanni at Bibona in 1386 [152]. The house at *Celle* in 1417, when the nearby church at Certalla was said to have been destroyed completely for eighty years, was presumably at

143. Ms : *Subarella*. Dedicated to San Giovanni, 1420 : *supra*, p. 120.
144. San Jacopo and San Giorgio, Arezzo, were separate preceptories in 1385 : Malta, Cod. 281, fol. 79v.
145. Sant'Angelo, Capraia, 1420 : Malta, Cod. 344, fol. 170v-171.
146. A Hospitaller house in 1306 : *Cartulaire*, n° 4850.
147. Arch. Vat., Reg. Vat. 114, fol. 61-61v ; Reg. Aven. 39, fol. 706-706v ; Paatz, *op. cit.* note 43, V, p. 97-99.
148. Siena, Archivio di Stato, Capitoli 171, n° 31. Sant'Angelo *sub terra* near Capalbio, 1420 : Malta, Cod. 344, fol. 171-171v.
149. Delaville Le Roulx, *op. cit.* note 24, p. 76 ; Pauli, *op. cit.* note 60, II, p. 104-107 ; cf. E. Coturri, "I Templari in Valdinievole : la *Mansio Templi* del Colle di Buggiano", in *I Templari : mito e storia, op. cit.* note 7, p. 331-335.
150. *Supra*, p. 121.
151. Malta, Cod. 317, fol. 170-170v.
152. Malta, Cod. 281, fol. 14v-15v, 36-36v, 38v, 54, 76-76v, 92v.

Cigoli [153]. These places, probably not normally preceptories, corresponded in part to places listed in the papal accounts of 1302/1303 : the *Hospitale S. Iohannis de Ceuli* or Cigoli in the Diocese of Lucca, and in the Diocese of Volterra the hospitals of San Giovanni *de Turre* which was possibly at Poggibonsi, of San Giovanni at Bibona just south of Cecina and of San Giovanni at Péccioli, and also the *mansio Templi de Montelopio cum domo de Certalla* [154]. The hospital at Croce Brandegliana near Pistoia was mentioned in 1409 [155], as in 1420 was the *domus* of Vignale in the *comitatus* of Piombino [156]. Obviously, other places remain unidentified. There were also Hospitaller houses and possessions in Sardinia which depended on the Priory of Pisa ; some, including San Leonardo delle Sette Fontane near Santulussurgiu, came from the Templars [157].

Templar houses within the Hospitaller Priory of Pisa, not all of which passed to the Hospital, included [158] : Aquapendente ; Arezzo, Santa Margherita [159] ; *Caporsoli*, possibly the *hospitalis* of Montorsoli near Florence ; *Cerbaria* near Lucca ; Certalla ; Civitavecchia, San Giulio and Santa Maria ; Colle di Buggiano in the Valdinievole ; Corneto, San Matteo ; Florence, San Jacopo ; Frosini near San Galgano [160] ; Grosseto, San Salvatore or San Leonardo ; Lucca, San Pietro ; Montefiascone, San Benedetto ; Montelepio ; Pisa, San Sepolcro ; Pisa, Santa Sofia [161] ; Pistoia, the *hospitalis* of Croce Brandegliana ; Pitigliano [162] ; San Gimignano, San Jacopo ; Santa Maria in Capità at Bagnoregio ; Siena, San Pietro in Camollia ; Valentano, Santa Maria ; and Vignale near Piombino [163].

153. Malta, Cod. 340, fol. 167v-169v.

154. *Rationes Decimarum, op. cit.* note 11, II, p. 201, 258.

155. Malta, Cod. 335, fol. 136v.

156. Malta, Cod. 344, fol. 171v.

157. Not studied here ; references in F. BRAMATO, *Storia dell'Ordine dei Templari in Italia : le fondazioni*, Rome, 1991, p. 73, and V. ATZENI, "Templari e Cavalieri Ospedalieri di S. Giovanni in Sardegna", in *Humana Studia*, 2, 1950, p. 362-380.

158. This list, incomplete and in part debatable, is based on GILMOUR-BRYSON (*op. cit.* note 15), SZABÒ (art. cit. note 7), BRAMATO (*op. cit.* note 157), and *supra* ; the southern limits of the priory were uncertain. BRAMATO, *ibid.*, p. 73, accepts the Templar house at Sovana as proposed in CAPONE, *op. cit.* note 13, p. 129.

159. As San Giorgio : *supra*, p. 119.

160. M. BORRACELLI, "La Magione Templare di Frosini e l'importanza delle strade che vi convergevano", in *I Templari : mito e storia, op. cit.* note 7, p. 311-324.

161. TOLAINI, *op. cit.* note 68, p. 123-124, note 260.

162. In 1441 the Hospitaller preceptory of *la badia alavina de Pitiliano* in the Priory of Pisa had recently been in secular hands, quite possibly since 1312 or earlier : Malta, Cod. 355, fol. 127v. It was probably the presumed Templar house (of Santa Maria ?) in Vinea near Pitigliano : B. CAPONE, L. IMPERIO and E. VALENTINI, *Guida all'Italia dei Templari*, Rome, 1989, p. 151-153. That a Templar was castellan of the papal castle at Ponte dell'Abbadia does not (*contra* CAPONE, *op. cit.* note 13, p. 148-155) show that the castle belonged to the Templars.

163. BORRACELLI, art. cit. note 160, p. 316.

XVIII

THE HOSPITALLER PRIORY OF VENICE IN 1331[1]

The systematic reconstruction of the medieval history of the Order of Saint John in Italy has never been attempted, though there is a considerable, if often unsatisfactory, body of published work[2]. The surviving sources are both fragmentary and dispersed, while existing articles and monographs are almost exclusively concerned with local themes and are based on only a portion of the materials still available; they scarcely add up to a history of the Hospital in Italy or in any one of the seven priories of the Italian province. Fragments of the late-medieval archives of the Venetian priory survive in well over 900 *filze* which, however, largely contain post-medieval materials such as estate books, accounts and leases[3]. A further 22 *filze* recently detached from the prioral archive are in Padua, Archivio di Stato, Commenda di Malta, and another 30 *buste* concerning the Preceptories of Montebello, Longara and Villaga are in Vicenza, Archivio di Stato, Corporazioni Religiose Soppresse, Buste 3065-3094[4]. The study of the relations between the government of Venice and the Hospital at Rhodes bears only marginally on the affairs of the priory in the period before the Terraferma came largely under Venetian rule after about 1405[5], so that it is important to make use of documents in the papal registers[6], in the numerous local archives spread across North-East Italy, in those parts of the Hospital's central archive from Rhodes now preserved on Malta[7], and elsewhere. Since the southern areas of the Venetian priory have been more extensively studied in print[8], those to the north receive special attention below.

From these materials it is largely possible to identify Hospitaller preceptories, churches and other buildings, to establish which possessions belonged to the Templars before passing to the Hospital in or after 1312, and to study estate management, relations with the lay authorities and other matters demanding extensive local research. The sources could also be used to illuminate themes, such as prices and agrarian practices, which are not connected exclusively with Hospitaller history. The three texts presented below are used merely to outline an answer to two fundamental questions on which the Hospital's rulers, whether at Rhodes or elsewhere, needed precise information: how many *domus* or preceptories did the priory of Venice contain and what was their taxable income? The texts provide a cross-section of the priory at one given moment in 1331, and they supply details of the preceptors who held some, though not all, of the houses; the list of estimated incomes, which seems almost complete, included almost every house. The brief introduction and the gazetteer leave much work still to be done and will require considerable amendment and expansion. The gazetteer establishes basic information on each house, but each single commandery could eventually receive a separate study of its own and the present purpose is rather to build up a picture of the priory, its extent and structure. Such information should in turn be fitted into the information available from inquests into other priories, most notably those conducted in 1338 and 1373[9]. Unfortunately, only one inquest for a diocese within the Priory of Venice, that for Treviso, survives from the great papal inquest of 1373[10].

Certain technical difficulties baffled even contemporaries. There was recurrent confusion between the Hospital as an order, a hospital, a hospice and a *hospicium* or house, while a single hospital could serve the poor, the sick, the aged and the passing pilgrim. The Templars possessed *hospitales* which, like some Templar preceptories, were sometimes dedicated to San Giovanni, and long before 1312 the Hospital held houses and churches dedicated to San Giovanni del Tempio which were, confusingly, never Templar possessions[11]. The boundaries of priories and preceptories could change, and so could their titles; a preceptory was sometimes termed a *prioratus*; a preceptor might hold two or more preceptories; a *domus* or *mansio* could be reduced in status so that it became a *membrum* of another preceptory, and preceptories were sometimes united in one or split into more than one; furthermore, a preceptory might include a parish or hospital, and these sometimes had titles or dedications which differed from that of their preceptory. Such complications were especially frequent in the decades following 1312 when the Hospital was absorbing the Templars' properties and many changes were being made.

The Templars' archives did not survive, and the sources and bibliography available for the systematic study of the Italian Temple are scanty[12] while much recent work by Italian «templaristi» is inspired by esoteric as well as scientific concerns. The works of Bianca Capone should be used with some caution but they do provide little known texts, maps, illustrations and valuable topographical locations; unfortunately, they tend to present general bibliographies rather than precise documentation for particular points[13]. The «templaristi» are apt to turn local traditions into facts, to misinterpret toponyms such as «Tempio» and «Mason», and mistakenly to attribute Templar origins to Hospitaller houses; the supposed «preceptory» at Grignano near Trieste and its «passage» to the Hospital provide a good example[14]. It is often considered, erroneously, that the term «Mason» or «Magione» necessarily indicates a Templar house and that «Commenda» always represents a Hospitaller origin, while Hospitaller establishments with the dedication San Giovanni del Tempio have systematically been listed as Templar houses[15].

* * *

The Hospitaller and Templar orders emerged in Jerusalem in the years following the Latin conquest of 1099. The Templars were an association of knights and others concerned to protect the holy places and pilgrims travelling to visit them. The Hospitallers originally maintained a hospital in Jerusalem and cared for the poor, but during the twelfth century they too became primarily a military organization involved in an armed struggle against the infidel. Whether priests, *milites* or sergeants, their *fratres* were all religious who took vows of poverty, chastity and obedience, and who lived according to rules and statutes granted by the pope to whom they owed an ultimate obedience. Both orders received extensive properties and privileges in the West which included houses, churches, urban properties and, above all, rural estates; these provided centres for the recruitment and maintenance of brethren and furnished the funds for their hospices, hospitals and other charitable activities together with a surplus for the *responsiones*, the dues sent to finance the struggle in the East. These properties were arranged in preceptories each of which normally formed part of a priory, and the priories were grouped in provinces which corresponded after about 1310 to the *langues* or nations at Rhodes, but it was the preceptory, with its house, church and cemetery, which was the focus of the material and spiritual life of the *fratres* and their point of contact with the Western public.

The uneven distribution of the Hospital's estates and the way in which they were divided into preceptories of varying size and wealth depended in part on the vagaries of donors and the endowments they made. In Central and Southern Italy, as across much of Western Europe, Hospitaller preceptories were predominantly agricultural units and some were far from any sizeable town[16], but in Northern Italy the *domus* itself was frequently located within or just outside a town, and many were situated along or very close to the Via Emilia, that long straight highway running south-eastwards across the plain of Northern Italy, and on other ancient Roman roads which led from the Alpine passes to Venice or other ports of embarkation for the East, or to Rimini and thence to Rome. Many houses therefore served not only as centres of activity for the *fratres* and as hospices for the poor, sick or elderly but also as stopping places for pilgrims and crusaders, and for the Hospitallers themselves as they moved to or from the East[17]. Properties could be purchased, sold or exchanged so that they were more conveniently distributed, and the location of a *domus* consisting of scattered estates was not necessarily central to them but might well be placed at some distance from them in or near a town. By no means all preceptories were situated along the main routes leading eastwards[18], but the town or suburban preceptory with urban as well as rural properties was especially common in North-East Italy. There was probably little direct farming of the Hospitallers' estates in the Priory of Venice, and the archives contained numerous leases of farms and vineyards, especially where lands lay in mountainous parts[19].

During the twelfth century in particular there was a widespread movement both to found and to give service in hospitals and hospices, especially in the towns. Such hospices were often small and poorly endowed, and many were served by men and women who took no vows and who followed no formal rule or constitution so that their hospices eventually fell into difficulties which tempted bishops and others to assign them to a well established major order such as the Hospital. Occasionally the Hospitallers also received a parish with care of souls. The bishop sometimes had to intervene to settle subsequent conflicts as, for example, when the Hospital's priests imparted the last rites to the dying and attempted to secure legacies to the detriment of the secular clergy[20]. Bishops and monasteries transferring properties to the Hospital might take care to reserve their rights. Thus in 1335 when the Archbishop of Ravenna granted the Hospitallers, who previously had no house in that city, the parish church of San Giorgio *in Porticu* in the centre of Ravenna with all its rights, he insisted that the priest in charge should not be a Hospitaller and that the bishop was to institute him; that, notwithstanding the Hospital's privileges, the priest was to respect the bishop's interdicts, attend his synods and pay whatever dues were owed, including a pound of wax each year to symbolize the bishop's overlordship; and that the wishes of Ranuccio *de Mattagliatis*, who had endowed the church, be respected[21]. Thus, although the Hospitallers had to send their *responsiones* to the East and were therefore generally exempt from ecclesiastical taxation, certain houses and churches did pay a variety of dues some of which were listed in the accounts of the papal collectors[22].

The Hospitallers acquired lands in various ways, the greatest single accession being that which came from the Templars in and after 1312. Donations varied greatly. The Marchese of Este bequeathed the Hospital a number of properties across a wide area in 1142[23], but it remains uncertain what, if anything, the Hospitallers eventually received from him. At Prata the local lay lords were buried in the Hospitaller church. Extensive property in and around Treviso was acquired in 1315 in exchange for the former Templar Preceptory at Valeggio south-west of Verona, a transfer justified on the grounds that Valeggio lay more than three

days' journey from Venice so that property there would be difficult to adminis-
ter[24]. None the less, a few preceptories were at a considerable distance in Istria
and Tirol. In the Priory of Venice the *domus* often had mixed origins in a number of separate donations or rearrangements of properties. The typical preceptory
consisted of a residence and a church with stables, a cemetery and sometimes a
hospice. A grandiose urban palace might have a courtyard, while rural houses
would have granaries, mills and dovecotes. In North-East Italy the preceptory
was seldom fortified and normally had no secular jurisdiction or seignorial
rights, though at San Quirino near Pordenone the Hospital received the whole
villa or village from the Temple. Exemptions were most frequently ecclesiastical. There were often rural chapels and oratories, and sometimes one or more
parishes. Most preceptories were dedicated to a saint, much the most common
patrons being Saint John and the Virgin. Hospitals in the West were increasingly
taken over by the communal authorities but, somewhat unusually, some of those
in the Venetian priory maintained their charitable functions during the fourteenth
century.

Many houses and hospices were established along the major roads. On the
Via Emilia there were preceptories, some of course Templar in origin, at Milan,
Piacenza and Firenzuola in the Priory of Lombardy; then there were houses near
Fidenza, where the Via Francigena struck southwards from the Emilia, and along
the Emilia at Parma, Calerno, Reggio, Modena, Sanguinario, Ponte S. Am-
brogio, Bologna, Borgonovo, Imola, Faenza, Forli, Ponte Ronco, Cesena and
Rimini where the Via Emilia reached the sea and the borders of the Priory of
Rome. Another string of preceptories ran from Bologna to Ferrara, Rovigo,
Padua, Mestre and Venice, while others followed the route from Verona to Montebello, Vicenza, Padua and Venice. From Venice there were land and water
routes to Treviso, and beyond Treviso there was a scatter of preceptories in Fri-
uli, Istria and the Alps. Other houses were close to these routes without being on
them, and some were far away from the main highways but on lesser roads, at
bridges or in passes; sometimes the house had obligations to maintain the bridge.
The *domus* might be just outside a town by a gate, in the enclosed *borgo* or suburb, or in the main city. Some towns had two or more preceptories, and these
could be alongside the Via Emilia as it ran through the town as, for example, at
Bologna, Parma and Forli[25].

* * *

The Hospital was established in Venice itself possibly by 1123, and by 1180
there was apparently a Prior of Venice with extended jurisdictions[26]. In 1180 the
Hospitaller Fr. Archimbaldo *prior domus Venezie* was at Imola setting up a

house there[27]; in 1181 he was *prior Sancti Egidii de Venecia*[28] and in 1187 *magister Hospitaliorum Italiae*[29]. In that last year Iohannes de Balda, acting for the Master of the Hospital and for the Prior of Venice, received land at Venice *in fossa putrida* on which to construct a church and an *ospitalis*[30]. This may have been the site known by 1267 as S. Giovanni, S. Egidio having meanwhile disappeared[31]. There was a Hospitaller Prior of *Longobardia* in 1176, and in 1198 Fr. Simone *de Levata* held the joint Priory of Lombardy and Venice[32]. From that time donations and foundations were increasing throughout North-East Italy. There was a Prior *Guillielmus* in 1214[33], a Prior *Guglielmus de Vultalbio* in 1235[34], and at least between 1263 and 1293 the Prior of Venice was Fr. Engheramo *de Gragnana*[35]. Fr. Guglielmo Bolgaroni was vice-prior in 1296[36]; a Fr. Rodolfo was vice-prior in 1298[37]; Fr. Engheramo *de Gragnana* was prior in 1301[38]; and Fr. Gregorio *de Parma* was prior in 1304[39] and 1306[40]. By 17 October 1312 Fr. Leonardo *de Tibertis* was Prior of Venice and acting as the Hospital's procurator at the papal *curia*[41]. He was replaced in 1330 by his kinsman Fr. Napoleone *de Tibertis* who governed the priory until about 1364[42]. The latter's successor was the Florentine Fr. Bartolomeo Benini[43]. On 26 May 1365, following Benini's resignation, he was succeeded by Fr. Giovanni da Rivara[44], a noble from Piedmont[45]. Apparently, not one of these priors was a Venetian[46].

Fr. Leonardo *de Tibertis* was an outstanding administrator who was employed for many years to settle the Hospital's financial and organizational problems throughout Western Europe. In 1327 he went to England where he so successfully restored a disastrous financial situation that the English Hospitallers chose him as their prior[47]. He remained Prior of Venice until 24 October 1330 when he was formally named Prior of England[48]. The new prior Fr. Napoleone *de Tibertis*, who had been Preceptor of Faenza in 1317[49], was named prior on 24 October 1330[50]. Fr. Napoleone was active in Italian affairs. Thus in 1339 he was papal rector in the provinces of Campagna and Marittima and also a senator of Rome[51]; he was much involved in military matters and administration outside his priory[52]. His family came from Monteleone di Spoleto where he established a house for female Hospitallers[53]; he also founded the hospice of Santa Caterina adjoining the Order's house in Venice[54].

Fr. Leonardo *de Tibertis* had struggled with debts caused by the expenses incurred for the conquest of Rhodes, which was completed by 1310, by the extravagances of the Master Fr. Foulques de Villaret, who was deposed in 1317, and by the costs of acquiring and absorbing the properties of the Templars following their dissolution in 1312. In the Priory of Venice many of the Templès lands were secured without serious difficulties[55]; the Templars attempted to resist in Venice itself, but the government ensured that the Hospital received the Templar house of Santa Maria *in capite Brolii* near San Marco and in 1324 it purchased the whole property, which included a cemetery, from the Hospitallers[56]

THE HOSPITALLER PRIORY OF VENICE IN 1331

In 1317 a special levy, apparently to be raised by pledging movable and immovable properties, was imposed on each priory. The total required was very approximately 207,000 florins of which 37,100 florins, or roughly 18 per cent, was to come from the Italian priories and preceptories; the Venetian quota was 4000 florins which was approximately 11 per cent of the Italian total and which compared with 4000 florins from the Priory of Capua and 6000 each from the Priories of Lombardy, Pisa, Rome and Barletta. The Priory of Venice owed 700 florins a year of *responsiones*, equivalent to 6 per cent of the Italian total of 11,800 florins and to less than one per cent of the grand total of 81,200 florins[57]. By November 1322 it had become clear that ordinary taxation and special levies could not resolve the problem, and Pope John XXII licensed the Hospitallers, acting in accord with the bishop and subject to various limitations, to lease or sell property in places where they held two houses in order to raise 20,000 florins in addition to the annual *responsiones* of about 50,000 florins in order to finance an Eastern expedition of 100 brethren as well as to repay their general debts which still stood at 193,000 florins. In July 1323 the Master instructed the Prior of Venice to raise 2144 florins to help repay 10,000 florins owed to Giovanni di Paolo da Spoleto, and one result was a series of leases and sales made by the Vice-Prior Fr. Bono from Città di Castello, Preceptor of Santa Maria di Valverde, and other brethren at Reggio where the Hospital had received various Templar properties[58].

In 1330 a chapter-general arranged once again for extensive taxation to pay off the Hospital's debts. The priories were to provide a total annual *responsiones* of just over 92,400 florins together with a special tax totalling some 82,000 florins; of these sums, the Venetian priory was due to pay 800 florins a year of *responsiones* and a special levy of 1070 florins; both figures represented just over one per cent of the respective totals[59]. The letter appointing Fr. Napoleone *de Tibertis* as prior insisted that he pay 1870 florins by 24 June 1331 and 800 florins of *responsiones* on each 24 June thereafter[60]. The resulting *extimum* or list of estimated incomes of individual preceptories drawn up and sealed at the prioral chapter at Venice on 5 April 1331 envisaged a total income of 3939 florins but how much of that could be drawn on for taxation was not made clear. These incomes were presumably calculated before the *responsiones* were deducted but whether the estimates took count of other expenditures was not stated. There were probably all sorts of incomes in kind and produce, such as chickens and eggs, which were not estimated as cash profit, but there was no indication whether expenses for the upkeep of houses and the maintenance of the brethren and their households, the service of churches, legal fees, charitable contributions and suchlike outgoings had also to be met from the sums estimated[61]. A few preceptories were apparently not listed[62]. Estimated incomes varied greatly; they could be as low as 10 florins at Croce Pecorino and 12 at Montebello, or as high as 200 florins at Calerno and Campania. Of 67 preceptories, about 45 had incomes of 60 florins or less. In addition each priory owed a sum, which for the Italian priories varied in 1311 between 25 and 50 florins, as the *pitancia*, the monies destined to support the brethren of the Italian province resident at Rhodes[63]. These were not included in the *responsiones*. The estimates of 1331 suggest that, very approximately, the former Templar properties, perhaps representing between 20 and 25 out of some 74 preceptories, would have accounted for at least 1400 out of the total of 3939 florins, that is for at least a third of the total[64]. The suppression of the Temple had increased the priory's incomes by roughly 50 per cent.

Preceptors were frequently moved from one *domus* to another[65]. They seldom, if ever, belonged to grand families, and none of the 52 brethren listed in 1331 was demonstrably a Venetian. The prior and one preceptor belonged to the Tiberti family from Monteleone above Spoleto, while three preceptors came from Spoleto and one each from Perugia and Rieti. Fr. Francesco *de Gragnana* was presumably a kinsman of the former prior with that name. Some preceptors were given a single name which provided no indication of their family or place of origin, and others were described as from towns such as Bologna, Ferrara, Modena and Parma, all within the priory; two northern preceptors were known as *theotonicus*, and the rest had names of no special distinction. The Hospital's own documents seldom distinguished between priests, *milites* and sergeants, though a Fr. Atto was described as *miles* in 1312[66], as were Fr. Pietro Giovannelli *Mercadantis* in 1333 and Fr. Martino de *Muusis*, Preceptor of S. Giovanni at Imola, in 1341[67]. The Tiberti must have been *milites*, and a Fr. Ignazio, son of Count Alberigo da Faenza, was a leading Hospitaller in 1344[68]; Federico *de Bonacossis de Manta* was due to be received as a *miles* in 1352[69]. Not all preceptors were present at the prioral chapter of 1331; other brethren may have been ill, on Rhodes or Cyprus, aboard ship in transit or otherwise absent. They were not necessarily in the East. Fr. Gregorio *de Parma* was Prior of Pisa in 1317[70]. Fr. Napoleone *de Tibertis*, Preceptor of Faenza, Fr. Tebaldino *de Vignali*, Preceptor of Treviso, and Fr. Paolo da Modena, Preceptor of the Temple at Forlì, were representing their priory at a Hospitaller assembly in Avignon in 1317[71]. Fr. Paolo da Modena became Preceptor first of Erfurt and then of Topstädt in 1317 and 1318, and was Prior of Saxony and Thuringia from 1320 to 1324[72]. In 1313 Fr. Masino *de Jugulo*, Preceptor of Parma, was collecting monies in Denmark as the Hospital's procurator in Scandinavia[73]. Fr. Pietro dei Pattarini da Imola, a member of the lesser urban nobility in that town who was *iuris utrius professor*, had been *podestà* of Viterbo; from 1323 he accompanied the Master, acting as his unofficial chancellor at Avignon, Paris and elsewhere, becoming Prior of Rome in 1327 and dying at Florence in 1330[74].

Some brethren held more than one preceptory, so there were fewer preceptors than there were preceptories, of which there were about seventy. The total number of brethren is not known; two texts of 1331 mentioned between them at least 54 brethren[75]. The more important of the *domus* housed several Hospitallers; thus an act of the Preceptor of S. Giovanni at Padua in 1323 was made with the consent of a Fr. Gerardo, *conventualis* of the house, of Fr. Jacopo, its *chapelanus*, and of Fr. *Bonensegna*, *custos* of the nearby *domus* of Bevadoro[76]. There may have been between one hundred and two hundred brethren in the Priory of Venice. A statute of 1302 required the seven priories of the Italian *langue* or province to provide thirteen out of a total of eighty *freres d'armes* for service in the Convent at Cyprus[77], so that two military brethren and possibly a priest may in theory have been the average contribution of an Italian priory. The number of brethren in the Rhodian islands after 1310 was certainly much greater than eighty, and in 1331 the Venetian priory may have provided some of them. The chapter-general held at Rhodes in 1337 called on that priory to send just one *frater* to the Convent and at least one was already there; that was Fr. Ruggero *de Parma*, who was not listed at the 1331 chapter in Venice but who was apparently at Rhodes from 1332 to 1340, by which time he was Admiral of the Hospital[78].

The preceptories of the Priory of Venice, unlike those of many other Hospitaller priories, were largely urban in character. There were rural houses, many – though not all – of them with small incomes, but many preceptories were located inside or just outside a town; some had a hospital or hospice, and some held considerable town properties. Rather than manage their estates directly, the preceptories apparently leased parcels of land on a variety of terms. They paid comparatively meagre *responsiones*. Their *fratres* were seldom of distinguished family and few served at Rhodes. It was mostly in the town, in their *contrada*, their *borgo*, their parish or their hospice that the Hospitallers of the Venetian priory fulfilled their role in society.

¹ I am extremely grateful for a grant from the Gladys Krieble Delmas Foundation which made much of the following research possible, and for the assistance provided by the Istituto Ellenico di Studi Bizantini e Postbizantini at Venice; Luciana Valentini most kindly identified numerous place names in the library of the British School at Rome; and Francesco Tommasi gave much helpful advice and information.

² Preliminary considerations in A. LUTTRELL, *Templari e Ospitalieri in Italia*, in *Templari e Ospitalieri in Italia: la chiesa di San Bevignate a Perugia*, ed. M. RONCETTI *et al.*, Perugia 1987.

³ Venice, Archivio del Gran Priorato di Venezia dell'Ordine di Malta [cited as Filza]; I am most grateful to the Grand Prior, Fr. Gherardo Hercolani, for permission to use this archive and to his staff for their assistance there. The archive is described in J. DELAVIL-LE LE ROULX, *Cartulaire général de l'Ordre des Hospitaliers de S. Jean de Jérusalem: 1100-1310*, 4 vols., Paris 1894-1906, 1, pp. cxx-cxxv, and in E. SCHERMERHORN, *Notes on the Commanderies of the Grand Priory of Venice...*, in *Archivum Melitense*, 9 (1934); G. SOMMI PICENARDI, *Dell'Archivio del Gran Priorato dell'Ordine Gerosolimitano in Venezia*, in *Monumenti Storici pubblicati dalla R. Deputazione Veneta di Storia Patria*, 4 ser.: *Miscellanea*, 11, Venice 1889, gives its history. Schermerhorn makes use of some early-modern *cabrei* and estate books, as does another brief work, C. GHINI, *L'Ordine Gerosolimitano di Rodi e di Malta nella Romagna: le Commende di Cesena, Rimini e Forlì*, Forlì 1975. Delaville's *Cartulaire* publishes comparatively few texts concerning the Venetian priory. Certain documents not yet traced in the prioral archive are cited below from summaries there in the Ms. *1757, Sommario o sia Ristretto delle Scritture*, vol. 1.

⁴ Cited as Filza Padova and Filza Vicenza. The provenance of the 14 *buste* entitled «Ordine di Malta» in Treviso, Archivio Vescovile, and of 83 *buste* entitled «Commenda di SS. Vitale e Sepolcro» in Verona, Archivio di Stato, seems uncertain. Other local archives contain further materials; *Cartulaire*, 1, pp. cxxiv-cxxv, lists some at Bologna, Modena, Parma, Ferrara and Venice.

⁵ A. LUTTRELL, *Venice and the Knights Hospitallers of Rhodes in the Fourteenth Century*, in *Papers of the British School at Rome*, 26 (1958).

⁶ Notably the records of the collectors of the papal tenths in *Rationes decimarum Italiae nei secoli XIII e XIV: Aemilia*, ed. A. MERCATI *et al.*, Vatican 1933, and *Venetiae-Histria-Dalmatia*, ed. P. SELLA, G. VALE, Vatican 1941.

⁷ Valletta, National Library of Malta, Archives of the Order of St. John of Jerusalem [cited as Malta, Cod.], Codd. 5820-5917 are *cabrei* from the Priory of Venice.

⁸ Most notably in the best introduction to the subject, in E. NASALLI ROCCA DI CORNE-LIANO, *Istituzioni dell'Ordine Gerosolimitano di Rodi e di Malta nell'Emilia e nella Ro-*

THE HOSPITALLER PRIORY OF VENICE IN 1331

magna. Contributo alla storia del diritto ospedaliero, in *Rivista di storia del diritto italiano*, 14 (1941), with information on local Hospitaller archives.

[9] A. LUTTRELL, *Papauté et Hôpital: l'Enquête de 1373*, in *L'Enquête pontificale de 1373 sur l'Ordre des Hospitaliers de Saint-Jean de Jérusalem*, 1, ed. A.-M. LEGRAS, Paris 1987.

[10] A. LUTTRELL, *The Hospitallers of Rhodes at Treviso: 1373*, in *Mediterraneo Medievale: Scritti in onore di Francesco Giunta*, 2, Soveria Manelli 1989, expanded and amended, with much prosopographical detail, in G. CAGNIN, *Templari e Giovanniti in territorio trevigiano (secoli XII-XIV)*, Treviso 1992.

[11] F. TOMMASI, *«Templarii» e «Templarii Sancti Iohannis»: una precisazione metodologica*, in *Studi Medievali*, 3 ser., 24 (1983).

[12] For the Templar possessions and their transfer to the Hospital, see R. CARAVITA, *Rinaldo da Concorrezzo arcivescovo di Ravenna (1303-1321) al tempo di Dante*, Florence 1964; see also F. BRAMATO, *Regesti diplomatici per la storia dei Templari in Italia*, in *Rivista del Collegio Araldico*, 78-80 (1980-1982); ID., *L'Ordine dei Templari in Italia: dalle origini al pontificato di Innocenzo III: 1135-1216*, in *Nicolaus. Rivista di teologia ecumenico-patristica*, 20 (1985); and above all ID., *Storia dell'Ordine dei Templari in Italia*, Rome 1991.

[13] B. CAPONE, *I Templari in Italia*, Milan 1977; ID., *Vestigia templari in Italia*, Rome 1979; ID., *Quando in Italia c'erano i Templari*, Turin 1981; B. CAPONE, L. IMPERIO, E. VALENTINI, *Guida all'Italia dei Templari: gli insediamenti templari in Italia*, Rome 1989.

[14] Cf. A. BUFFULINI, *Santa Maria di Grignano e i Templari*, in *Comunità religiose di Trieste: Contributi di conoscenza*, Trieste 1979.

[15] Eg. L. IMPERIO, *Insediamenti templari e itinerari di pellegrini tra il Piave e il Tagliamento*, in *Atti del II convegno di ricerche templari*, Turin 1984, p. 108.

[16] Eg. A. LUTTRELL, *Two Templar-Hospitaller Preceptories North of Tuscania*, in *Papers of the British School at Rome*, 39 (1971).

[17] For the background of developments in Northern Italy, see CARAVITA (cited in n. 12) and J. RILEY-SMITH, *The Knights of St. John in Jerusalem and Cyprus: c. 1050-1310*, London 1967. In addition to NASALLI (cited in n. 8), see A. COLOMBO, *I Gerosolimitani e i Templari a Milano e la via Commenda*, in *Archivio Storico Lombardo*, 53 (1926); G. BASCAPÈ, *Le vie dei pellegrinaggi medioevali attraverso le Alpi Centrali e la pianura lombarda*, in *Archivio Storico della Svizzera Italiana*, 11 (1936); ID., *L'Attività ospitaliera dell'Ordine di S. Giovanni Gerosolimitano nel Medio Evo: itinerarii ed ospizii dei pellegrini nell'Alta Italia*, in *Rivista Araldica*, 34 (1936); E. NASALLI ROCCA DI CORNELIANO, *Lineamenti dell'organizzazione regionale e della funzione assistenziale dell'Ordine Gerosolimitano degli Ospedalieri nel medioevo italiano*, in *Studi di storia e diritto in onore di Carlo Calisse*, 3, Milan 1940; L. TACCHELLA, *Il Sovrano Militare Ordine di Malta nella storia di Vicenza, Padova, Verona e Brescia*, in *Studi Storici Veronesi Luigi Simeoni*, 18-19 (1968/9); ID., *Il Sovrano Ordine Militare di Malta nella storia di Verona*, Genoa 1969; A. LUTTRELL, *The Hospitallers' Hospice of Santa Caterina at Venice: 1358-1451*, in *Studi Veneziani*, 12 (1970). The Hospital received many houses from the Templars who also maintained hospices along pilgrim routes: T. SZABO', *Templari e viabilità*, in *I Templari. Mito e storia: Atti del Convegno internazionale di studi alla Magione Templare di Poggibonsi*, Sinalunga-Siena 1989.

[18] That many Hospitaller and Templar *mansiones* were on Roman sites on a Roman road has often been noted but should not always be assumed. L. TACCHELLA, *La «Mansio» gerosolimitana di Gazzo di Pressana in territorio veronese*, in *Studi Storici Verone-*

si Luigi Simeoni, 26- 27 (1976-7), may have identified this *domus* correctly (though it was not a Templar house), but there is no evidence that it was a Roman *mansio*. A. CON- FORTI CALCAGNI, *Per la storia delle comunicazioni romane: una nuova via da Verona al- l'Adriatico*, in *Economia e Storia*, 2 ser., 2 (1981), cites TACCHELLA, p. 18, in support of her theory, whereupon L. TACCHELLA, *Le «Mansiones» giovannite di S. Giovanni di Lon- gara, di Vicenza e di Saianega di Sossano Vicentino*, in *Studi Storici Luigi Simeoni*, 35 (1985), p. 106 n. 3, speaks of the Hospitaller *domus* as «sulla romana Via Porcilano»; but that is a hypothesis.

[19] Best local analysis in CAGNIN (cited in n. 10), pp. 36-40; in general, A. LUTTRELL, *Les exploitations rurales des Hospitaliers en Italie au XIVᵉ siècle*, in *Les Ordres militai- res, la vie rurale et le peuplement en Europe occidentale (XIIᵉ- XVIIIᵉ siècles)*, = Flaran, 6, Auch 1984.

[20] N. GALASSI, *Dieci secoli di storia ospitaliera a Imola*, 1, Imola 1966, pp. 119-123.

[21] A. TARLAZZI, *Appendice ai Monumenti Ravennati dei secoli di mezzo del conte Marco Fantuzzi*, 1, Ravenna 1876, pp. 223-227; cf. E. NASALLI ROCCA DI CORNELIANO, *La Commenda di Ravenna dell'Ordine di Malta*, in *Rivista del Sovrano Militare Ordine di Malta*, 14 (1950).

[22] In addition to *Rationes* (1933) and (1941), see Treviso, Archivio Vescovile, Qua- ternus Collecta: 1330.

[23] A. GLORIA, *Codice diplomatico padovano*, 2, 2 parts, Venice 1879-1881, part 1, pp. 304-305.

[24] *Infra*, Doc. I.

[25] Cf. NASALLI (cited in n. 8), pp. 69- 71.

[26] CAGNIN (cited in n. 10), pp. 25, 56 n.84. The notes in G. SOMMI PICENARDI, in *Del Gran Priorato dell'Ordine Gerosolimitano in Venezia*, in *Nuovo Archivio Veneto*, ns. 7 (1892), pp. 142-144, are here revised entirely.

[27] GALASSI (cited in n. 20), 1, pp. 309- 310.

[28] R. MOROZZO DELLA ROCCA, A. LOMBARDO, *Documenti del commercio veneziano nei secoli XI-XIII*, 1, Rome 1940, pp. 320-321.

[29] *Chronicon Magni presbiteri*, ed. G. PERTZ, in *Monumenta Germaniae Historica: Scriptores*, 17, Hannover 1861, p. 508.

[30] F. CORNER, *Ecclesiae Venetae...*, 12, Venice 1749, p. 387. TOMMASI (cited in n. 11), p. 377, demonstrates that this text contains no mention of the Templars whose Venetian house was dedicated to S. Maria, yet it has always been regarded as Templar in origin: correct LUTTRELL (cited in n. 17), p. 373. CAPONE *et al.* (cited in n. 13), pp. 80-82, and BRAMATO, *Storia dell'Ordine dei Templari* (cited in n. 12), p. 63, wrongly interpret the land *in fossa putrida* as being given to the Temple and as becoming San Giovanni del Tempio and passing to the Hospital after 1312.

[31] TOMMASI (cited in n. 11), p. 377 n. 18.

[32] *Cartulaire* (cited in n. 3), 1, nos. 501 (1176), 1026 (1198).

[33] I. AFFÒ, *Storia della città di Parma*, 3, Parma 1793, p. 55 n.(a).

[34] NASALLI (cited in n. 8), p. 75.

[35] Filza 544 (1263). Engheramo, at times also Prior of Rome and Lombardy, was prior in 1293: J. DELAVILLE LE ROULX, *Les Hospitaliers en Terre Sainte et à Chypre: 1100-1310*, Paris 1904, p. 420.

[36] *... uiceprior dom[or]um prioratus Veneciarum dicti hospitalis citra Pad[...]*: Filza Padova 1. SOMMI PICENARDI (cited in n. 26), pp. 103-104, and DELAVILLE (cited in n. 35),

p. 420, wrongly give Bolgaroni as prior.

[37] ... *viceprior in prioratu Veneciarum*: Filza Padova 10.

[38] TACCHELLA, *Le «Mansiones»* (cited in n. 18), p. 160 n. 3. The summary of this text in *Cartulaire* (cited in n. 3), 4, no. 4547, gives «Girardo». Fr. Girardo *de Gragnana* was Prior of Pisa and a papal *cubicularius* in 1299, and later he was Hospitaller and in 1303 Marshal of the Hospital in Cyprus; *ibid.*, 3, no. 4471; 4, nos. 4586, 4620-4621, and TOMMASI (cited in n. 11), pp. 380-381. The Gragnana family may have come from Garfagnana in Northern Tuscany.

[39] *Dominus Gregorius prior provincialis domorum Hospitalis*, 1304: Treviso, Biblioteca Comunale, Ms. 109 vol. 4, f. 400r-406r.

[40] Filza Padova 7 (20 July 1306). He was *Gregorius de Parma, dignissimus prior Veneciarum* on 2 August 1306: G. MANTESE, *Memorie Storiche della Chiesa Vicentina*, 2-3, Vicenza 1954-1958, 2, p. 401 n. 9. He may have been the Prior of Venice at Rhodes in July 1310: F. AMADI, in *Chroniques de Chypre d'Amadi et de Strambaldi*, ed. R. DE MAS-LATRIE, 1, Paris 1891, p. 370.

[41] S. PAULI, *Codice Diplomatico del Sacro Militare Ordine Gerosolimitano, oggi di Malta*, 2, Lucca 1737, pp. 36-40. Fr. Niccolò della Mazza of Parma was Preceptor and not, as often supposed, Prior of Venice: CORNER (cited in n. 30), 12, pp. 242-245; Venice, Archivio di Stato, Commemoriali, 1, f. 193r-v.

[42] J. DELAVILLE LE ROULX, *Les Hospitaliers à Rhodes jusqu'à la mort de Philibert de Naillac: 1306-1421*, Paris 1913, pp. 77-78, 140, 145.

[43] *Ibid*, p. 145.

[44] Malta, Cod. 319, f. 204r-v.

[45] DELAVILLE (cited in n. 42), p. 197.

[46] The first Venetian prior was Fr. Angelo Marcello who was provided by his uncle Pope Eugenius IV in 1431: A. MARCELLO, *Documenti intorno ad Angelo e Lorenzo Marcello del S. M. O. Gerosolimitano priori di Venezia nel secolo XV*, Venice 1891.

[47] DELAVILLE (cited in n. 42), pp. 21- 22, 32-35, 37, 39 n. 5, 53-55, 68-69.

[48] Malta, Cod. 280, f. 4r, 5r. DELAVILLE (cited in n. 42), p. 77 n. 5, gives Fr. Napoleone as a nephew of Fr. Leonardo. Leonardo's *nepos*, Fr. Francesco *de Tibertis*, was lieutenant in the Preceptory of Bologna in 1314: Malta, Cod. 16 no. 11.

[49] C. FAURE, *Études sur l'administration et l'histoire du Comtat-Venaissin du XIIIe au XVe siècle: 1229-1447*, Paris-Avignon 1909, pp. 204-207.

[50] Malta, Cod. 280, f. 5r.

[51] DELAVILLE (cited in n. 42), pp. 77- 78.

[52] G. FALCO, *I Comuni della Campagna e della Marittima nel Medio Evo*, in *Archivio della R. Società Romana di Storia Patria*, 49 (1926), pp. 181, 183-184; E. DUPRÉ-THESEIDER, *Roma dal Comune di Popolo alla Signoria pontificia: 1252-1377*, Bologna 1952, pp. 505, 563-567: references most kindly supplied by Tersilio Leggio.

[53] Details in F. TOMMASI, *Il monastero femminile di San Bevignate dell'Ordine di San Giovanni Gerosolimitano (Secoli XIV-XVI)*, in *Templari e Ospitalieri* (cited in n. 2), pp. 54, 64-65.

[54] LUTTRELL (cited in n. 17), pp. 373- 375.

[55] CARAVITA (cited in n. 12), pp. 161- 162 *et passim*; ID., *La figura di Rinaldo da Concorezzo, arcivescovo di Ravenna, grande inquisitore per il processo ai Templari*, in *I Templari: Mito e Storia* (cited in n. 17). Temple goods consigned at Bologna in 1314 are listed in G. GHIRARDACCI, *Della Historia di Bologna*, 1, Bologna 1596, p. 576.

[56] CORNER (cited in n. 30), 12, pp. 241- 252, but wrongly stating there were two Templar houses in Venice.

[57] Extremely approximate calculations based on incomplete figures in Archivio Vaticano, Reg. Vat. 66, f. 307v- 309r, 335r-346r, partially and inaccurately summarized in *Jean XXII (1316-1334): Lettres communes*, ed. G. MOLLAT, 1, Paris 1904, nos. 4450-4472, followed, with further inaccuracies, in DELAVILLE (cited in n. 42), pp. 22-23; one full text in *Diplomatarium Danicum*, 2 ser., 7, ed. F. BLATT, K. OLSEN, Copenhagen 1956, pp. 369- 376.

[58] Malta, Biblioteca, Ms. 1474.

[59] Malta, Cod. 280, f. 4r-8r, transcribed, with errors, in G. TIPTON, *The 1330 Chapter General of the Knights Hospitallers at Montpellier*, in *Traditio*, 24 (1968), pp. 301-304. There are ambiguities in the text. DELAVILLE (cited in n. 42), p. 56, reports a total of 162,530 florins and 100 silver marks.

[60] *Infra*, Doc. III.

[61] LUTTRELL (cited in n. 9), pp. 31-34, discusses such accounts.

[62] *Infra*, pp. 30-33

[63] Text of 1311 listing Italian *pitancia* dues, in copy of 1442, in Malta, Cod. 355, f. 243r-243v; it inexplicably omits the annual figure, possibly 25 florins, for the Priory of Venice.

[64] These are hypothetical figures based on estimates; it seems possible that 38 preceptories were originally Hospitaller, 17 Templar and 19 mixed or uncertain, but it is not clear how many Templar properties were never acquired, or were alienated, or were wholly or partially merged into Hospitaller preceptories.

[65] Spoleto, Archivio del Duomo, Archivio Capitolare, Perg. 588 (transcribed by Francesco Tommasi), listed a group of preceptors in 1324; in 16 cases the preceptories they held in 1331 are known, and only five were then still in the same *domus* (assuming that *Acto de Baratis* of S. Trinità, Ferrara, in 1324 was not the *Acto de Marinis* of 1331).

[66] G. TIRABOSCHI, *Storia dell'Augusta Badia di S. Silvestro di Nonantola*, 2 vols., Modena 1784-1785, 2, pp. 408-410.

[67] GALASSI (cited in n. 20), 1, pp. 123 n. 1, 125 n. 1. The Fr. Giovanni *de Clarignano*, Preceptor of Longara in 1331, may have been the same who was *miles* in 1365: Filza Padova 10.

[68] ... *frater Dominus Ignatius quondam domini Comitis Alberici de civitate Faventia, visitator generalis Militum nobilium hospitalis S. Johannis gerosolimitani citra mare*: I. SCHUSTER, *Un Protocollo di notar Pietro Gregorio nell'Archivio di Farfa*, in *Archivio della R. Società Romana di Storia Patria*, 35 (1912), pp. 547-548. Fr. Bonacurso *de Albrigonibus* was Preceptor of Longara in 1306: Vicenza, Archivio di Stato, Corp. Relig. Ognissanti, Busta 2115.

[69] Malta, Cod. 318, f. 155v.

[70] MOLLAT (cited in n. 57), no. 4452.

[71] FAURE (cited in n. 49), pp. 204-207.

[72] DELAVILLE (cited in n. 42), pp. 39, 73, 75.

[73] *Diplomatarium Danicum* (cited in n. 57), 2 ser., 7, pp. 10-11, 38-40.

[74] A. LUTTRELL, *The Hospitallers in Cyprus, Rhodes, Greece and the West: 1291-1440*, London 1978, XV, pp. 410-413, 419-420.

[75] *Infra*, Docs. II-III.

⁷⁶ Filza Padova 1.

⁷⁷ *Cartulaire* (cited in n. 3), 4, no. 4574, § 14.

⁷⁸ Malta, Cod. 280, f. 29r (1332), 37r (1335), 41r, 42r (1337), 46r (1340); Fr. Ruggero da Parma was *retentus ad manum* of the Master, probably that is he was a member of his household, from 1332 to 1337. He died before 20 October 1347: Cod. 317, f. 164r-v. Fr. Giovanni Melengario, Preceptor of S. Giovanni, Padua, at the 1331 chapter, was *retentus* in the Priory of Venice in 1332 (f. 28r), but the significance of that is uncertain. 47 brethren, at least eight of them from Parma, were listed at a chapter in Venice in 1343: CAGNIN (cited in n. 10), pp. 92-94.

XIX

THE ITALIAN HOSPITALLERS AT RHODES :
1437-1462

by

Stanley FIORINI and Anthony LUTTRELL

The nature and organization of the individual "Langues" or provincial groupings among the Hospitallers of the Military Order of Saint John on Rhodes between 1309 and 1522 have scarcely been studied. This article presents two apparently unique texts which concern the Langue of Italy. Document I is a text of 1442 recopying bulls of 1312 and 1321 which are especially important as belonging to a period before 1346 for which the archives are virtually lost. Document III, of unknown provenance, is the text of a paper register of about 11 useful folios which was apparently reused from some other codex, since the first folio corresponds to an earlier folio 285 ; the entries are in various hands and in Italian or Latin. There is a set of registers for the Italian Langue running from 1564 to 1791 [1] and a register for the English Langue covers the years 1523 to 1567 [2]. The other Rhodian registers surviving on Malta contain numerous references to the Italian Hospitallers which could not, for reasons of space, be utilized to complete or annotate information given here, though limited identifications are provided in the indices [3]. Documents from the Langues were occasionally copied into the chancery registers, sometimes in order to record their confirmation ; thus in 1452

---

1. Valletta, National Library of Malta, Archives of the Order of St John, Cod. 2125-2157. The fundamental study is J. SARNOWSKY, "Der Konvent auf Rhodos und die Zungen (*lingue*) im Johanniterorden : 1421-1476", in *Ritterorden und Region - politische, soziale und wirtschaftliche Verbindungen im Mittelalter*, Z. NOVAK ed., Torun, 1995 (Ordines Militares Colloquia Torunensia Historica, 8).

2. Text in H. SCICLUNA, *The Book of Deliberations of the Venerable Tongue of England : 1523-1567*, Malta, 1949.

3. Much material from the Malta archives is in G. BOSIO, *Dell'Istoria della Sacra Religione et Illustrissima Militia di S. Giovanni Gerosolimitano*, II, 2nd ed., Rome, 1629, with index ; the second edition should be used. An important selection of these texts is published in Z. TSIRPANLIS, *Anekdota Eggrapha gia te Rodo kai tis Noties Sporades apo to Archeio ton Ioanniton Ippoton : 1421-1453* (Unpublished Documents concerning Rhodes and the South-East Aegean Islands from the Archives of the Order of St John : 1421-1453), Rhodes, 1995. For details and bibliography on some individual Italian commanderies, A. LUTTRELL, *The Hospitallers in Cyprus, Rhodes, Greece and the West : 1291-1440*, London, 1978, item x, and ID., *The Hospitallers of Rhodes and their Mediterranean World*, Aldershot, 1992, items XIII-XIV ; see also ID., "The Hospitallers of Rhodes between Tuscany and Jerusalem : 1310-1431", in *Revue Mabillon*, n.s., 3, 1992, pp. 117-138, and ID., "The Hospitaller Priory of Venice in 1331", in *Militia Sacra : gli Ordini militari fra Europa e Terrasanta*, E. COLI et al. eds., Perugia, 1994, pp. 101-143.

item XXI from the Italian records was copied, with only minor variations, into the Master's register [4].

When in 1442 the Prior of Rome, Fr. Battista Orsini, refused to pay the *pitancia* which his priory owed to the Italian Langue at Rhodes, the Council there referred the dispute to a commission which examined the magistral bulls of 1312 which had established the amounts due. These were copied from a bull of 1321 given, in the Master's absence, by his lieutenant, the Marshal Fr. Giraud de Pins, whose seal, which was attached to it, was described in 1442. The bulls of 1312 were actually notes of letters reflecting decisions taken in the Chapter General of April 1311 [5]. They had presumably been copied in 1321 from a register which contained the acts of Chapters General, or bulls issued by the Master, or both. Orsini lost his case and the proceedings were copied into the register for 1442 where they were validated by the Master and Convent. Perhaps as the result of some copying error, this version omitted any mandate for the Priory of Venice, which certainly collected *pitancia* dues [6].

*
* *

The brethren of a multi-national institution such as the Hospital had to live together in their central headquarters or Convent but they naturally tended to divide into groups according to their region of origin and its spoken language. The Order had evolved in Jerusalem following the first crusade of 1099, and during the following centuries its possessions in the West were gradually grouped into provinces such as those of Spain, France and Italy. Each Western province, except that of Auvergne which had only one priory, was composed of a number of priories, Italy having eight priories, one of which was that of Hungary. The system of Langues or "tongues" evolved in the East. At first it functioned particularly with regard to the composition of administrative bodies ; after the loss of Acre and the Convent's retreat to Limassol on Cyprus in 1291, a series of proposals for administrative reform made in 1295 envisaged a directorate of *diffinitores* representing each of the seven Langues [7]. A Langue consisted of its province's brethren in the Convent. It corresponded to but was largely distinct from its Western province, though there were ways in which individual priories were attached to their Langue ; for example,

4. Malta, Cod. 363, fol. 118v ; documents from magistral registers concerning disputes between Italian brethren are used in SARNOWSKY, *op. cit.*, pp. 52-53, 63, notes 67-70.

5. It is not known when registers of magistral bulls were first kept ; on early chancery practice at Rhodes, see LUTTRELL (1978), item XV, which remains incomplete. The earliest surviving register of acts of Chapters General is that for 1330-1344 : Malta, Cod. 280. On the *pitancia*, see SARNOWSKY, *op. cit.*, p. 61, notes 44-45.

6. Sixteen commanderies paid just over thirty florins to the Prior of Venice in 1415 : Venice, Archivio del Gran Priorato di Venezia dell'Ordine di Malta, Filza 774, II, fol. 9v-10. In 1443 the Priory of Auvergne was setting aside the incomes of two commanderies to provide 120 francs a year for its Langue's *pitancia* : Malta, Cod. 350, fol. 101.

7. Sources indicated in J. RILEY-SMITH, *The Knights of St John in Jerusalem and Cyprus : c. 1050-1310*, London, 1967, pp. 276, 283-286, 288, 296-297, 319, 328, 344 ; the origins of the Langues deserve further study.

XIX

brethren from any part of a Langue could in theory secure a commandery or a priory anywhere within their Langue's province in the West, and each priory was obliged to send a contribution or *pitancia* to sustain all the members of its Langue in the Convent.

Before 1291 many brethren at Acre lived in a single *auberge* in the suburb of Montmusart which was grand enough for the king to lodge in it in 1286 [8], and after 1291 they had a building at Limassol known as the *ostel de sains* in which certain brethren had their own rooms [9]. However, on arrival at Rhodes, which probably lacked any suitable large building, they occupied individual houses or rooms referred to in 1311 as *herbergies* and in 1357 as *haulberges* [10]. Gradually these houses, known as *ostels* or *hospicia*, became the property of the individual Langues, being exchanged and amalgamated until one house developed into the central *auberge* of each Langue [11]. These *auberges* were the buildings, perhaps with various dependent chambers or houses, such as the *belles salles* of 1480 in which the brethren of each Langue would meet and eat or the *hostelz* of the *nacions* mentioned in 1485 [12].

The Langues acquired property, furnishings and incomes, and had their own chief officer or *pillerius*, in the Italian case often the Admiral [Doc. III, item XVII], who sat as their representative on the Order's Council. From about 1330 it was understood that each Langue had the right to provide one senior official or *bailivus*, and in the case of Italy this was the Admiral [13]. The Langue had its chapel and chaplain [VIII], and its brethren could, but only with licence from the Master, meet to discuss their Langue's business, which in particular involved questions of seniority affecting appointments in the West and of the service or *caravana* which counted towards seniority. A statute, accepted in 1446 but never confirmed, showed that each *auberge* had its own servants, that brethren might eat or lodge there, that it was subsidized by the Order's Treasury, and that the Langues' decisions concerning seniority and appointments within each Langue were to be accepted by the Master and Council, except in relation to priories, to Conventual offices and to offices nominated by Chapter General [Doc. II]. Some of these and other matters were recorded in the Langue's register, with some brethren acting as procurators or keeping accounts ; the Langue also had its own notary and its own chaplain [VIII, XXX].

8. *Ibid.*, pp. 191, 248-250, 267.

9. K. SINCLAIR, "The Hospital, Hospice and Church of the Healthy belonging to the Knights of St John of Jerusalem on Cyprus", in *Medium Aevum*, 49, 1980, pp. 254-257 correcting previous interpretations of the phrase *ostel de sains*.

10. References in A. GABRIEL, *La cité de Rhodes : MCCCX-MDXXII*, 2 vols., Paris, 1921-1923, II, p. 37.

11. The evolution of the *auberge* of the Langue awaits study ; it probably appeared after about 1350 : A. LUTTRELL, "Rhodes Town : 1306-1350" (forthcoming).

12. References in GABRIEL, *op. cit.*, II, p. 38.

13. Texts in C. TIPTON, "The 1330 Chapter General of the Knights Hospitallers at Montpellier", in *Traditio*, 24, 1968, pp. 293-308.

The Hospitaller's Western Incomes for 1373/1374 as accounted at Avignon

Priory or Commandery	Responsiones	Taille	Arrears	Mortuaries	Spolia	Vacancies	Total
England	–	–	–	–	–	–	–
France	6,000	2,000	–	600	1,928	–	[10,528]
Aquitaine	2,670	–	–	–	–	–	[2,670]
Champagne	1,000	312	–	–	–	–	[1,312]
Auvergne	2,180	250	–	70	–	–	[2,500]
S. Gilles	3,919	1,000	530	1,939	–	–	[7,387]
Toulouse	1,646	246	305	301	–	–	[2,498]
Catalunya	2,742	1,711	950	–	–	–	5,403
Amposta	917	–	1,500	–	–	–	2,417
Navarre	500	231	–	–	–	–	731
Castile	–	–	–	–	–	–	–
Portugal	–	–	–	–	–	–	–
Lombardy	–	–	41	–	217	–	258
Pisa	922	288	–	–	–	–	1,210
Rome	–	288	–	–	–	–	288
Messina	–	–	–	–	–	–	–
Naples	692	346	–	–	–	–	1,038
Alife (scambi)	–	–	–	–	–	–	–
Capua	692	231	–	39	–	–	963
S. Eufemia	–	–	–	–	–	–	–
Venosa	346	115	–	–	–	–	461
Monopoli	–	–	–	–	–	–	–
Barletta	–	–	–	–	–	–	–
Venice	922	288	–	–	–	–	1,210
Hungary	–	–	–	–	–	–	–
Alamania	1,012	344	–	–	–	–	1,356
Bohemia	–	–	–	–	–	–	–
	[26,160]	[7,650]	[3,326]	[2,949]	[2,145]	[–]	[42,230]

The Hospitaller's Western Incomes for 1374/1375 as accounted at Avignon

Priory or Commandery	Responsiones	Taille	Arrears	Mortuaries	Spolia	Vacancies	Total
England	–	–	–	–	–	–	–
Ireland	–	–	–	–	–	–	–
France	6,250	1,250	–	1,042	–	1,317	9,859
Champagne	1,042	312	–	–	–	–	[1,354]
Aquitaine	1,250	–	–	–	–	–	[1,250]
Auvergne	2,000	500	–	–	–	–	[2,500]
S. Gilles	4,548	852	646	650	–	893	7,589
Toulouse	817	178	380	–	–	–	1,375
Catalunya	2,900	1,769*	–	–	–	–	[4,668]
Amposta	916	1,327*	–	–	–	–	2,243
Navarre	500	337*	–	–	–	30	867
Rome	922	288	–	–	–	–	[1,210]
Venosa	342	114	–	–	–	–	[456]
Pisa	922	288	–	–	–	–	[1,210]
Alamania	1,000	459	100	–	–	–	[1,559]
Bohemia	1,200	612*	2,008	–	–	–	[3,820]
Hungary	300	–	–	–	–	–	[300]
Venice	800	382	–	–	–	–	[1,182]
Barletta	2,000	1,024*	–	–	–	–	[3,024]
Monopoli	400	229*	553	–	–	–	[1,182]
Messina	–	1,182*	–	–	–	–	[1,182]
Lombardy	–	–	–	–	–	–	–
Castile	–	–	–	–	–	–	–
Portugal	–	–	–	–	–	–	–
	[28,109]	[11,103]*	[3,687]	[1,692]	[–]	[2,240]	[46,830]

*Includes sums paid for the Master's passage to Rhodes.

The Langues could function in various ways to regulate quarrels within regional groups at the Convent, to facilitate relations between the brethren at Rhodes and those in the West, and to limit the French monopoly of office at Rhodes by providing for positions to be shared or alternated between Langues [14]. They also provided a channel for the supply of resources to the Convent whose fundamental requirements from the Western provinces were men and, above all, money. Each *domus*, that is each commandery or preceptory, owed a general tax, the responsions, plus extraordinary imposts, the *spolia* of deceased brethren, vacancies, *mortuaria* and so forth, all normally paid to the prior who was responsible for transferring them to the Conventual Treasury. Sometimes, as for Lombardy in 1441, the Treasury could by-pass the prior and collect responsions through its own receiver [xviii]. Incomes varied from year to year. In 1373/4 the Italian priories paid about an eighth of the Western total, but in 1374/5 it was much higher at 9446 florins or about on fifth of a total of 46,830 florins received at Avignon as shown in the tables on the preceding pages [15].

The Italian case was complicated by the anomalous existence of five rich commanderies which were exempt from prioral jurisdiction and paid their responsions and other dues directly to the Treasury. Each of these was a capitular commandery or *preceptoria* granted not by the Langue but, technically at least, through the Chapter General [xvii]. All commanders owed a small sum as the *pitancia* which supported the brethren of their Langue in the Convent. The way in which the *pitancia* for the Italian Langue was divided among the priories was fixed in 1311 at 215 florins, or maybe 239 if the Priory of Venice was due to pay 24 florins as in 1442 [xxvi], and that was confirmed following a dispute in 1442 [Doc. I]. In 1462 the Prior of Venice sent to the Langue 24 florins as part of his priory's *pitancia* [xxvi].

The number of Hospitallers needed to control and defend the Rhodian islands and their inhabitants was not great. The statutes of 1467 envisaged a theoretical complement of 350, with 300 knights, 30 chaplains and 20 sergeants. The Italian presence, in which the *milites* from the Priories of Venice and above all of Lombardy predominated, was projected at 47, or less than an eighth, to be divided as follows [16] :

---

14. E.g. in 1373 the Italian and Provençal Langues agreed to share certain benefices in the Kingdom of Naples and in the Priories of Capua, Barletta and Hungary : J. Delaville Le Roulx, *Les Hospitaliers à Rhodes jusqu'à la mort de Philibert de Naillac : 1310-1421*, Paris, 1913, pp. 174-175, and R. Valentini, "Un Capitolo Generale degli Ospitalieri di S. Giovanni tenuto in Vaticano nel 1446", in *Archivio Storico di Malta*, 7, 1936, pp. 134-135.

15. A. Luttrell, "The Hospitallers' Western Accounts : 1373/4 and 1374/5", in *Camden Miscellany*, 30, London, 1990, pp. 8-9 [11,193 is here corrected to 11,103] ; these accounts were certainly incomplete.

16. Text in Gabriel, *op. cit.*, II, pp. 226-227. The Italians provided 70 out of 551 brethren in 1513, roughly the same proportion : Bosio, *op. cit.*, II, p. 610. In 1459 it was estimated that there should be 335 brethren in the East : Malta, Cod. 282, fol. 76.

Priory	Knights	Chaplains	Sergeants	Total
Barletta and Capua	6	2	1	9
Lombardy	11	1	1	13
Messina	4	1	1	6
Pisa	4	1	1	6
Rome	4	1	–	5
Venice	7	1	–	8

There were at least fifteen members of the Italian Langue in residence in 1431 [17] and in 1442 twenty-six were present to vote in the *auberge* [XIX], but presumably there were others elsewhere on Rhodes, on Cyprus or Kos, or in Saint Peter's Castle at Bodrum on the mainland near Kos, while a few other Italians may have been Conventual chaplains or members of the Master's household. In 1441 the Italian Langue employed a French Hospitaller as its chaplain [VIII]. The names of Ceva, Carretto, Grimaldi, Doria, Airasca, Valperga, Piossasco and Scalenghe were among those which reflected the predominance of Lombards, Ligurians and Piedmontese in the Convent. Many Hospitallers, especially those who were priests, never went to the East at all. Others were probably sent to Rhodes in uncoordinated ways. Some went to seek promotion but others resisted. In 1411 six Hospitallers of the Priory of Venice met in Treviso where they named four brethren from whom the prior was to select just one to send to Rhodes. One of the six, Fr. Angelo de Rossi, was among the four selected and he at once produced a series of excuses : *inter alia*, he had already spent ten years serving the Prior of Venice in Rome ; his brother had a large family which would suffer from his absence ; he was engaged in a lengthy lawsuit which might be lost in his absence to the detriment of the Order ; and he himself was poor and in great need of money [18].

Each Langue constituted a corporation with a juridical personality. It could hold and lease property, receive incomes and endowments, appoint procurators, establish foundations, maintain records and so on. The Italian Langue owned *hospitia*, or houses, and was already altering and amalgamating them by 1348 [19]. The location of its *auberge* is unknown, but by 1480 it was in the north-east of the *castello* near the chapel of Saint Dimitri [20]. The Italian Langue was also responsible for the hospice of

17. Malta, Cod. 351, fol. 112.
18. Text in LUTTRELL (1992), item I, p. 11.
19. Malta, Cod. 317, fol. 232v.
20. GABRIEL, *op. cit.*, II, pp. 62-63. In 1436 the Italians in the *fabrica* or *domus* of their *albergia* had opened a window overlooking the *auberge* of France (which stood on the north side of the modern Knights Street) : text in TSIRPANLIS, *op. cit.*, pp. 278-279. In 1433 there was a house in *strata maiori dicta mal canthune per quam itur ad albergiam fratrum dominorum lingue Italie* : Malta, Cod. 350, fol. 13.

Santa Caterina in the *borgo* which had been founded in 1391 by the Neapolitan Fr. Domenico de Alamania²¹. When Roberto da Sanseverino, Count of Caiazzo, visited Rhodes in 1458, he and his companions were received by some twenty Italian Hospitallers and lodged in that hospice²². An *auberge* might contain lodgings²³ but basically it was for the brethren to eat and meet while they slept in separate houses²⁴. The chapel must have possessed liturgical books and furnishings²⁵ while the *auberge* would have owned beds, linen, pots, pans and so on²⁶ ; the Italians had plate and metal utensils [vii, xiv]. An *auberge* would have its horses and at least one slave²⁷, while the Italians' properties included gardens, a vineyard, a warehouse and mills [i-vi, xxiii].

The Langue's obligations naturally included duties of defending the islands. The Italian Tower at Bodrum was built by Fr. Angelino Muscetula, then captain of the castle, in 1436²⁸. In 1465 the Italians were responsible for a sector in the south-eastern part of the walls of Rhodes²⁹. In 1445 they were arranging to construct and pay for a tower in that area, at the end of the street of the Genoese [xxiv] ; this may have been an Italian quarter of the *borgo*. At a later date the Italian Tower was next to the Koskino Gate³⁰. In 1445 the Italian Langue appointed procurators to find and contract with master masons, who were presumably Greeks such as the *protomaistro murador* Manolo Constanti to whom in 1457 an inscription in Italian and Greek was placed on the new town wall he had built³¹. The tower must have formed part of an overall fortification scheme. There seems to have been no regular obligation to serve at sea, but the Italian Langue had to provide four brethren to perform their *caravana* on Kos and four at Bodrum ; individuals could pay for a substitute or compound for 40 florins [ix-xiii, xxvii-xxxiii] ; the number

21. GABRIEL, *op. cit.*, II, pp. 102-106, 227-228.

22. The count was invited by the Admiral, Fr. Sergio de Seripando, to stay in his *caxa*, which Sanseverino confusingly called *lo albergo de Italiani*, but he seems not to have done so : ROBERTO DA SANSEVERINO, *Viaggio in Terra Santa*, G. MARUFFI ed., Bologna, 1888, pp. 54-56.

23. The unconfirmed statute of 1446 stated that brethren might stay (*hospitentur*) in their *auberges* : Doc. II.

24. GABRIEL, *op. cit.*, II, pp. 37-38. In 1433 the Langue of Spain had *camere* in which its brethren resided : text in TSIRPANLIS, *op. cit.*, pp. 255-256.

25. See the list of possessions in the *Auberge* of Spain in 1530: Malta, Cod. 414, fol. 179.

26. E.g. texts in SCICLUNA, *op. cit.*, pp. 12, 75.

27. Text of 1357 in A. LUTTRELL, *Latin Greece, the Hospitallers and the Crusades : 1291-1440*, London, 1982, item VI, pp. 86-87.

28. A. MAIURI, "I Castelli dei Cavalieri di Rodi a Cos e a Budrûm (Alicarnasso)", in *Annuario della R. Scuola archeologica di Atene*, 4-5, 1921-1922, pp. 298-300.

29. Text in GABRIEL, *op. cit.*, I, pp. 143-144.

30. Little survives of the original tower which was later rebuilt : *ibid.*, I, pp. 55-57.

31. Text *ibid.*, I, p. 98 ; on the Greek masons at Rhodes, *ibid.*, I, p. 113, and A. LUTTRELL, *The Later History of the Maussolleion and its Utilization in the Hospitaller Castle at Bodrum* (= *The Maussolleion at Halikarnassos. Reports of the Danish Archaeological Expedition*, II/2), Aarhus, 1986, pp. 160-161, note 84. The text of 1445 throws unique light on the fortification process.

due to serve at Bodrum had risen to seven or eight by 1462 [xxix] [32]. These details were carefully recorded since the *caravana* counted towards seniority.

The most disputed issue was naturally that of benefices. Exactly how priories and commanderies were acquired was a matter of continual legislation and particular negotiation which varied from time to time and from priory to priory, but at least a portion of appointments was reserved to brethren who served in the Convent [33]. In about 1390 Philippe de Mézières, who knew Rhodes well, declared it a scandal that Hospitallers spent five years there to secure a good benefice and then retired to a comfortable commandery in the West, but in reality he was describing a system which was well understood and which worked reasonably satisfactorily [34]. Seniority, *ancianitas*, was a ceaseless preoccupation, as the Italian records made clear, especially as a means to the first commandery, which was achieved through seniority and was known as *de chiuimento* [xx] or *cabimento*. Even the receiver in Lombardy who had never been to Rhodes but was in Conventual service was granted such seniority [xviii]. There were other paths to advancement : through princely or papal influence or provision [35], through magistral grace or nomination to a *camera* or office in the Master's gift [xx], or through a commandery in *ius patronatus* in the gift of the founding family [36]. By statute, brethren who recovered property of the Order which had passed into secular hands could retain it for life [xx]. In the case of Fr. Battista Orsini, his powerful family influence allowed him to exploit this statute as a way of building up considerable wealth in Central Italy [xvi-xvii] [37].

From about 1420 there were increased pressures for a stricter interpretation of the requirement that *milites* should be of noble or knightly birth [38]. An unconfirmed statute of 1446 laid down that knights were not to be received until investigations into their family and their personal merits had been conducted in their priory ; they were also to pay or give a surety for the *passagium* to Rhodes which was in effect an entrance payment [39]. Most brethren entered the Hospital while in the West but

32. In 1459, 335 brethren were needed in the East, including 50 at Bodrum, 25 on Kos and 40 on the galley *della guardia* : Malta, Cod. 282, fol. 76-80v. Those on Kos were owed *lor soldaya de lor carauane* in 1447 : text in Tsirpanlis, *op. cit.*, pp. 462-463. In about 1460, of 62 brethren on two Hospitaller galleys in action against the Turks, only three were Italians : New York, Pierpont Morgan Library, Glazier Collection, G. 55, fol. 141-141v.

33. Appointments to the Aragonese priory are studied in Luttrell (1978), item xi, and M. Bonet Donato, *La Orden del Hospital en la Corona de Aragón : Poder y Gobierno en la Castellanía de Amposta (ss. XII-XV)*, Madrid, 1994.

34. A. Luttrell, "Rhodes : base militaire, colonie, métropole de 1306 à 1440", in *Coloniser au Moyen Age*, M. Balard, A. Ducellier eds., Paris, 1995, pp. 238-240.

35. E.g. A. Luttrell, "Del Carretto, Daniele", in *Dizionario Biografico degli Italiani*, XXVI, Rome, 1988, pp. 394-397.

36. E.g. F. Tommasi, "Il Monastero femminile di San Bevignate dell'Ordine di San Giovanni Gerosolimitano (secoli xiv-xv)", in *Templari e Ospitalieri in Italia : la chiesa di S. Bevignate a Perugia*, M. Roncetti et al. eds., Perugia, 1987, pp. 53-78.

37. On Orsini, texts of 1434 and 1444 in Luttrell (1978), item x, pp. 115-117, 123-124.

38. Luttrell (1982), item i, pp. 264-265.

39. Malta, Cod. 1698, fol. 75v.

some were received in the Convent, as in the case of Fr. Marioto di Giovanni Martellini of Florence who was accepted in 1452 but was obliged within one year to produce certificates attesting his knightly estate from his prior and from three or four other brethren [xxi]. Some brethren belonged to Italian families ruling Aegean islands ; the register recorded Fr. Fantino Quirini of Stamphalia [xxv], Fr. Antonio Corogna of Siphnos [xxx] and three members of the Crispo family who were Dukes on Naxos [xxvi, xxx]. The question of whether Fr. Silvestro de Cocovaginis, Commander of Orte, could "wear gold" [xix] suggests he was a sergeant being granted a knightly privilege [40]. There was no clear division between those who made, or planned to make, a career primarily in the West and others whose ambitions centred on the alternative hierarchy of the Convent where a Hospitaller might acquire or lease a house and country garden while securing office and income. Of those Italians mentioned in their Langue's register some had considerable education. Fr. Giovanni de Norcia was a *decretorum doctor* and Fr. Michele de Castellacio was *utriusque iuris doctor*, a judge of appeals at Rhodes and Commander of San Antonio on Naxos ; Fr. Antonio Morosini was simultaneously a *miles*, a doctor of canon law, Commander of Treviso and Bishop of Santorini in the Aegean. Fr. Melchiore Bandini was Chancellor of the Order. In the East Fr. Giorgio de Monteafia, Fr. Angelino Muscetula, Fr. Roberto de Diana and others became Captains of Bodrum, while Fr. Giorgio de Monteafia, Fr. Angelino Muscetula and Fr. Fantino Quirini were among those who served as Admiral. Fr. Roberto de Diana briefly governed Rhodes as the Master's lieutenant in 1438. On Rhodes Fr. Giovanni Papa was Captain of the Marine Gate [xxix] and Fr. Giovanni Caraffa became *Bayliuo* of the *Comerchio* [iii]. Fr. Fantino Quirini was Commander of Kos and *appaltator* of the island of Nisyros ; he was endlessly involved in the affairs of the Hospital's lesser islands. Many brethren secured commanderies in Italy and some became priors. For example, Fr. Giuliano Benini and Fr. Giorgio de Monteafia were Priors of Pisa, Fr. Fantino Quirini, Fr. Roberto de Diana and Fr. Battista Orsini were Priors of Rome, and Fr. Giovanni Caraffa was Prior of Capua [41].

Down to 1374 the Southern French virtually monopolized the Mastership and many other offices on Rhodes, and even thereafter the three French Langues of Provence, Auvergne and France retained their predominance. However in 1433, following the formal creation of a German Langue in 1428, the Germans began, with Italian and Spanish support, to attack the lucrative French control of the office of Treasurer. The Chapter General held at Rome in 1446 produced passionate rows as the four non-French Langues assaulted the French. Among the Italians

---

40. There are indications that military sergeants serving in the Convent were considered as *milites*. An inquest of 1373 listed six sergeants as *Fratres sargandi, qui ultra mare vocantur milites* : text in A.-M. LEGRAS, *L'Enquête pontificale de 1373 sur l'ordre des Hospitaliers de Saint-Jean de Jérusalem*, I, Paris, 1987, p. 149.

41. Texts in TSIRPANLIS, *op. cit.*, pp. 194, 288, 334-335, 352-355, 637-639 : on Quirini, *ibid., passim* ; on Morosini, LUTTRELL (1992), item xiv, pp. 767-768 ; on Bandini, ID. (1982), item ii, pp. 146, 149-150, item iii, pp. 67-68 ; on Caraffa, Malta, Cod. 283, fol. 2v.

present were Fr. Fantino Quirini, Fr. Gaspare Airasca, Fr. Giuliano Benini and others with grievances acquired at Rhodes. The most extreme, Fr. Giorgio Piossasco, spoke *verba obprobriosissima et vilissima* against the French, while Fr. Melchiore Bandini wrote down most of the proceedings [42]. In 1467, by which time the Spanish Langue had been divided into the two Langues of Aragon and Castile, the Italians secured a triumph. The Master, Fr. Ramon Zacosta, died in Rome following a Chapter General held there, and Pope Paul II insisted on naming the new Master after consulting twenty-three Hospitallers present in Rome. Seven of these were Italians, five of whom, including Fr. Melchiore Bandini and the Admiral Fr. Cencio Orsini, voted for Fr. Battista Orsini ; Orsini did not vote for himself and the Italian Prior of Hungary voted for the Prior of Pisa. Eight votes were cast for Fr. Raymond Riccardi, Prior of Provence, but two German, one English and one Portuguese votes also went to Orsini. By one vote the Italians, somewhat luckily, secured the Mastership [43].

42. Texts in VALENTINI, *op. cit.*, a fundamental study of the politics of the Langues ; see also LUTTRELL (1995), pp. 238-240.

43. Malta, Cod. 283, fol. 1-1v, reported, not quite accurately, in BOSIO, *op. cit.*, II, pp. 309-310.

DOCUMENT I

Text of 1442 recopying bulls of 1312 and 1321

National Library of Malta, Archives of the Order of St John, Cod. 355, fol. 243-243v.

Cum certa contemptio siue controuersia exorta esset inter venerabiles fratres lingue Italie in sacro conuentu Rhodi residentes actores ex una racione, et causa pitanciarum eisdem fratribus rationaliter debitarum, et venerabilem dominum fratrem Baptistam de Ursinis, prioratus Vrbis priorem, se deffendentem partibus ex altera, coram reuerendissimo domino Magistro ac venerando suo consilio in quo interfuerunt reuerendi ac venerabiles fratres Fochaldus de Rochechoart, Francie prior ac reuerendissimi domini Magistri locumtenens, Johannes Morelli ecclesie dicti conuentus Prior, Guido de Domaniaco Hospitalerius, Philipus de Ortaliis Drapperius, Vgo Midilton Turchpilerius, memorati conuentus baiuliui, Johannes de Vilaguto castellanie Emposte castellanus, Guillermus de Verna Admoree, Johannes de Villafrancha Maioricarum, baiuliui capitulares, Guillermus de Lastico dicti reuerendissimi domini Magistri senescallus, Guido de Luriaco Gebenensis ac domini Manescalli, Johannes Scot Sauonensis ac domini Admirati, Johannes Truller Interlossen ac domini magni baiuliui, Fulcus de Pontes locumtenens Magni Preceptoris, Petrus Prunet pilerius albergie Magne Prouincie, Johannes Perrinus Gombremontis ac domini Thesaurarii generalis, baiuliuorum locumtenentes ac domorum premissarum preceptores, dicte partes videlicet procuratores fratrum dicte venerande lingue actores et dictus reuerendus dominus prior se deffendentes personaliter constituti post multa hinc inde petita pariter et obiecta tandem a dictis procuratoribus ad victoriam actionis eorundem fuit quoddam instrumentum siue bulle patentes exhibite cum quadam bulla cerea in cera viridi sculpta infra casea cere albe cuius sigilli erat forma equi currentis circumcirca littere dicebant : Sigillum fratris Geraldi Maneschali Hospitalis Iherusalem. Non rase non canzellate aut in structura aliqualiter lazerate, sed sane clare integre ac omni prorsus vicio et suspicione carentes, quarumquidem litterarum tenor sequitur, et est talis, videlicet :

Nouerint vniuersi presentes litteras inspecturi ac eciam audituri quod nos, frater Geraudus de Pinibus sancte domus Hospitalis sancti Johannis Jherusolimitani Marescallus, conuentus cismarini et domini Magistri humilis locumtenens in cunctis partibus cismarinis, testimonio presencium litterarum testificamur et dicimus quod nos, ad instanciam et requisicionem religiosorum in Christo nobis carissimorum fratrum lingue Italie in dicto conuentu comorancium, vidimus contineri in quibusdam cartulariis seu registris cancellarie Rhodi dicte domus notas infrascriptas quarundam litterarum quas venerabilis et religiosus vir frater Fulco de Vilareto, olim Magister dicte domus, mandauit quibusdam prioribus Ytalie et Apulie iuxta ordinacionem dudum factam per dictum tunc Magistrum et conuentum cismarinum in eorum capitulo generali in Rhodo celebrato anno domini M° III^c vndecimo, decimo kalendas madii prout in eisdem registris continetur, quarum notarum tenores de uerbo ad uerbum secuntur, sub hiis verbis : § Item mandatum fuit per dictum dominum Magistrum priori Lombardie vel eius locumtenenti quod transmictat citra mare annis singulis fratribus lingue Ytalie in conuentu cismarino comorantibus viginti quinque florenos auri quos ex dicto prioratu habere debent ipsi fratres quolibet anno pro eorum pitancia prout ordinatum extitit in capitulo generali proxime celebrato et quod idem prior dictos florenos colligat et recipiat a preceptoribus prioratus predicti. Datum Rhodi, die decima mensis januarii anno Domini M° III^c vndecimo. § Item mandatum fuit priori Pisarum uel eius locumtenenti quod transmictat citra mare quolibet anno fratribus lingue Ytalie in conuentu cismarino comorantibus triginta florenos auri quos ex dicto prioratu habere debent ipsi fratres singulis annis pro eorum pitancia prout ordinatum extitit in capitulo generali proxime celebrato et quod dictus prior ipsos florenos colligat et recipiat de preceptoribus prioratus predicti. Datum Rhodi, die decima mensis januarii anno Domini millesimo III^c vndecimo. § Item mandatum fuit priori Vrbis vel eius locumtenenti quod fratribus lingue Ytalie in conuentu cismarino comorantibus transmictat quolibet anno viginti quinque florenos auri quos habere et recipere debent pro eorum pitancia annis singulis ex prioratu predicto et quos idem prior exhigat et recipiat a preceptoribus prioratus predicti iuxta ordinacionem factam in generali capitulo proxime celebrato. Datum Rhodi, die decima mensis januarii anno Domini millesimo III^c vndecimo. § Item similiter mandatum factum est priori Capue vel eius locumtenenti quod mictat citra mare quolibet anno fratribus lingue Ytalie in conuentu Rhodi sistentibus viginti quinque florenos auri quos ipsi fratres habere debent ex dicto prioratu annis singulis pro pitancia eorundem prout ordinatum extitit in generali capitulo proxime celebrato et quod prefatus prior ipsos florenos exigat et recipiat a preceptoribus prioratus predicti. Datum Rhodi, die decima mensis januarii anno Domini millesimo III^c vndecimo. § Item preceptum factum est priori Baroli uel eius locumtenenti quod transmictat quolibet anno citra mare fratribus lingue Ytalie in conuentu Rhodi comorantibus, quinquaginta florenos auri quos ipsi fratres quolibet anno habere debent pro eorum pitancia ex prioratu predicto prout extitit in proximo preterito generali capitulo ordinatum, et quod idem prior dictos florenos exigat et recipiat a preceptoribus prioratus memorati. Datum Rhodi, die decima mensis januarii anno Domini millesimo III^c vndecimo. § Item simile mandatum factum est preceptori Sancte Trinitatis de Venusii vel eius locumtenenti de transmictendis quolibet anno citra mare fratribus lingue Ytalie in conuentu cismarino sistentibus triginta florenos auri quos habere debent ipsi fratres annis singulis ex dicto prioratu pro eorum pitancia iuxta ordinacionem factam in generali capitulo proxime celebrato. Datum Rhodi, die decima mensis januarii anno Domini millesimo III^c vndecimo. § Item mandatum fuit priori Messane vel eius locumtenenti quod transmictat citra mare anno quolibet fratribus lingue Ytalie in conuentu Rhodi comorantibus triginta florenos auri quos ipsi fratres habere debent annis singulis ex dicto prioratu pro eorum pitancia prout ordinatum extitit in generali capitulo proxime celebrato et quod idem prior dictos florenos exigat et recipiat a preceptoribus prioratus predicti. Datum Rhodi, die decima mensis januarii anno Domini millesimo CCC undecimo. In quorum omnium testimonium et certitudinem pleniorem nos, locumtenens predictus, sigillum cereum officii nostri dicte marescallie presentibus duximus appendendum. Datum Rhodi, die quinta decima mensis nouembris anno Domini millesimo trescentesimo vicesimo primo, quinte Indicionis.

Postulantes procuratores prefati, nomine ac vice lingue predicte Ytalie, dictas litteras admicti earumque vigore dictum venerabilem priorem et alios in eisdem expressatos tamquam veros priores et preceptores ac veros debitores fratrum dicte lingue ad soluendum pitancias antedictas compelli debere presente dicto venerando priore et dicente dictas litteras non esse amictendas neque earundem virtute compelli posse vt ab adversariis suis petitur actento maxime quod suo tempore dictum onus prioratui predicto Vrbis impositum non existit remictens se ad iudicium et cognicionem supradicti reuerendissimi domini Magistri ac sui prefati reuerendi consilii vtrum dicte littere sunt amictende uel ipse eciam earundem virtute cogi compellique possit. Quiquidem reuerendissimus dominus Magister ac domini de consilio supradicti, partibus ad sufficienciam auditis, comiserunt dictam eorum causam audiendam et refferendam reuerendis religiosis dominis fratribus Johanni Morelli, antedicti conuentus Priori, et Johanni de Villaguto, castellanie

Emposte castellano. Qui domini auditores ipsis partibus vocatis pariter et auditis donec aliquid dicere et allegare voluerunt, ac de tota causa supradicta debite certificati (*sic*) relacionem fecerunt decima septima mensis augusti M° IIII° XLII coram predictis reuerendissimo domino Magistro et suo venerando consilio de omni jure actione racione et causa parcium predictarum relacionem plenissimam fecerunt.

Quiquidem reuerendissimus dominus Magister et premissi in dicto consilio congregati audita relacione dictorum commissariorum et auditorum in presencia parcium predictarum facta et ab ipsis partibus ratificata dicentes se se nichil aliud dicere aut allegare velle postulantes declaracionem et diffinicionem supradicte eorum contempcionis, et partibus extra locum se positis, ac omnibus visis et consideratis que videnda et consideranda fuerunt declarauerunt et sumauerunt vnanimiter nemine discrepante peticionem dictorum procuratorum nomine dicte lingue fore iustam et racionabilem et maxime propter tenorem instrumenti siue litterarum antedictarum in quibus apparet dictum venerabilem priorem et ceteros priores cum preceptoriis fore veros debitores tamquam puri gubernatores et legitimi rectores prioratuum et preceptoriarum in dictis litteris expressatorum, declarantes instrumentum siue litteras antedictas ac omnia et singula in eisdem contenta fore bonas et bona validas et valida ac in omnibus et per omnia eisdem fides dari debere plenissima secundum seriem stabilimentorum ac laudabilium consuetudinum Religionis eisdem tamquam bonas et validas approbantes et ratificantes et ad cautelam in presenti registro per me canzellarium registrari. Mandantes ad cautelam dicte lingue Italie et dictorum procuratorum eius nomine presencium petencium et postulancium et ad cautelam, etc. Neque intendimus propter hanc nostram declaracionem pitanciarum supradictarum aliquid detrahere seu in aliquo preiudicare iuribus nostri comunis thesauri que hab[er]i in prioratibus prefatis et preceptoriis eorundem neque responsionibus siue loco responsionum quinto uel decimo ordinato et imposito in nostro generali capitulo Rhodi celebrato neque oneribus impositis et imponendis consuetis solui annuatim per priores supradictorum prioratuum et per preceptores domorum seu baiuliarum eorundem prioratuum. Die et anno infrascripto fuit extractum de canzelarie in forma sequenti videlicet :

Nouerint vniuersi et singuli presentes pariter et futuri quod nos, frater Johannes de Lastico, etc. et nos conuentus Rhodi domus eiusdem, ad instanciam et requisicionem venerabilium ac religiosorum in Christo nobis precarissimorum fratrum Fantini Quirini conuentus nostri Rhodi Admirati ac baiulie nostre Langonis, etc. preceptoris, nec non Baptiste de Vrsinis prioratus nostri Vrbis prioris, ceterorumque preceptorum et fratrum venerabilis lingue Ytalie, de registris nostre cancellarie extrahi fecimus fideliter de uerbo ad uerbum ea que secuntur, videlicet : Cum certa contemptio siue controuersia exorta esset inter venerabiles fratres lingue Ytalie, etc. vt supra infine vero sequ[enti]. Nos vero supradicta omnia et singula ratificantes aprobantes et confirmantes quia diligenti facta collatione cum registris nostre cancellarie effectualiter concordare inuenimus ; ideo, in testimonium veritatis et robur premissorum, bulla nostra comunis plumbea presentibus est appensa. Datum Rhodi in nostro conuentu, die XVII setambris M° IIII° XLII.

DOCUMENT II

The Unconfirmed Statute of 1446 concerning the Auberges at Rhodes
National Library of Malta, Archives of the Order of St John, Cod. 1698, fol. 81-81v.

De hospiciis seu albergiis fratrum Conuentus.

Baiuliui omnes fratribus sue lingue hospicium prebeant, haberint in nostro conuentu domum sibi et fratribus aptam, in qua preceptores et fratres conuentuales sub obediencia eorum commedant et hospitentur, sed ipsi baiuliui ueluti patres fratres suos beneuolencia et caritate tractent, et expensas conpetentes faciant, et in statu honesto et fratribus condecenti teneant, a nostro comuni thesauro pro fratribus at seruitoribus eorum sue lingue frumentum et mense necessarias expensas recipiant, sed quocies necessitas exegerit vniuscuiusque lingue fratres pro comunibus negociis illius impetrata et obtenta a magistro licencia cum suo baiuliuo seipsos fratres congregabunt, uocatis sue lingue prioribus et preceptoribus in conuentu residentibus convocatis, ad quam uocatocium (*sic*) ire tenebuntur, ibique vnicuique suam ancianitatem et jura licebit allegare. Sed Baiuliui auditis omnibus magistro et consilio quod a maiori illorum parte conclusum fuerit, curabunt nunciare ipseque magister et consilium habito ad nostra stabilimenta recursu, quod canonicum et iustum fuerit debebit (*sic*) approbare, exceptis prioratibus baiuliatibus conuentus et baiuliatibus capitularibus super quibus ad magistrum et consilium deliberacio spectat.

DOCUMENT III

Deliberazioni della lingua d'Italia a Rodi : 1437-1462
National Library of Malta, Biblioteca, Ms. 728 [1].

[I] M CCCC XXXVII, die secundo mensis madii.

Nos frater Gaspar Ayrasca et frater Johannes de Marchis de Nursia, procuratores et procuratorio nomine lingue Ytalie, procurantes meliorationem et utilitatem dicte lingue, habentes et considerantes utilitatem et meliorationem dicte lingue, inuenimus quamdam vineam positam et situatam in contrata Parambolini fore et esse propter vetustatem ipsius aliqualiter deterioratam, quare facientes iuxta posse nostrum maximam inquisitionem super meliorationem et utilitatem dicte lingue, inuenimus quemdam probum virum Michaelem Saguli, iardinarium, cum quo habita [spec]iali concordia et dispositione fuimus contenti dare tradere et consignare sibi dictam vineam ad habendum, tenendum, fructandum et meliorandum donec et quousque diem suum clauderit extremum et vita ipsius Michaelis tantum et quod post mortem ipsius dominium[a] dicte vinee et meliorationem ipsius sit et esse debeant dicte lingue Italie sine aliquali solutione pro melioratione predicta, cum [condi]tione aposita quod ipse Michael predictus teneatur et debeat annuatim, toto tempore vite sue et eius vita durante, solvere asperos sex cum dimidio moneta curentis tunc temporis in civitate Rhodi et hoc in festo beate

---

1. The modern pencil enumeration of entries in Roman capitals is indicated in the left hand margin.

Virginis de mense septembris, predicta obseruare promitit et attendere dictus Michael ad penam duorum ducatorum auri tociens quociens contrauenerit impredictis, que pena soluta uel non soluta rata et firmata, etc.

a. et *deleted*.

[ii] M CCCC XXXVIII°, die prima aprilis.

Venerabiles fratres lingue Ytalie existentes in unum in eorum hospicio, de licencia reuerendi domini locumtenentis unanimiter congregati, de eorum bona spontanea voluntate tradiderunt et concesserunt religioso domino fratri Melchiori Bandino, cancellario conuentus Rhodi et preceptor Nursie et Mugnani dicte lingue, eorum jardinum positum in contrata Chiporie qui anthiquitus vocabatur Periuoli tu Nipoti, cum infrascriptis pactis et condictionibus videlicet, quod dictus dominus frater Melchior teneat possideat et usufructet antedictum jardinum pro suo libero voluntatis ipsum locando at affictando personis sibi placitis non tamen ipsum aliquo modo pignorando uel alienando, uel extra dictam linguam quomodolibet trasferendo, et fructus ipsius percipiat et soluere donec vitam duxerit in humanis, reseruato tamen quod si dictus dominus frater Melchior accesserit ad partes ponentis seu alibi causa comorandi extra conuentum eo tunc teneatur et debeat dictum jardinum dimittere dicte lingue et quandocumque dictus dominus frater Melchior reuerteretur ad dictum conuentum, reddat et capiat dictum jardinum sicut per prius ipsum habebat, soluendo anno quolibet in festo beate Marie de mense augusti procuratoribus fratrum dicte lingue pro ipsa lingua recipientibus florenos Rhodi curentes octo. Et quando ipsum jardinum dimittet non possit repetere expenssas per ipsum factas in dicto jardino.

[iii] Die xii jullii M CCCC LVI.

La venerabile lingua de Italia sia dato in affitto e pro nome de afitto lo sopra ditto jardino che tenea lo ditto fra Melchior Bandino al venerabile religioso fra Johann Caraffa, bayliuo del comercho de Rh[od]io, per anni cinque incommin-çando lo afito al primo zorno de agosto proximo ch'e da uenir M CCCC [LVI], in quello modo e forma che teneua lo ditto fra Melchior Bandini pagando neti florini otto ogni anno.

[iv] M CCCC XL. die primo septembris.

In Dei nomine amen. Venerabiles domini fratres Leonelus de Ceua et Johannes de Marchis de Nursia, procuratores lyngue Italie, de voluntate et consensu domini admirati et tocius lingue, locauerunt quamdam eorum appothecam que est in castro Jani [...]ª, barbitonsori, per florenos XII pro quolibet anno ad annos tres, Et quia quia solueret pro reparatione dicte domus ducatos quatuor, fuit contentum inter dictas partes quod quolibet anno computaretur et defalcaretur ducatus unus et unus tercius de dictis XII florenis, usque ad annos tres predictos.

a. *Blank*.

[v] Nota che adi iii del mese de marzo delanno de M CCCC XLI li venerabili religiosi frar Lafranchin de Captaneis de Casalegio e frar Lodouico dela Torre, como procuratori dela lingua de Italia, de consentimento e volunta de ladmirayo e de tuti li frati dela lingua predicta, apaltano a Costa Ypsiquidali la possession de Mortona posta nelisola de Rhodes a termine de anni tre, acominzando al primo de de aprile proximo venente, per floreni ventidoyª, zoe XXII de Rhodes lanno, apagar de tre mesi in tre mesi. Et e tenuto el dicto Costa a miliorar e non pezorar la dicta possession. E lo dicto Costa confesso hauer hauto imprestito dali dicti procuratori, ducati X, zoe dece de Rhodo, li quali promese de render ali procuratori de la ditta lingua che sera in quello tempo quanto lassara la dicta possession, in capo deli dicti anni III com apar di zo per scrittura del comercho lanno e lo zorno com e scritto di sopra.

Item, nota che adi XII de marzo lanno ut sopra, li sopradicti procuratori, frar Lafranchino e frar Lodouico, imprestano al sopradicto Costa Ipsiquidali floreni VI de Rhodo azoche mecta in ordine et reconzo el molino dela detta possession de Mortona. E che non son tenuti ad imprestarli piu altri denari a cason de ditto molino. Et esso Costa se obligo arender li dicti floreni VI a requista deli detti procuratori. Oltra di zo se bisognasse el ditto molino altra despesa el ditto Costa de spender de suo proprii denari. E la fine la spesa fatta se de detrare dila summa delo fitto deve dar ogni anno, come di zo apar per uno scritto fatto de volunta del detto Costa.

a. *Ms* : Vintididoy.

[VI]   Item, nota che adi X del mese di nouembre de lanno mille CCCC XLII el venerabile religioso frar Zeorzio Arcor, come aprocurador dela lenga di Italia, aue apaltato e affitato per anni X proximi dauenire a Dimitrio Damaschino un molin dela dita lenga al molo del porto posto a raxon di firini VIII siue octo lanno franchi e neti e ogni spexa sopra del dito Dimitri, a fare page IIII lanno chome dusanza chome piu largamente apar per scrittura del comerchio, e che lo debia render meliorato e piasente a zascuna persona che lo volesse affitare.

[VII]   Nota che adi XVIII del mese de marzo, lanno de la natiuitate M CCCC XLI, son imprestate le infrascripte cose al venerabel religioso frar Zorzo de Montafia, comendator de Ferara e capitaneo del castel San Piero, per la lingua de Italia, zoe per consentimento de ladmiralio e de tuti li frati dela dicta lingua :

Primo, taze VI de argento
Item, culiari IIII dargento
Item, scutele XII de stagno
Item, stagnate II de stagno da vino
Item, mo[...]pa II de aqua de stagno.

[VIII]   Adi primo de marzo 1441, noy procuratori dela lingua de Italia, frar Lafranchino Captanio e frar Lodouico de la Torre, habiamo fatto rasone cum fra Andrea, capellano de la dicta lingua, per lo seruitio dela capella dela lingua predicta posta in lo albergo de Italia, per mesi IIII, zoe de nouembrio, decembrio, zenar e febrar de M CCCC XLI. E a receuuto per li ditti mesi floreni de Rhodo IIII, zoe quatro. E de acordio se cassato de offitiar dicta capella.

Nota che adi primo de marzo, lanno desopra, habiamo tolto in scambio del dicto frar Andrea, et per capellano de dicta capella, frar Johan Belloso, de la lingua de Franza, capellano.

[IX]   M CCCC XLIIII. Carauana del Castel San Piero.

F[rar] Michael de Valperga   per un anno
F[rar] Petro Chanal   per un anno
F[rar] Bertholomeo deli Obici   per un anno
F[rar] Antonio de Arascha   per mesi VIIII et mezo.

           M CCCC XLIIII. Carauana del Lango.

F[rar] Arnaldino Prouana   per mesi IIII e mezo
F[rar] Matioto Filingeri   per anno uno
F[rar] Galliazo da Alemania   per anno uno
F[rar] Sinibaldo de Norsia   per mesi VII e mezo.

[X]   Anno M CCCC XLIIII et die VIII del mese de nouembre, li venerabili religiosi frar Bertholameo de Gozonibus da Osmo, locumtenente de monsignor lo armirayo, e frar Georgio de Plozascho, comandator de Yurea, elleti per li frari de la lingua e per lo infrascripto venerabil frar Bertholameo de Chanizanis, comendator de San Sepulcro de Florentia, per le soe charauane del Castel San Pietro e del Lango, hano indicato el ditto comendatore de Florentia deue pagar per ditte charauane florini quaranta, zoe XL de Rhodi, al San Johanne del mese de jugno da M CCCC XLVI. Et in testimonio, obligando tuti soy beni presenti et avinidori, se soto scritto ditto comendator de Florentia, de soa propria mano.

Io, frar Bartholomeo predecto, sono contento aquanto di sopra e scripto e a fede di cio mi sono soscripto di mia propria mano detto di anno e mese. Presente fra Piero Pelegrino e fra Mario procuratori di deta lingua e consentienti[a].

a. *Sentence in different hand.*

[XI] M CCCC XLV. Carauana del Castel San Piero.

F[rar] Antonio de Ayrascha	per mesi II e mezo
F[rar] Bertholameo de Senis	per anno I°
F[rar] Michael de Castellano	per anno I°
F[rar] Roberto de Diana	per anno I°
F[rar] Jo[hann]e de Ceua	per anno I°

M CCCC XLV. Carauana del Lango.

F[rar] Michel de Valper[ga]	per anno I°
F[rar] Petro Chanal[a]	per
F[rar] Arduino de Marzenach[b]	

a. *This line deleted.* — b. *The whole passage of four lines* M CCCC XLV (...) Marzenach *was incomplete and was cancelled.*

[XII] Anno M CCCC XLI et die XIII mensis septembris.

Essendo lo venerabel religioso frar Achiles Pecora de Senis, comendator de San Mano e di Sancto Johanne del Ponte Arigo etc. obligato a far soa charauana nel Castel San Piero e nel isola de Lango, lo ditto frar Achiles e la lingua de Italia inseme congregata forno contenti che ditto frar Achiles pagasse per le ditte soe charauane florini quaranta, zoe XL de Rhodo, li quali florini XL li venerabili religiosi signori frar Laffranchino de Captanei de Casalegio, comendator de Nouayra etc. e frar Antonio de Auria, comendator de Taurino, procuratori de ditta lingua confessono hauer hauti e receuuti in pecunia numerata dal prefato frar Achiles numerante e pagante a nome e per le ditte charauane. E pero li ditti procuratori, a nome de ditta lingua, quietano, absolueno e liberano lo dicto frar Achiles dale dicte charauane del Castel San Piero e de Lango, si che da mo auanti non sia piu tenuto ni obligato ale ditte charauane. E a perpetua memoria le sopradicte cose son state scritte nel presente libro, etc.

[XIII] M CCCC XLIII. Carauane Castri Sancti Petri.

Frar Matioto Frangier	per anno uno
Frar Sinibaldo de Schalisco	per anno uno
Fra Oldouino de Valperga	per anno uno
Fra Andrea dela Crose	per mese VI

Carauana del Lango.

Frar Johan de Vintimilia	per anno I°
Fra Simonino } Fra Arnaldino Prouana }	per anno I° mesi VII e mezo

[XIV] Die XXVI decembris 1441[a].

Venerabiles domini fratres Leonellus de Ceua et Johannes de Nursia, procuratores lingue, de mandato reverendi domini admirati et de licencia tocius lingue, dederunt stanea infrascripta domino Johanne Querino, domino de Stampalea, ad aptandum ea in Veneciis.

Et primo, plati fracti XXI
Item, scutelle fracte XXIIII
Item, salerios fracte II
Item, scutelini II
Item, staninos magnos III et unam de aqua
Item, mensuras de vino III
Item, incissorias
Item, quarte de stagno
Sunt omnia rotulli decem et nouem, onquie nouem.

   a. *Entry cancelled because items returned.*

[xv]   MCCCC XLII, die VIII mensis junii.

Venerabiles religiosi fratres Achiles del Pecora et Georgius de Alchur, procuratores venerabilis lingue Italie, confessi fuerunt se habuisse et recepisse per manus domini Karoli Maurozeni nomine spectabilis viri domini Johannis Quirini, comitis Stampalea, supradictas pecias stagni videlicet, vireos III pro vino, duos magnos et unum mediocrem, et vireos tres pro aqua, quartos duos pro vino, XII platellos magnos, XVIII scutellas, XII salseria, XII talliera siue incisora, quadra[gin]ta, saleria XII. In summa rotoli XVIII, onchie III. Et ideo cassata fuit supradicta scriptura.

[xvi]   De ordinatione prioratuum [preceptoriarum] et similium cum suis dependentibus.
M IIII^c XXXIIII, die v junii.

Reverendus dominus frater Angelinus Mussetula, dignus Admiratus conuentus Rodi, ceterique domini fratres lingue Italie residentes in dicto conuentu existentes, congregati in eorum albergia de licencia reuerendissimi domini Magistri, ut moris est, pro negociis eorum lingue disponendis et ordinandis, ordinauerunt et admiserunt ad requisicionem et supplicacionem domini fratris Baptiste de Ursinis, preceptoris Castri Araudi prioratus Pisarum, quod cum ipsa preceptoria Castri Araldi est grauata expensis multis propter custodiam castri quod est situatum in loco in quo est semper et continue est confluentia gentium armorum et detentum temporibus retroactis tyrannice per seculares, quod preceptoriole videlicet Sanctus Johannes de Suarella et Sanctus Manus, scite et posite in territorio patrimonii Sancti Petri in Tussia, cum omnibus pertinenciis suis in prioratu Pisarum post obitum fratrum Achille de Senis et Johannis de Urbe Veteri, preceptorum ipsarum preceptoriarum, vel quocumque alio modo vacauerint, sint et esse debeant annexe, incorperate dicte preceptorie Castri Araldi et membri ipsius preceptorie, et hoc vigore stabilamenti nouiter facti per reuerendissimum dominum nostrum Magistrum d[ominum] fratrem Anthonium Fluviani in capitulo generali Rodi celebrato de M CCCC XXXIII ita quod hoc tota lingua consentiit, sic tamen quod responsiones ordinarie dicti castri et ipsarum preceptoriarum in aliquo non diminuantur.

[xvii]   Die III julii M CCCC XXXIIII.

Transactum et concordatum fuit per dominos admiratum et fratres lingue Italie nemine ipsorum discrepante existentes congregatos in eorum albergia, ut moris est, de licencia reuerendissimi domini Magistri [et] quod dominus frater Baptista de Ursinis, preceptor Castri Araldi, gubernator et administrator prioratus Urbis, recuperando preceptoriam Venosii quandocumque et qualitercumque^a habere debeat de gratia eandem preceptoriam Venosii, ita quod una cum illa possit et valeat aliam dignitatem Religionis obtinere, quamvis illa preceptoria Venosii est preceptoria per capitulum, et quod non possit sibi in aliquo prejudicare dicta concessio de presenti neque in futurum, ymo quod qualiter aliam dignitatem una cum dicta preceptoria Venosii habere et obtinere possit et valeat, cum sibi

conceditur illa de gratia speciali ipsius lingue, videlicet per reuerendos dominos
fratrem Angelinum Mussetula, admiratum, pillerium et caput ipsius lingue,
Robertum de Dyana priorem Urbis, Hectorem de Alamania preceptorem Neapolis,
Johannem Scot, Anthonium Morezinum, Petrum Peregrini, Nicolaum Daschum,
Guillelmum de Aragonia, Jacobum de Achioles, Godfredum Rane, Georgium de
Pusasco, Gasparem de Arasca, Petrum Morezinum, Bartholomeum Sanzio,
Jacobellum de Monopolo dicte lingue residentes in conuentu Rodi, fauentes ipsam
linguam seu saniorem et majorem partem ipsius lingue Italie.

    a. *After* qualitercumque : ipse *deleted.*

[xviii]   M CCCC XLI, die primo mensis augusti, de comuni consensu omnium
venerabilium fratrum venerabilis lingue Italie, insimul congregatorum unanimiter
et nemine discrepante, fuit concessa ancianitas fratri Antonio de Casalibus,
receptori responsionum prioratus Lombardie, quod non obstante quod numquam
ad conuentum uenerit nec ibi moram traxerit, ipse frater Antonius habere debeat
ancianitatem existendo in ipso prioratu acsi in dicto conuentu moram traxisset
admicti que debeat ad preceptorias, honores et beneficia, secundum stabilimenta
et consuetudines Religionis cum pro tempore casus acciderit. Et ad memoriam
perpetuam voluerunt dicti procuratores quod predicta ancianitas in presenti libro
scriberetur.

[xix]   Anno M CCCC XLII, de mense nouembris, fo congregata la venerabel
lingua de Italia nel albergo consueto, de licentia et voluntate del reuerendissimo
monsignor lo Maestro. Etia[m] per casone de dar licencia a frar Siluestro de
Cocouaginis, comendator de Horta, de posser portar oro, forno in dicta lingua frari
XXVI deliquali XIII forno di voluta e consentiendo che alora, e avanti, ditto frar
Siluestro possa portar oro, como frar chavalier, non prejudicando a nisuno
benefitio ni offitio o dignita de frar chaualier, e XIII forno de opinione simile ma
la remetiuano al capitol generale proxime venente, doue simil cose se costumato de
concedere.

[xx]   Anno M CCCC L, adi xxviiii de marzo, fo passato per tuta la lingua
concordeuelmente, essendo capo de ditta lingua fra Johan Karaffa locotenente de
monsignor lo admirayo, che fra Georgio de Monteafia, comendatore de Ferrara, e
fra Laffranchino Captanio, commendatore de Nouayra, permutasseno le commen-
darie loro, zoe frar Georgio la comandaria di Pavia, la qual hauia per collacione de
Magistro, cum la comandaria de Castelnouo Tartonese che tenia fra Laffranchino
de gratia di lingua e leuata de man de seculier, non intendendo che sia per via de
chiuimento, ma per via de permutatione e collatione, in quella forma che tuti doy
teniuano le ditte comandarie auanti la presente permutatione. Essendo procuratore
de la lingua fra Lodouico dela Torre e fra Jacobo de Alexandra.

[xxi]   Die viiii de decembre M CCCC LII. Congregata la venerabile lingua de
Italia, in la albergia costumata, de licentia del reuerendissimo in Christo patre
monsignor lo Maestro, per lo reuerendo signor fra Georgio de Monteafia, del
conuento de Rhodes admirayo, e comparuto Marioto de Johani Martellini da
Firenza, dimando che piazasse al ditto monsignor lo admirayo e ditta lingua de
acceptarlo per fra chaualier in lor compagnia. La qual lingua, ouer signori frari de
ditta lingua hano passato in questo modo, zoe che lo ditto Marioto debia prouar
infra uno anno autenticamente per testifficatione de monsignor de Pisa, fra
Julliano Benigno, e di tre o quatro frari del ditto priorato che luy sia tale quale se
apartene ali stabilimenti de esser fra chaualier. E se in caso infra lo ditto anno non
lo prouasse luy Marioto se sotomette spontaneamente a tute quelle pene dano li
stabilimenti. El qual anno cominci a correre dal jorno chel ditto Marioto pilliara
lo habito. Item e passato che cum ditta conditione ditto Marioto habia labito dela
Religione e sia fra chaualler de ditta lingua. Scritta fo questa presente scrittura

inpresentia de li venerabili frari Johan Molleti e fra Toma Chamot procuratori de ditta lingua.

[xxii] M CCCC XXXVI, die xxi januarii.

Ex comissione domini admirati et tocius lyngue, fratres Johannes Scotto et Nicolaus de Aschio, ad videndum computa et rationes fratris Andree Saluagii et fratris Alefranchini de Casalegio, de procuratione anni preteriti, de omnibus administratis per eos. Et qui frater Andreas dedit seu reddidit in manibus fratrum Georgi de Plosesco et Petri Pauli de Dugnano, procuratores anni presentis, ducatos septem de Rhodo et asperos XVI. Et dictus frater Alefranchinus reddidit in manibus dictorum procuratorum ducatos quatuor asperos decem et dinarios duos.

M CCCC XXXVII, die ii mensis madii.

Ex comissione domini admirati et tocius lingue, domini fratres Nicolaus de Asculo et Johannes de Marchis de Nursia ad videndum computa et rationes dominorum fratrum Georgii de Ploçasco et Petri Pauli de Dugnano, de procuratione anni preteriti, de omnibus administratis per eos, habitis et receptis per procuratores tunc temporis ordinatos in presentia dictorum restituerunt tam in pecuniis quam etiam argentis, masariciis et aliis rebus, absoluerunt predictos procuratores ab omnibus gestis et administratis per ipsos.

[xxiii] M CCCC XLII, die xix nouembris.

Ex comissione domini locumtenentis reuerendi domini admirati et totius lingue, fratres Georgius de Plozasco, preceptor Yporesie, et Johannes Sidor, preceptor Rendatii, ad videndum computa et rationes fratris Lanfranquini ex Captaneis de Cassalegio et Ludouici de la Torre, de procuratione anni preteriti, de omnibus administratis per eos. Qui procuratores visis et bene calculatis omnibus rederunt et pro resto computorum tradiderunt et consignauerunt in manibus fratrum Achilis de Pecora, preceptoris Sancti Mani etc., et Georgii de Arcatoribus, per manus ser Marchi Bello, florenos Rhodi curentes LXXXI et unum denarium et per manus fratris Melchioris Bandini, canc[ellarii], pro zardino florenos VIII. Quorum prefatus dominus locumtenens et lingua dictos procuratores et administratores quitauerunt et absoluerunt et per quitos et absolutos fieri voluerunt de omnibus et singulis per ipsos administratis et in eorum procuratione contentis.

[xxiv] M CCCC XLV, adi vii del mese de jugno.

Nel albergo de Itallia consueto, de licentia del reuerendissimo monsignor lo Maestro, for[no] congregati li venerabili frari de ditta lingua nel conuento de Rhodo comoranti. E de comuna concordia e consentimento e passato, e hano constituiti suoy procuratori e de la dicta lingua li honorabeli religiosi signor frari Gotifredo Rana, Antonio de li Signori e Sinibaldo de Sebalischi de dicta lingua, aliquali hano dato amplissima possanza, baylia e auctorita tanto bastante quanto alor sia possibile, de cerchar maistri murat[or]i cum li quali habiano contratar patezar e composarse per edificar la torre, la qual ditta lingua ha determinato de fare e fabricare ad honor de dicta lingua, presso ala muraia de Rhodo, uerso la ruga ouer la strata de Zenoesi, e affitare la opera de ditta torre a quelo pretio che alor procuratori parera cum piu auantazo de ditta lingua, e a fermar ditti pacti e compositione cum dicto (sic) magistri muratori per scrittura autenticha solemnemente, in maynera e modo che per questa causa non habia piu casone de assunarse ditta lingua.

Anchora e passato e confermato la taxa che passata in altra lingua tenuta proximamente, e imposita sopra li frari de ditta lingua comorante al conuento, secondo che particularmente apare in scriptis, e pero schoder e recuperar ditta taxa per casone dela fabrica de ditta torre dali frari sopraditti, son stati ordenati procuratori lo sopraditto fra Gotifredo e frar Jacobo de Fonssaro, ali quali hano datto plenissima possanza per poter schoter ditta taxa dali ditti frari, per ogni via melior. E che tuto homo che contradicesse a pagar la taxa aluy imposta, lo possan constrenger per via dela rason e justitia, azo che la ditta opera per lor manchamento non se resti de fare e adimplire.

Anchora hano ordinati auditori de conti de li procuratori de dicta lingua, dal tempo passato fin al presente jorno, li sopraditti frar Antonio de Signori e frar Sinibaldo, cum plena possanza de veder et examinar ditti conti e azeptarli e refutarli secondo che alor parera. E visti e auditi dicti conti debeno referir a ditta lingua.

[xxv] M CCCC XLV, adi xxiii octobris, li venerabili religiosi fra Johannes Sidot et fra Johannes Borgesii, procuratori dela venerabile lingua, a nome de dicta lingua hano confessato hauer hauto e receuuto dal reuerendo signor monsignore lo admirayo, misser fra Fantino Quirini, ducatos CC de Rhodi, li quali ha donato liberalmente ala dicta lingua per constructione dela noua torre de Italia. E pero hano quitato dicto monsignor lo Admirayo per imperpetuum secondo che apare per mano de Eliseo, notario de nostra lingua, e in testimonio questo resta scritto in lo libro presente de dicta lingua.

[xxvi] Die xxiii mensis octubris M° CCCC° LXII, in Rhodi, in la lingua de Ytalia, fra Johanne Crispo et fra Bernardo Peruzi, procuraturi de la predicta venerabile lingua de Ytalia, confessano hauir receputi da fra Petro Morsini, mandati et scossi dal reuerendo monsignor lo prior de Venecia, per parte dele pietancie delo priorato de Venecia, florini vintiquatro de Rhodes, de li quali florini XXIIII quitano et absolglino lo dicto priore.

[xxvii] Adi 10 delo mese di nouembro, facimo assapir per la presente scripta come toccando la carauana de lo Lango lo presenti anno de 1461 ad fra Dioniosio de Crapania la lingua de gratia le la donata pagando per reparacione de dicta lingua florini sedeci deli qual florini 16 de pago incontenenti in contanti florini 10. Resta a dar florini 6.

Li signori procuratori dela lingua, zoe frare Bernardo Perutii et Johanne Crespo, confesseno hauer receputo florini VI dal sopraditto fra Dionisio pro resto dela sopra ditta scrittura, dela qual quantitate de florini XVI quitano lo ditto frare Dionisio.

[xxviii] Die xii mensis januarii M CCCC LXII. Nota sia come frare Johanne de Monteaffia sia dato et pagato per la sua carauana, la qual li tochaua al Castel San Piero del anno sopradritto, florini XVI, li quali sono sopra una camera che teneua frare Tineto Ro[m]er che staua in compagnia de frare Princiual Vagnon, per la qual cosa la venerabel lingua de Ytalia quita lo ditto frare Johanne per la ditta carauana del ditto anno.

[xxix] La carauana del Castel San Piero per lo anno M CCCC LXII.

Primo, F[rar] Johanne de Aspria, anno uno   sive I°
F[rar] don Henrico de Centellis, comandator de Pollizo, anno uno   siue I°
F[rar] Princiualo Vagnon, anno uno   siue I°
F[rar] Marco Taparello, anno uno   siue I°
F[rar] Leone de Belloch, anno uno   siue I°
F[rar] Luchino de Castelazo, anno uno   siue I°
F[rar] Henrico de San Martin, anno uno   siue I°
F[rar] Matheo de Vintimillia, anno uno   siue I°
F[rar] Francesco Motela, mesi doy   siue II mesi

Die xviii mensis januarii, anno quo supra, congregata la venerabile lingua come e de costuma, sopra le carauane, la qual venerabile lingua dimandaua chel venerabile religioso frare Johanne Papa, capitaneo dela porta dela marina, deuesse fare sua carauana, lo qual venerabile frare Johanne Papa se leuo, dicendo come in tempo de frare Fantino Quirino, quondam Admyraio del conuento de Rhodo, li fo comandato ditta carauana, lo qual quondam frare Fantino, comandator de Lango et Admirayo, li dono ditta carauana, sopra lequal cose metendo la mano sua sopra la croce çuro, come cusi fo, la e qual lingua vedendo suo sacramento la donado et estada contenta che habia fato sua caraua[na].

[xxx]   La carauana delo Lango del anno M CCCC LXII.

Primo, frare Marco Crespo, anno uno   siue I°
Frare Anthonio de Coronia, anno uno   siue I°
Frare Nicolino Crespo, anno uno   siue I°
Frare Ludovico de Scalengis[a], mesi[b] noue   siue VIIII

    a. *After* Scalengis : anno *deleted.* — b. *After* mesi : uno *deleted.*

[xxxi]   Nota come adi xxiii mensis jullii, frare Nicolao de Ferraria ha pagato ala venerabile lingua de Ytalia ali signori procuratori per la sua carauana cheli tocha lanno che auenire, zoe lanno LXIII, alo Lango, fl[oreni] X, per li quali lo quitano.

[xxxii]   Die xxiii mensis jullii, anni supradicti, frare Johanne de Monteaffia tiene una camera dela lingua de Italia, la qual haueua habuta da frare Tineto Romer per florini VIII, laqual camera, perche lui e per andare in ponente, quita essa ala venerabile lingua, per la qual cosa per ditta quitatione de essa camera la ditta lingua de Ytalia se chiama contenta dela carauana la qual die fare esso frare Johanne alo Lango, lanno M CCCC LX [...] et si lo quita per essa carauana.

[xxxiii][a]   Questo di viiii° di nouembre M CCCC L°XII, frare Roggieri dalla Casa, perche se ne via in ponente per sua bisogni, a pagato alla lingua in mano di frar Johann Crespo, procuratore della lingua, per la sua carouana del Castello Sanpiero chelli toccaua questo anno [florini] sedici, zoe fl° XVI, per ditta carouana del Castello.

Et per la carouana de Lango, in caso non ci fussi quando ha a tocare, promette per lui frare Troiolo da Monte Mellino, viuendo dicto frare Roggieri.

    a. *Item XXXIII entirely deleted.*

ADDENDA ET CORRIGENDA

Not included among the seventy-eight items now reproduced in four *Variorum Reprint* volumes or among other publications listed in the 'Addenda et Corrigenda' section of the 1992 *Variorum* volume are the following items concerning the Hospitallers:

'Emphyteutic Grants in Rhodes Town: 1347–1348', *Papers in European Legal History: Trabajos de Derecho Histórico en Homenaje a Ferran Valls i Taberner*, ed. M. Peláez, v (Barcelona, 1992); 'Les Hospitaliers à Chypre et à Rhodes: 1291–1522', in *L'Ordre de Malte dans les Pays-Bas Méridionaux (XIIe–XVIIIe siècles)*, ed. M. Forrier (Brussels, 1993); 'Malta and Rhodes: Hospitallers and Islanders', in *Hospitaller Malta, 1530–1798: Studies on Early Modern Malta and the Order of St John of Jerusalem*, ed. V. Mallia-Milanes (Malta, 1993); 'The Military Orders: 1312–1798', in *The Oxford Illustrated History of the Crusades*, ed. J. Riley-Smith (Oxford, 1995); 'Ta Stratiotika Tagmata', in *Istoria tes Kyprou*, ed. T. Papadopoulos, iv part 1 (Nicosia, 1995); 'The Earliest Templars', in *Autour de la Première Croisade*, ed. M. Balard (Paris, 1996); 'The Earliest Hospitallers', in *Montjoie: Studies in Crusade History in Honour of Hans Eberhard Mayer*, ed. B. Kedar *et al.* (Aldershot, 1997); 'To Byzantio kai oi Joannites Hippotes tes Rodou: 1306–1409', *Symmeikta*, xi (1997); 'El Final de la Dominació catalana d'Atenes: la Companyia navarresa i els Hospitalers', *L'Avenç* [Barcelona], ccxiii (1997); 'The Hospitallers and the Papacy: 1305–1314', in *Forschungen zur Reichs-, Papst- und Landesgeschichte: Peter Herde zum 65. Geburtstag*, ed. K. Borchardt - E. Bünz, ii (Stuttgart, 1998); 'The Latin East', in *The New Cambridge Medieval History*, vii: *c.1415–c.1500*, ed. C. Allmand, (Cambridge, 1998); 'The Hospitallers' Early Written Records', in *The Crusades and their Sources: Essays Presented to Bernard Hamilton*, ed. J. France – W. Zajac (Aldershot, 1998); 'La Funzione di un Ordine Militare: gli Ospedalieri a Rodi (1306–1421)', in *I Cavalieri di San Giovanni e il Mediterraneo: I Convegno Internazionale di Studi Melitensi* (Taranto, 1998); 'English Contributions to the Hospitaller Castle at Bodrum in Turkey: 1407–1437', in *The Military Orders*, ii: *Welfare and Warfare*, ed. H. Nicholson (Aldershot, 1998).

The following amendments make special use of *The Military Orders*, ii: *Welfare and Warfare*, ed. H. Nicholson (Aldershot, 1998).

I The Genoese at Rhodes, 1306–1312

p. 746: The text of 27 May 1306 is republished with minor amendments in A. Luttrell, 'To Byzantio kai oi Joannites Hippotes tes Rodou: 1306–1409', *Symmeikta*, xi (1997), pp. 210–13.

For the Western background, add A. Luttrell, 'The Hospitallers and the Papacy: 1305–1314', in *Forschungen zur Reichs-, Papst- und Landesgeschichte: Peter Herde zum 65. Geburtstag*, ed. K. Borchardt – E. Bünz, ii (Stuttgart, 1998); the demonstration (p. 616) that Clement V did not grant the Hospital an 'exemption' on 17 April 1309 reinforces the considerations in L. García-Guijarro Ramos, 'Exemption in the Temple, the Hospital and the Teutonic Order: Shortcomings of the Institutional Appproach', in *The Military Orders*, ii, pp. 291–2. For other recent viewpoints, S. Menache, *Clement V* (Cambridge, 1998), and *idem*, 'The Hospitallers during Clement V's Pontificate: The Spoiled Sons of the Papacy?', and M. Barber, 'The Trial of the Templars Revisited', both in *The Military Orders*, ii.

II Gli Ospitalieri di San Giovanni di Gerusalemme dal Continente alle Isole

p. 79: The texts cited probably do not permit the implication that the Templars were in 1300–1302 transferring their general headquarters from Limassol to the island of Ruad.

III The Greeks of Rhodes under Hospitaller Rule, 1306–1421

p. 208, n. 86: for 'Cod. 325' read 'Cod. 352,'

Add important observations and texts in Z. Tsirpanlis, *Anekdota Eggrapha gia te Rodi kai tis Noties Sporades apo to Archeio ton Iohanniton Ippoton: 1421–1453* (Rhodes, 1995).

VI The Building of the Castle of the Hospitallers at Bodrum

Add B. Arbel – A. Luttrell, 'Plundering Ancient Treasures at Bodrum [Halikarnassus]: A Commercial Letter Written on Cyprus, January 1507', *Mediterranean Historical Review*, xi (1996); A. Luttrell, 'English Contributions to the Hospitaller Castle at Bodrum in Turkey: 1407–1437', in *The Military Orders*, ii. At p. 160, n. 84: add F. Karassava-Tsilingiri, 'Fifteenth-Century Hospitaller Architecture on Rhodes: Patrons and Master Masons', ibid.

IX The Spiritual Life of the Hospitallers of Rhodes

See the important contribution by A. Forey, 'Literacy and Learning in the

Military Orders during the Twelfth and Thirteenth Centuries', ibid. Two recent works, *Juan Fernández de Heredia y su Epoca: IV Curso sobre Lengua y Literatura en Aragón*, ed. A. Egido – J. M. Enguita (Zaragoza, 1996), and J. M. Cacho Blecua, *El Gran Maestre Juan Fernández de Heredia* (Zaragoza, 1997), are stronger on the philological than the historical side.

p. 91, n. 17: Supra, pp. 83–4.
p. 93, n. 62: delete '55, plate 32.'
p. 95, n. 107: for 'Ragney' read 'Reaney'

X The Hospitallers' Medical Tradition: 1291–1530

The remark (p. 68) that the Munich manuscript contains no indication that it was describing the Hospitallers' hospital is incorrect: B. Kedar, 'A Twelfth-Century Description of the Jerusalem Hospital', and also S. Edgington, 'Medical Care in the Hospital of St. John in Jerusalem', both in *The Military Orders*, ii.

p. 67, last line: for '1189' put '1181'.
p. 73, in. 56: add Z. Tsirpanlis, 'Gnosta kai Agnowsta euale Idrumata ste mesaionike Pole tes Rodou (14os-16os ai.),' in *Phileremou Agapesis: Timetikos Tomos gia ton Kathalete Agapeto G. Tsopanake* (Rhodes, 1997).
p. 73, n. 59: for 'p. 64' read 'p. 69'

XI The Hopitallers' Western Accounts: 1373/4 and 1374/5

See now J. Sarnowsky, '"The Rights of the Treasury": The Financial Administration of the Hospitallers on Fifteenth-Century Rhodes, 1421–1522', in *The Military Orders*, ii.

p. 9, line 7: for '[11,193]*' put '[11,1031*'
p. 12, line 5: for 'dei' put 'del'.
p. 12, line 12/13: for '1 ij dr.' put 'iiij dr.'
p. 13, line 34: delete 'el'
p. 15, line 6: for 'Costantinoble' put 'Constantinoble'
p. 15, line 28: 'los quals fueron embiados'
p. 17, line 8: for 'Baubure' put 'Bauburc'
p. 17, line 27: for 'Items' put 'Item'
p. 20, line 18: for '.iij. flor.' put '.iiij. flor.'
p. 20, line 26/27: delete 'Item pago alos . . . papa xcv flor'.

XII The Hospitaller Province of Alamania to 1428

Add L. Jan – V. Jesensky, 'Hospitaller and Templar Commanderies in Bohemia and Moravia: their Structure and Architectural Forms', and K. Borchardt, 'The Hospitallers in Pomerania: Between the Priories of Bohemia and *Alamania*', both in *The Military Orders*, ii. J. Mol, 'The Beginnings of the Military Orders in Frisia', ibid., p. 315, argues convincingly that the phrase *commendator domus* referred not to a single regional commander for Frisia (as suggested above at XII, p. 33) but to all the Frisian commanders.

p. 39, n. 48: read '*A Jerusálem Szent János-Lovagrand Magyarországon*, 2 vols., Budapest 1925–1928'

XIII   The Structure of the Aragonese Hospital, 1349–1352

passim: for 'Añiés' read 'Aniés'

p. 319, n. 21: to read: 'Miret, p. 384; B. Alart, *Suppression de l'Ordre du Temple en Roussillon*, Bulletin de la Société Agricole, Scientifique et Littéraire des Pyrenées Orientales, 15 (1867), p. 81, n. 2.'

p. 230, n. 3: That Fr. Fortuner de Glera was a priest and not, as often asserted, a knight is confirmed in R. Sáinz de la Maza Lasoli, *El Monasterio de Sijena: Catálogo de Documentos del Archivo de la Corona de Aragón*, ii (Barcelona, 1998), p. 46. That Sancha de Azlor was Prioress of Sigena by 19 August 1367 (ibid., ii, p. 74) in theory restricts the dating of the Sigena *retable*, in which Fr. Fortuner appears as donor, to a period from August 1362 to August 1367, since the frame bears the arms of Sancha's predecessor, Toda Pérez de Alagón.

p. 320: The suggestion that Fr. Juan Fernández de Heredia was illegitimate is disproved by the fact that Urraca Maça de Vergua, the wife of his father Garcia Fernández de Heredia, was his mother, as show by a supplication of 1345 in Archivio Vaticano, Suppliche 10, f. 30 (kindly communicated by Karl Borchardt).

p. 320, n. 24: for 'Infra, p. . . . ' put 'Madrid, Carp. 706 no. 33.'

p. 328: for further *freyras*, see Sáinz de la Maza, *passim*.

See also M. Bonet Donato, *La Orden del Hospital en la Corona de Aragón: Poder y Gobierno en la Castellania de Amposta (ss. XII–XV)* (Madrid, 1994).

XIV   The Economy of the Fourteenth-Century Aragonese Hospital

See also P. Ortega, 'Rentas del Castellán de Amposta (Orden del Hospital) en las Encomiendas de Ascó, Caspe y Miravet a principios del siglo XV', in *Miscel.lània de Textos Medievals*, viii (Barcelona, 1996).

XVI   Gli Ospedalieri e un Progetto per la Sardeqna, 1370–1374

For similar schemes, E. Lourie, 'Conspiracy and Cover-Up: the Order of Montesa on Trial (1352)', in *Iberia and the Mediterranean World of the Middle Ages: Essays in Honor of Robert I. Burns S.J.*, ed. P. Chevedden *et al.* (Leiden, 1996).

XVIII   The Hospitaller Priory of Venice in 1331

Major additions are G. Cagnin, *Templari e Giovanniti in Territorio trevi-giano (secoli XII–XIV)* (Treviso, 1992), G. Cagnin *et al.*, *Santa Maria Nova di Soligo* (Treviso 1994), with important studies on its frescoes, and M. Mariani, 'Gli Ordini Ospitalieri in Romagna', in E. Caruso *et al.*, *Pellegrini, Crociati et Templari* (Castrocaro Terme, 1994).

INDEX

This necessarily selective and incomplete index lists only people and places, including Hospitaller houses and brethren; it excludes many brethren and preceptories from the Priories of *Alamania*, Bohemia and Hungary (item XII), Aragon (XIII), Pisa (XVII) and Venice (XVIII), and from the Italian *langue* between 1437 and 1462 (XIX), as also many Genoese (item I) and Rhodian Greeks (III). 'Fr.' and *soror* indicate Hospitallers. References to the Addenda et Corrigenda are indicated by the abbreviation Add. (e.g. Add. 4 means Addenda et Corrigenda page 4).

Printed and bound by CPI Group (UK) Ltd, Croydon, CR0 4YY

17/10/2024

01775690-0009